FOUNDATIONS IN CLINICAL PHARMACY PRACTICE

Mr. Sri Venkatesh Uriti
Mr. Venkateswarlu Garla
Miss. Pratiksha P. Alabade
Dr. Sridhar Babu Gummadi
Dr. Shivkumar Shete

ISBN: 9788198765703

Scan to view online

Editors

Mr. Sri Venkatesh Uriti

Mr. Venkateswarlu Garla

Miss. Pratiksha P. Alabade

Dr. Sridhar Babu Gummadi

Dr. Shivkumar Shete

First Edition: 2025
ISBN: 9788198765703

Maximum Retail Price: Rs. 1000/- (Inclusive of all taxes)

Published by ThinkPlus Pharma Publications,
Door No. 9-15/1, Indrapalem, Kakinada, AP-533006, India
Website: www.books.jopir.in

Cover Page Illustration: Kiran Priyam Kumar Sarella

Printed at Tarangini Printing Works, Subhadra Arcade, Bhanugudi, Kakinada, AP-533003, India.

DEDICATION

This textbook is dedicated to the patients who have inspired us to continually improve pharmaceutical care, the students who represent the future of our profession, and the countless healthcare professionals who collaborate daily to advance patient-centered care. Your stories, challenges, and triumphs drive our commitment to excellence in pharmacy practice.

We also dedicate this work to the educators and mentors who have shaped our understanding of clinical pharmacy and instilled in us the passion for evidence-based practice and lifelong learning. Your wisdom continues to guide the evolution of pharmacy education and practice.

It is dedicated to the patients whose needs remain at the center of our professional purpose, reminding us that behind every prescription is a person deserving of our best care and to all who strive to advance the science and practice of pharmacy in service of human health and wellbeing.

"May this book serve as a trusted companion in your professional journey"

CONTENTS

ACKNOWLEDGMENTS

The creation of this textbook on clinical pharmacy practice is a result of the culmination of knowledge, experience, and dedication from numerous individuals and organizations. The editors wish to express their profound gratitude to:

The contributing authors, whose expertise, diligence, and commitment to pharmacy education have made this textbook possible. Each chapter reflects countless hours of research, writing, and revision to ensure accuracy and relevance to contemporary practice.

Our academic institutions and clinical practice sites for providing the environments where many of the concepts in this book are taught, refined, and implemented.

The reviewers who meticulously examined each chapter, offering invaluable feedback that enhanced the clarity, accuracy, and educational value of the content.

The publishing team, whose expertise in design, layout, and production transformed the manuscript into the finished work before you.

Our colleagues and staff members who provided administrative support, encouragement, and understanding throughout the development process.

The patients who have shared their healthcare journeys with us, providing the real-world context that brings clinical pharmacy to life.

Finally, we acknowledge our families and friends whose unwavering support and patience during the long hours of writing and editing made this work possible.

While it is impossible to name everyone who contributed to this endeavor, please know that your support has been essential and deeply appreciated.

ACKNOWLEDGEMENTS

CHAPTER 1

PRINCIPLES OF CLINICAL PHARMACY

Author

Mr. Sri Venkatesh Uriti, Associate Professor, Department of Pharmacology, Sri Sivani College of Pharmacy, Etcherla, Srikakulam, Andhra Pradesh, India

Abstract

Clinical pharmacy has evolved from traditional dispensing functions to direct patient care, emphasizing medication optimization through collaborative practice. Pharmacists now serve as essential healthcare team members across diverse settings including hospitals, ambulatory clinics, community pharmacies, and long-term care facilities. Core competencies encompass medication therapy management, clinical decision-making, patient education, and systems-based practice. The profession requires advanced knowledge in pharmacotherapy, pathophysiology, pharmacokinetics, and communication skills. Interprofessional collaboration with physicians, nurses, and allied health professionals has become fundamental, with pharmacists contributing specialized medication expertise while respecting team dynamics. This patient-centered approach has demonstrated significant improvements in medication safety, therapeutic outcomes, healthcare costs, and quality measures, positioning pharmacists as indispensable members of modern healthcare teams focused on optimal medication use.

Keywords: *Medication Therapy Management, Collaborative Practice, Pharmaceutical Care, Clinical Competencies, Interprofessional Teams*

Learning Objectives

After completion of the chapter, the learners should be able to:

- Trace the historical evolution of clinical pharmacy from traditional dispensing roles to direct patient care functions.
- Describe the core responsibilities of clinical pharmacists across various healthcare settings including medication therapy management, education, and quality improvement.
- Compare and contrast clinical pharmacy practice across different settings including hospitals, ambulatory clinics, community pharmacies, and long-term care facilities.
- Demonstrate the essential competencies required for clinical pharmacy practice including pharmacotherapy knowledge, clinical problem-solving, and communication skills.
- Apply principles of interprofessional collaboration to optimize patient outcomes through effective team-based care.
- Evaluate the impact of clinical pharmacy services on healthcare quality metrics, patient outcomes, and healthcare costs.

EVOLUTION OF CLINICAL PHARMACY

Clinical pharmacy practice evolved from traditional product-focused pharmacy functions to direct patient care activities beginning in the 1960s. This transformation emerged in hospital settings where pharmacists began leaving the dispensary to provide medication consultations on patient care units. Early pioneers including Paul Parker at the University of Kentucky and Charles Walton at the University of California, San Francisco established the first clinical pharmacy programs, expanding pharmacist responsibilities beyond medication preparation to include therapeutic recommendations, patient monitoring, and education.

Academic and Training Developments

Educational reform paralleled practice evolution, with pharmacy curricula shifting to incorporate clinical sciences alongside traditional pharmaceutical chemistry and compounding. The transformation of pharmacy education culminated in the adoption of the Doctor of Pharmacy (PharmD) as the sole professional degree, becoming mandatory for all US pharmacy schools by 2000. Postgraduate residency training expanded significantly, with PGY1 residencies providing general clinical training and PGY2 programs offering specialized experiences in areas including critical care, oncology, and ambulatory care.

Table 1.1: Evolution of Clinical Pharmacy Practice

Time Period	Practice Focus	Milestones	Impact on Patient Care
1960s	Drug distribution	Unit dose systems, medication profiles	Improved medication accuracy
1970s	Clinical services	Pharmacokinetic monitoring, drug information	Direct patient care involvement
1980s	Pharmaceutical care	Patient outcomes, responsibility for drug therapy	Problem identification and resolution
1990s	Evidence-based practice	Integration of research evidence, outcomes research	Data-driven interventions
2000s	Medication therapy management	Comprehensive medication reviews, collaborative practice	Formalized direct patient care services
2010s	Provider status recognition	Billing privileges, expanded prescriptive authority	Autonomous practice development
2020s	Technology integration	Telehealth services, AI decision support, precision medicine	Enhanced access and personalization

Professional Recognition Milestones

The establishment of Board of Pharmacy Specialties certification in 1976 provided formal recognition of specialized clinical knowledge, beginning with Nuclear Pharmacy and expanding to currently include 14 specialty areas. Collaborative practice legislation, first enacted in Washington state in 1979, provided legal authority for pharmacists to perform patient care functions through formal agreements with physicians. Medicare recognition of Medication Therapy Management services in the 2003 Medicare Modernization Act represented a landmark in payment for clinical pharmacy services outside hospital settings.

Evidence Base Development

Research documenting clinical pharmacy impact developed from early descriptive reports to sophisticated controlled studies demonstrating improved outcomes and cost-effectiveness. Landmark studies including the Asheville Project demonstrated significant improvements in chronic disease outcomes through pharmacist interventions. Meta-analyses have consistently shown clinical pharmacist services reduce medication-related adverse events by approximately 30-50%, improve therapeutic outcomes in numerous disease states, and provide positive return on investment through reduced healthcare utilization.

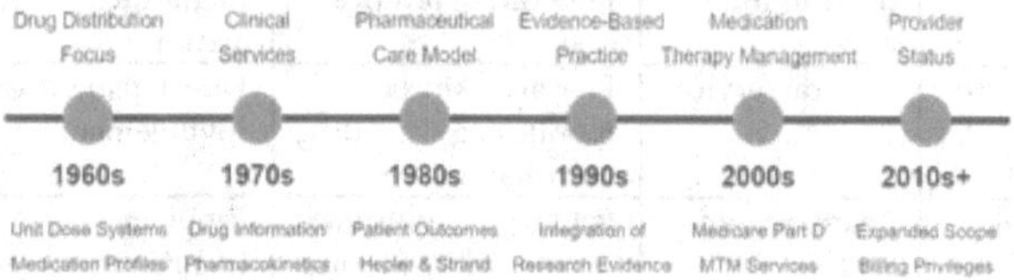

Figure 1.1: Evolution of Clinical Pharmacy Practice

International Expansion

Clinical pharmacy practice expanded globally, though with significant variation in implementation speed and scope. The United Kingdom, Canada, and Australia developed advanced practice roles similar to the United States, while other countries incorporated clinical elements more gradually. International organizations including the International Pharmaceutical Federation (FIP) have promoted clinical pharmacy development worldwide through practice standards, educational frameworks, and knowledge transfer initiatives.

ROLES AND RESPONSIBILITIES

Clinical pharmacists provide comprehensive medication management through systematic approaches including thorough medication history taking, therapy assessment, monitoring plan development, and follow-up evaluation. Patient assessment includes gathering relevant clinical data, performing targeted physical examinations when appropriate, and interpreting laboratory and diagnostic findings related to medication therapy. Medication therapy planning involves developing evidence-based recommendations for initiating, modifying, or discontinuing medications based on individual patient factors and therapeutic goals.

Prescribing Activities

Pharmacist prescribing authority varies across practice settings and jurisdictions, ranging from independent prescribing to various collaborative models. Collaborative practice agreements establish protocols allowing pharmacists to initiate, modify, or discontinue medications within defined parameters and patient populations. Dependent prescribing includes activities such as therapeutic interchange, dose adjustments, and renewal of chronic medications under physician authorization. Protocol development for prescribing activities requires careful delineation of patient eligibility, assessment requirements, documentation standards, and communication expectations.

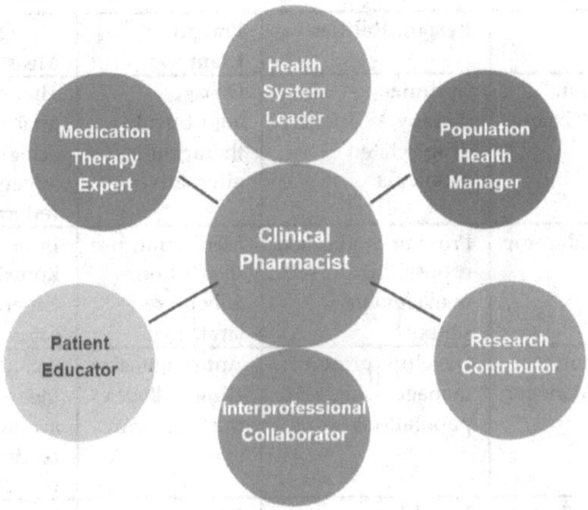

Figure 1.2: Roles and Responsibilities of Clinical Pharmacists

Education and Counselling

Patient education encompasses medication information delivery, self-management training, and health literacy-appropriate counseling addressing administration techniques, expected effects, potential adverse reactions, and monitoring parameters. Healthcare provider education includes formal presentations, guideline development, and point-of-care information provision about new medications, complex pharmacotherapy, and emerging evidence. Student and trainee precepting involves structured learning experiences for pharmacy students, residents, and other healthcare professions students, integrating clinical teaching with patient care responsibilities.

Population Health Management

Disease state management programs implement systematic approaches to optimizing care for specific conditions including diabetes, hypertension, anticoagulation, and asthma through evidence-based protocols, regular monitoring, and structured follow-up systems. Medication use evaluation identifies patterns of suboptimal therapy across patient populations, developing targeted interventions addressing systematic issues rather than individual cases. Quality measure improvement develops and implements strategies to enhance performance on standardized metrics including HEDIS measures, CMS star ratings, and accreditation standards.

Table 1.2: Clinical Pharmacist Roles and Responsibilities

Role	Responsibilities	Practice Examples	Outcome Measures
Medication Therapy Expert	Optimize drug therapy, identify drug-related problems	Dosage adjustments, therapeutic alternatives	Therapeutic goal achievement, adverse event reduction
Patient Educator	Provide medication counseling, self-management support	Medication use instruction, adherence strategies	Improved knowledge, adherence rates
Population Health Manager	Develop protocols, manage high-risk populations	Anticoagulation clinics, diabetes management	Quality measure achievement, readmission reduction
Health System Leader	Develop medication-use systems, formulary management	Policy development, guideline implementation	Cost containment, medication safety metrics
Research Contributor	Generate and apply evidence, quality improvement	Clinical trials participation, outcomes research	Publication output, practice advancement
Interprofessional Collaborator	Provide expertise to healthcare teams	Rounds participation, collaborative practice	Team satisfaction, care coordination metrics

Research and Scholarship

Practice-based research investigates clinical questions emerging from patient care, developing evidence to optimize medication use and document clinical pharmacy value. Quality improvement projects systematically enhance medication-related processes through structured methodologies including Plan-Do-Study-Act cycles and root cause analysis. Scholarly dissemination communicates clinical innovations, research findings, and practice advancements through peer-reviewed publications, professional presentations, and clinical guideline development.

PRACTICE SETTINGS

Inpatient clinical pharmacy services address the medication needs of hospitalized patients through direct involvement in multidisciplinary care teams. General medicine practice consists of comprehensive medication management for patients with diverse medical conditions, emphasizing safe transitions of care, appropriate empiric therapy, and medication reconciliation. Specialized practice areas including critical care, emergency medicine, and surgery require additional expertise addressing unique patient populations and medication management challenges.

Ambulatory Care Practice

Primary care settings integrate clinical pharmacists within medical home teams, providing chronic disease management, comprehensive medication reviews, and coordination with community pharmacies. Specialty clinics engage pharmacists in focused practice areas including anticoagulation, diabetes, hypertension, and heart failure through collaborative practice models supporting disease-specific management. Patient-centered medical homes formally incorporate pharmacists as core team members addressing medication optimization across conditions rather than through siloed disease management programs.

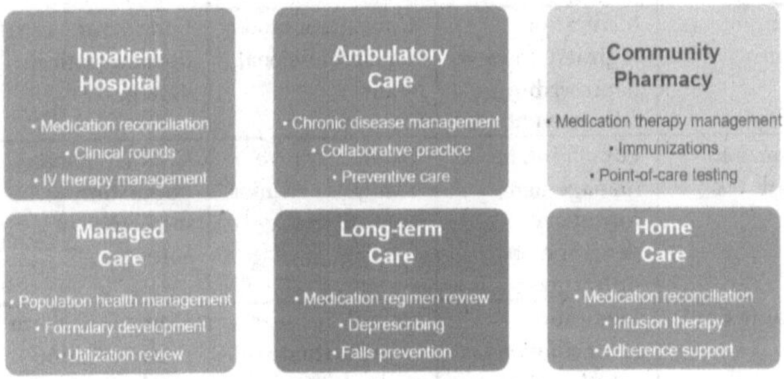

Figure 1.3: Clinical Pharmacy Practice Settings

Community Pharmacy Clinical Services

Enhanced medication therapy management transforms traditional dispensing-focused community pharmacy into clinical care centers through structured assessment, care planning, and follow-up services. Disease-specific programs implement targeted interventions for conditions including diabetes, asthma, and hypertension through regular monitoring, education, and collaborative care coordination. Vaccination services expand public health impact through immunization assessment, administration, and documentation, significantly increasing vaccination rates in communities with active pharmacy-based immunization programs.

Table 1.3: Clinical Pharmacy Practice Settings

Practice Setting	Clinical Activities	Team Structure	Documentation Systems
Inpatient Hospital	Medication reconciliation, rounds participation, IV therapy management	Interprofessional teams, unit-based practice	Electronic health record, clinical documentation systems
Ambulatory Care Clinic	Chronic disease management, preventive care, medication adjustment	Collaborative practice with physicians, team-based care	Electronic health record, patient registry systems
Community Pharmacy	Medication therapy management, immunizations, point-of-care testing	Independent practice, technician support	Pharmacy management systems, documentation platforms
Long-term Care	Medication regimen review, deprescribing, falls prevention	Consultant model, interprofessional team	Long-term care documentation systems
Managed Care	Population health management, formulary development, utilization review	Administrative teams, clinical committees	Claims databases, population management software
Home Care	Medication reconciliation, infusion therapy, adherence support	Remote teams, coordination with home health	Home care documentation platforms

Managed Care Organizations

Formulary management engages clinical pharmacists in medication selection, utilization criteria development, and evidence evaluation to optimize both clinical and economic outcomes across covered populations. Medication utilization review identifies patterns requiring intervention, including potentially inappropriate prescribing, drug-drug interactions, and adherence challenges. Clinical program development creates initiatives addressing specific therapeutic challenges, medication safety concerns, or quality improvement opportunities across member populations.

Specialized Settings

Home care pharmacy provides medication management for patients receiving home-based services, addressing complex regimens, infusion therapies, and transition challenges. Long-term care consultant pharmacy services implement systematic medication reviews, appropriate prescribing initiatives, and regulatory compliance programs for institutional settings. Specialty pharmacy practice manages complex, high-cost medications for conditions including oncology, rheumatology, and neurology through enhanced clinical monitoring, adherence support, and outcomes tracking.

CORE COMPETENCIES

Therapeutic expertise requires comprehensive understanding of pharmacology, disease pathophysiology, and evidence-based treatment guidelines applied through clinical decision-making. Specialized knowledge development maintains current expertise within practice areas through continuous learning, literature evaluation, and application of emerging evidence. Knowledge translation converts complex pharmacotherapeutic information into practical clinical applications adaptable to specific patient circumstances and preferences.

Critical Thinking and Problem Solving

Clinical reasoning employs systematic approaches to patient assessment, therapeutic planning, and monitoring through organized frameworks rather than intuitive or haphazard processes. Evidence evaluation applies critical analysis to research literature, assessing study validity, results significance, and applicability to specific clinical scenarios. Complex case management addresses multifaceted medication challenges including polypharmacy, multiple comorbidities, and competing therapeutic priorities through structured approaches balancing evidence, patient factors, and risk-benefit assessment.

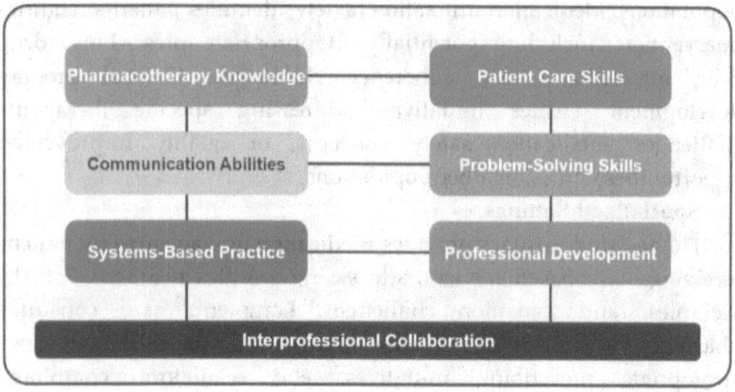

Figure 1.4: Core Competencies and Interprofessional Practice

Communication Skills

Patient-centered communication adapts information delivery to individual needs, health literacy levels, and learning preferences while employing techniques including teach-back verification, plain language, and cultural sensitivity. Interprofessional communication utilizes structured formats including SBAR (Situation-Background-Assessment-Recommendation) to convey clinical recommendations clearly and persuasively to other healthcare providers. Documentation creates comprehensive, clear records of clinical assessments, interventions, and follow-up plans within shared health records accessible to all team members.

Systems-Based Practice

Healthcare delivery knowledge applies understanding of various practice models, payment systems, regulatory requirements, and quality metrics influencing medication management across settings. Resource stewardship balances clinical needs against cost considerations, selecting therapeutically appropriate options with favorable economic impact when multiple alternatives exist. Process improvement identifies systematic medication use challenges and implements structured changes enhancing safety, efficiency, and effectiveness beyond individual patient interventions.

Leadership and Management

Team development builds effective clinical pharmacy services through staff recruitment, performance evaluation, and continuous professional development support. Program implementation transforms concept into operational reality through careful planning, resource allocation, stakeholder engagement, and outcome evaluation. Change management successfully navigates resistance to new practices through strategic approaches addressing organizational culture, incentive alignment, and barrier identification.

Table 1.4: Core Competencies for Clinical Pharmacists

Competency Domain	Skills	Assessment Methods	Development Strategies
Pharmacotherapy Knowledge	Disease state management, medication expertise	Board certification, knowledge examinations	Continuing education, structured training
Patient Care Skills	Assessment, care planning, monitoring	Direct observation, chart review	Preceptorship, simulation training
Communication Abilities	Patient counseling, interprofessional communication	Observed encounters, team feedback	Communication workshops, practice feedback
Problem-Solving Skills	Clinical reasoning, therapeutic decision-making	Case presentations, clinical scenarios	Case-based learning, journal clubs
Systems-Based Practice	Healthcare systems navigation, quality improvement	Project outcomes, system metrics	Leadership development, quality training
Professional Development	Self-assessment, continuous improvement	Portfolio review, reflection exercises	Mentorship, professional engagement

INTERPROFESSIONAL PRACTICE

Patient care teams integrate clinical pharmacists with physicians, nurses, and other healthcare professionals through structured collaboration rather than episodic consultation. Shared decision-making distributes clinical responsibilities based on professional expertise rather than traditional hierarchical models, with pharmacists assuming accountability for medication-related outcomes. Care coordination synchronizes interventions across team members and care settings, preventing fragmentation and duplication while ensuring comprehensive patient management.

Collaborative Relationship Development

Professional role understanding demonstrates knowledge of each discipline's unique and complementary contributions to patient care, recognizing both capabilities and limitations. Trust building establishes credibility through consistent demonstration of clinical competence, reliable follow-through, and patient-centered focus rather than professional territoriality. Conflict resolution addresses inevitable disagreements through constructive approaches focusing on patient needs rather than personal or professional differences.

Communication Strategies

Structured interactions establish consistent frameworks for clinical discussions, including team rounds, case conferences, and standardized consultation processes. Information sharing protocols determine appropriate content, timing, and methods for communicating medication-related information across team members. Electronic health record utilization optimizes shared documentation platforms for communicating assessments, recommendations, and follow-up plans accessible to all team members.

Educational Initiatives

Cross-disciplinary learning creates opportunities for shared knowledge development through joint continuing education, case discussions, and collaborative learning projects. Student interprofessional experiences integrate learners from multiple healthcare disciplines in shared clinical activities, developing collaborative skills alongside profession-specific competencies. Faculty development prepares clinical teachers to model effective interprofessional practice while facilitating learning across disciplinary boundaries.

Practice Advancement

Collaborative practice agreements formalize pharmacist-physician partnerships through written protocols defining clinical activities, decision-making parameters, and mutual responsibilities. Scope of practice expansion advocates for appropriate legal and regulatory frameworks supporting team-based care models utilizing all professionals at their highest capabilities. Outcomes documentation systematically collects evidence demonstrating the value of interprofessional models compared to traditional siloed approaches, supporting both practice advancement and sustainable payment models.

Table 1.5: Impact of Clinical Pharmacy Services on Healthcare Outcomes

Service Type	Clinical Outcomes	Economic Outcomes	Patient Experience Outcomes
Comprehensive Medication Management	22-30% reduction in medication errors, 15-20% improvement in therapeutic goal achievement	$3-5 ROI per dollar invested, 20-30% reduction in medication costs	40% improvement in medication understanding, 25% increase in satisfaction
Transition of Care Services	30-40% reduction in readmissions, 25% decrease in medication discrepancies	$1,500-3,000 savings per averted readmission	35% improvement in care coordination perception
Disease-Specific Management	15-25% improvement in clinical markers, 30% reduction in disease-related complications	20-35% reduction in disease-related healthcare costs	45% improvement in disease self-management confidence
Medication Safety Programs	50-70% reduction in adverse drug events, 40% decrease in high-risk medication errors	$5-7 ROI per dollar invested in safety initiatives	30% increase in safety perception ratings
Collaborative Practice Models	25-40% improvement in therapeutic goal achievement	30% reduction in total healthcare costs for managed conditions	50% improvement in care team satisfaction

Summary

• Clinical pharmacy evolved from product-focused to patient-centered care, emphasizing therapeutic outcomes rather than just medication dispensing.

• Core responsibilities include medication therapy management, therapeutic drug monitoring, patient education, and serving as drug information specialists.

• Clinical pharmacists practice in diverse settings including hospitals, ambulatory care clinics, community pharmacies, long-term care facilities, and specialty practices.

• Essential competencies include pharmacotherapy knowledge, clinical decision-making, communication skills, and evidence-based practice application.

• Interprofessional collaboration is fundamental, requiring pharmacists to work effectively with physicians, nurses, and other healthcare providers to optimize patient care.

• Professional development through continuing education, specialization, and board certification is crucial to maintain and advance clinical practice skills.

• Legal and ethical considerations guide the scope of clinical pharmacy practice and patient care responsibilities.

Multiple Choice Questions

1. Which of the following best describes the evolution of clinical pharmacy in the 1970s?
   A) Focus on drug distribution systems and medication profiles
   B) Introduction of pharmacokinetic monitoring and clinical services
   C) Development of pharmaceutical care as a practice philosophy
   D) Integration of pharmacists into team-based care models
2. The MOST distinctive feature that separates clinical pharmacy from traditional pharmacy practice is:
   A) The authority to dispense medications
   B) Taking direct responsibility for medication outcomes

C) Knowledge of pharmacology and therapeutics
D) Ability to counsel patients on medication use

3. In which practice setting would a clinical pharmacist most likely perform real-time interventions during interprofessional rounds?
A) Community pharmacy
B) Acute care hospital
C) Managed care organization
D) Pharmaceutical industry

4. Which core competency is MOST essential for a clinical pharmacist working in a collaborative practice agreement?
A) Sterile compounding technique
B) Clinical decision-making skills
C) Inventory management
D) Dispensing accuracy

5. When establishing an interprofessional practice model, the clinical pharmacist should FIRST focus on:
A) Demonstrating cost savings
B) Building relationships and trust with team members
C) Developing protocols and guidelines
D) Implementing documentation systems

6. Which statement best describes the medication expert role of clinical pharmacists in healthcare teams?
A) Pharmacists replace physicians in prescribing decisions
B) Pharmacists focus exclusively on cost-effective alternatives
C) Pharmacists provide medication expertise while respecting team dynamics
D) Pharmacists primarily serve as drug information resources when consulted

7. A clinical pharmacist is establishing services in a new practice setting. Which of the following should be the FIRST priority?
A) Developing a revenue model
B) Assessing medication-related needs of the patient population
C) Creating a documentation system
D) Establishing dispensing protocols

8. Which of the following best represents the impact of the pharmaceutical care movement on clinical pharmacy?
   A) Increased focus on product preparation and distribution
   B) Shift toward patient-centered care and outcomes responsibility
   C) Greater emphasis on business management skills
   D) Reduced need for clinical knowledge
9. The clinical pharmacist's role in population health management primarily involves:
   A) Dispensing medications to large patient groups
   B) Identifying and addressing medication-related needs across populations
   C) Managing pharmacy benefits for insurance companies
   D) Conducting large-scale clinical trials
10. Which of the following best describes effective interprofessional practice involving clinical pharmacists?
    A) Pharmacists function independently from other healthcare providers
    B) Pharmacists serve primarily as technical consultants on medication issues
    C) Pharmacists integrate into teams with shared goals and mutual respect
    D) Pharmacists focus exclusively on medication dispensing and distribution

Self-Assessment Questions

1. Describe three key milestones in the evolution of clinical pharmacy practice from the 1960s to the present day, and explain how each has shaped modern practice.
2. Explain the core responsibilities of a clinical pharmacist and how they differ from traditional dispensing roles.
3. Compare and contrast the clinical pharmacist's role in at least two different practice settings (e.g., acute care vs. ambulatory care).
4. Identify and explain three core competencies essential for clinical pharmacy practice and why each is important for effective patient care.
5. Describe specific strategies that clinical pharmacists can use to establish effective interprofessional relationships with physicians, nurses, and other healthcare providers.
6. Explain how the concept of pharmaceutical care transformed the profession of pharmacy, and how it relates to current clinical pharmacy practice.
7. Discuss the impact of collaborative practice agreements on expanding the clinical pharmacist's scope of practice.
8. Explain the significance of board certification in clinical pharmacy practice and its value to patients, healthcare organizations, and pharmacists.
9. Describe how technology has changed clinical pharmacy practice over the past decade and potential future impacts.
10. Discuss the economic value of clinical pharmacy services and how pharmacists can demonstrate their impact on healthcare outcomes

Bibliography

1. Hepler CD, Strand LM. Opportunities and responsibilities in pharmaceutical care. Am J Hosp Pharm. 1990;47(3):533-543.
2. American College of Clinical Pharmacy. The definition of clinical pharmacy. Pharmacotherapy. 2008;28(6):816-817.
3. Saseen JJ, Ripley TL, Bondi D, Burke JM, Cohen LJ, McBane S, et al. ACCP clinical pharmacist competencies. Pharmacotherapy. 2017;37(5):630-636.
4. Carter BL. Evolution of clinical pharmacy in the USA and future directions for patient care. Drugs Aging. 2016;33(3):169-177.
5. Zellmer WA. The future of health-system pharmacy: opportunities and challenges in practice model change. Ann Pharmacother. 2012;46(4):S41-S45.
6. Chisholm-Burns MA, Kim Lee J, Spivey CA, Slack M, Herrier RN, Hall-Lipsy E, et al. US pharmacists' effect as team members on patient care: systematic review and meta-analyses. Med Care. 2010;48(10):923-933.
7. Joint Commission of Pharmacy Practitioners. Pharmacists' patient care process. 2014. Available from: https://jcpp.net/wp-content/uploads/2016/03/PatientCareProcess-with-supporting-organizations.pdf
8. Weber E, Hepfinger C, Koontz R, Cohn-Oswald L. Pharmacy professionals' attitudes and perceptions toward culturally competent care. J Pharm Pract. 2022;35(1):86-91.
9. Reeves S, Pelone F, Harrison R, Goldman J, Zwarenstein M. Interprofessional collaboration to improve professional practice and healthcare outcomes. Cochrane Database Syst Rev. 2017;6(6):CD000072.
10. Sorensen TD, Pestka DL, Brummel AR, Rehrauer DJ, Ekstrand MJ. Seeing the forest through the trees: improving adherence alone will not optimize medication use. J Manag Care Spec Pharm. 2016;22(5):598-604.

CHAPTER 2

PATIENT CARE PROCESS

Author

Mr. Vijay Anand Kada, PharmD Scholar, Department of Pharmacy Practice, Pydah College of Pharmacy, Kakinada, Patavala, Andhra Pradesh, India

Abstract

The systematic patient care process provides a comprehensive framework for delivering clinical pharmacy services through five interconnected steps. Assessment techniques encompass medication history collection, laboratory data interpretation, and symptom evaluation to identify medication-related problems. Care planning involves prioritizing identified problems, establishing measurable outcomes, and developing patient-specific interventions considering efficacy, safety, and feasibility. Implementation strategies include direct interventions, prescriber recommendations, patient education, and care coordination. Monitoring evaluates therapy effectiveness, adverse effects, and adherence through appropriate parameter selection and follow-up scheduling. Documentation using standardized formats captures clinical reasoning, interventions, and outcomes through problem-oriented approaches, SOAP notes, and care plans. This standardized process ensures comprehensive pharmaceutical care delivery, facilitates communication with healthcare teams, demonstrates value, and improves patient outcomes through systematic medication management addressing both actual and potential drug therapy problems.

Keywords: *Pharmaceutical Care Plan, Medication Therapy Management, Drug Therapy Problems, Patient Monitoring, Clinical Documentation*

Learning Objectives

After completion of the chapter, the learners should be able to:

- Conduct comprehensive patient assessments integrating medication histories, laboratory data, and physical findings to identify medication-related problems.
- Develop patient-specific care plans with measurable goals, appropriate interventions, and monitoring parameters addressing identified medication-related needs.
- Implement pharmaceutical care interventions through direct patient care, interprofessional collaboration, and health system initiatives.
- Design appropriate monitoring plans with specific parameters, timeframes, and thresholds for evaluating therapeutic outcomes and adverse effects.
- Create comprehensive documentation that effectively communicates clinical findings, interventions, and follow-up plans using standardized formats.
- Apply the systematic patient care process across diverse practice settings and patient populations to ensure comprehensive medication management.

PATIENT ASSESSMENT TECHNIQUES

Patient interview techniques elicit complete medication information through structured questioning that progresses from current prescribed medications to non-prescription products, supplements, and intermittently used therapies. Open-ended inquiry employs questions including "What medications do you take and how do you take them?" rather than closed questions like "Do you take your medications as prescribed?" to reveal actual usage patterns. Brown bag review examines all medications physically brought by patients, revealing discrepancies between prescribed and actual regimens while identifying duplicate therapies, expired medications, and storage issues. Reconciliation with multiple sources validates patient-reported information against prescription records, discharge summaries, previous histories, and caregiver reports to construct a complete medication profile beyond any single source.

Clinical Data Collection

Medical record review systematically examines relevant components including problem lists, progress notes, laboratory data, diagnostic results, and consultation reports to establish clinical context for medication assessment. Targeted physical assessment performs focused examinations relevant to medication therapy including vital sign measurement, cardiovascular assessment, respiratory evaluation, and neurological screening when appropriate to the clinical situation. Point-of-care testing utilizes immediately available diagnostic capabilities including glucose monitoring, INR determination, lipid measurement, and A1C testing to assess current status and guide therapeutic decisions without delayed laboratory processing.

Table 2.1: Patient Assessment Components and Methods

Assessment Component	Information Sources	Elements	Documentation
Medication History	Patient/caregiver interview, prescription records, previous records	Current medications, past medications, allergies/ADRs, adherence	Comprehensive medication list with doses, frequencies, indications
Medical History	Patient interview, medical records, provider communication	Chief complaint, past medical history, review of systems	Chronological disease progression, current status of conditions
Laboratory and Diagnostic Data	Electronic health record, lab reports, diagnostic imaging	Relevant lab values, diagnostic test results, trending data	Baseline values, significant changes, correlation with therapy
Physical Findings	Direct patient examination, provider notes	Vital signs, targeted organ system assessment, general appearance	Objective data, changes from baseline, medication-related findings
Psychosocial Assessment	Patient interview, social work notes, care team input	Health beliefs, social support, financial resources, functional status	Barriers to care, adherence factors, support needs
Lifestyle Factors	Patient interview, dietary records, activity logs	Diet, exercise, substance use, sleep patterns	Impact on therapy, modification targets, patient priorities

Subjective Information Gathering

Symptom assessment evaluates patient-reported experiences that may represent either medication effects or underlying disease manifestations requiring distinction through systematic questioning about timing, characteristics, alleviating factors, and exacerbating conditions. Medication experience exploration examines patient perceptions of treatment effectiveness, adverse effects, and burden, recognizing that subjective experience significantly influences adherence and treatment decisions beyond objective clinical parameters. Health beliefs assessment explores patient understanding of their conditions, treatment goals, and medication expectations, recognizing that interventions misaligned with patient beliefs face significant implementation barriers regardless of clinical appropriateness.

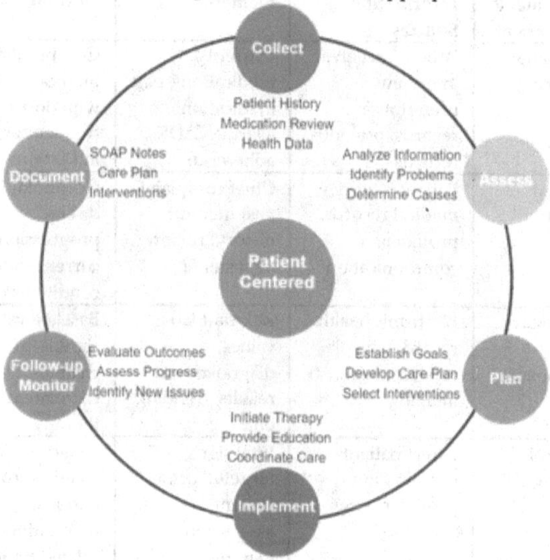

Figure 2.1: The Pharmacist's Patient care Process

Adherence Evaluation

Pattern identification distinguishes between different non-adherence types including unintentional (forgetting, misunderstanding, complexity) versus intentional (concerns about necessity, side effects, costs) through targeted questioning about specific adherence challenges. Barrier assessment examines practical obstacles including physical limitations, financial constraints, health literacy challenges, and regimen complexity contributing to medication underuse. Measurement tools employ validated instruments including the Morisky Medication Adherence Scale, Brief Medication Questionnaire, or Adherence to Refills and Medications Scale to quantify adherence issues consistently across patients and over time.

Problem Identification

Medication therapy problems classification categorizes identified issues into established frameworks including indication (unnecessary therapy or untreated condition), effectiveness (incorrect drug or dosage), safety (adverse effects or interactions), and adherence problems to ensure comprehensive assessment beyond symptom management. Prioritization methods rank identified problems based on factors including clinical severity, patient concerns, contribution to current symptoms, and feasibility of intervention rather than addressing issues in order of discovery. Root cause analysis examines underlying factors rather than superficial manifestations, distinguishing between symptoms requiring symptomatic treatment versus those indicating need for therapy modification or discontinuation.

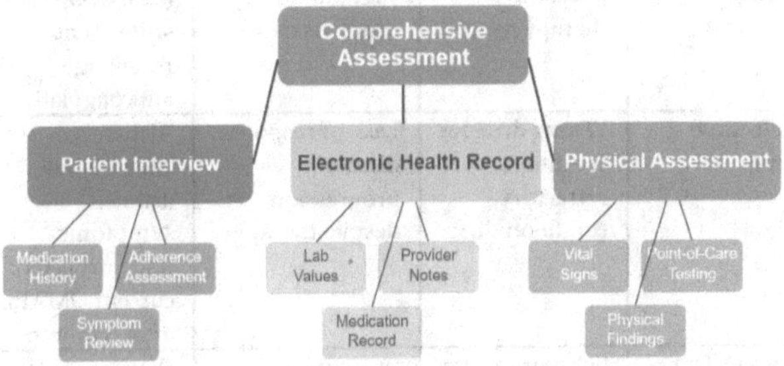

Figure 2.2: Assessment Techniques and Data Sources

CARE PLANNING

Measurable outcome identification establishes specific, quantifiable targets including laboratory parameters, symptom scores, functional capabilities, or quality of life measures rather than vague goals like "improvement." Timeframe establishment defines expected intervals for initial response, maximal effect, and reassessment points based on pharmacokinetic, pharmacodynamic, and disease progression considerations. Collaborative determination involves patients in goal-setting discussions, ensuring targets reflect patient priorities and preferences rather than solely provider-determined endpoints, significantly improving adherence to recommended therapies.

Table 2.2: Common Drug Therapy Problems and Assessment Findings

Drug Therapy Problem	Definition	Indicators	Examples
Unnecessary Drug Therapy	Medication without valid indication	No current diagnosis justifying therapy, duplicate therapy	"Patient taking two ACE inhibitors (lisinopril and enalapril) prescribed by different providers"
Need for Additional Therapy	Untreated condition, preventive therapy needed	Untreated diagnosis, suboptimal prophylaxis	"Patient with atrial fibrillation (CHA_2DS_2-VASc score=4) not receiving anticoagulation"
Ineffective Drug	Wrong drug for condition, refractory condition	Lack of response, disease progression despite therapy	"Patient's rheumatoid arthritis symptoms uncontrolled on current DMARD after 3 months"
Dosage Too Low	Subtherapeutic dose, drug interaction reducing effect	Inadequate response, subtherapeutic levels	"Vancomycin trough 8 mcg/mL (target 15-20 mcg/mL for endocarditis)"
Adverse Drug Reaction	Undesirable effect, unsafe drug	Symptoms of ADR, contraindicated medication	"Patient experiencing persistent dry cough on lisinopril therapy"
Dosage Too High	Excessive dose, impaired clearance	Toxicity symptoms, supratherapeutic levels	"Digoxin dose not adjusted for CrCl 25 mL/min; level 2.3 ng/mL"
Nonadherence	Failure to take medication as prescribed	Refill records showing gaps, patient-reported barriers	"Patient taking metformin once daily instead of twice daily due to GI side effects"

Therapeutic Alternatives Evaluation

Evidence-based assessment examines available research supporting various treatment options, considering quality of evidence, magnitude of effect, consistency across studies, and applicability to specific patient populations. Patient-specific factor consideration incorporates individual characteristics including age, comorbidities, concurrent medications, genetic factors, and past treatment responses that may influence therapy selection beyond population-based guidelines. Benefit-risk analysis systematically weighs potential advantages against possible harms for each therapeutic option, recognizing that guideline-recommended therapies may have unfavorable risk-benefit profiles for specific patients despite general population appropriateness.

Selection of Interventions

Medication therapy recommendations develop specific suggestions for initiating, modifying, or discontinuing medications based on assessment findings and therapeutic goals. Non-pharmacological interventions identify appropriate lifestyle modifications, dietary changes, physical activity recommendations, and self-management strategies complementing pharmacotherapy rather than operating in isolation. Referral determinations identify situations requiring additional expertise from medical specialists, other healthcare disciplines, or community support services based on identified needs beyond the pharmacist's scope.

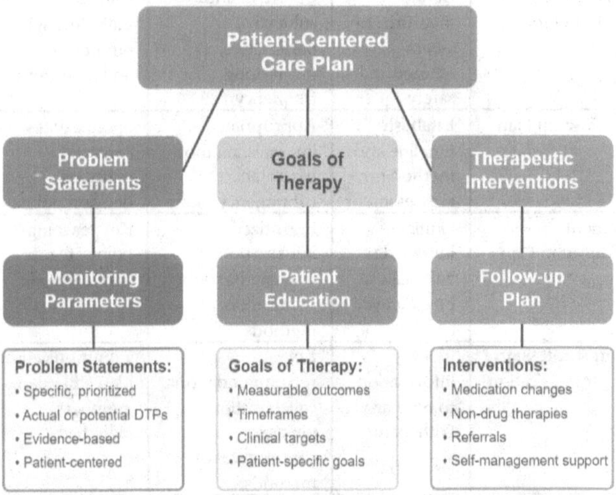

Figure 2.3: Components of a Patient-Centered Care Plan

Individualized Care Plan Development

Therapy customization adapts standard treatment approaches to individual circumstances including dosage adjustments for organ function, administration timing modifications for daily routines, and formulation selection based on swallowing capability or absorption considerations.

Table 2.3: Components of a Detailed Care Plan

Care Plan Element	Purpose	Considerations	Documentation Format
Problem Statement	Define drug therapy problems requiring intervention	Prioritization, clinical significance, patient perspective	Numbered problems with specific descriptions
Goals of Therapy	Establish desired outcomes for interventions	Measurable parameters, timeframes, patient-centered outcomes	Short-term and long-term goals with metrics
Interventions	Detail specific actions to resolve problems	Specificity, practicality, evidence basis	Action steps with responsible parties
Monitoring Parameters	Define measures to assess efficacy and safety	Objective and subjective parameters, monitoring frequency	Clinical indicators with target values and timeframes
Follow-up Plan	Establish timeline and method for reassessment	Appropriate intervals, method of contact, contingency plans	Specific dates, contact methods, decision points
Patient Education Plan	Outline knowledge and skills to be conveyed	Prioritized information, learning barriers, verification methods	Key teaching points, teach-back elements
Interprofessional Communication	Identify information to be shared with team	Key recommendations, collaboration needs, communication methods	Communication plan with team members identified

Regimen simplification identifies opportunities to reduce complexity through once-daily alternatives, combination products, synchronized administration times, or therapeutic class consolidation when appropriate. Patient preference integration incorporates patient-identified priorities, treatment limitations, and quality of life considerations into final recommendations rather than focusing exclusively on physiological outcomes.

Patient Education Planning

Educational needs assessment identifies knowledge gaps, misconceptions, and specific learning requirements based on health literacy, previous experience, and complexity of the medication regimen. Teaching method selection determines appropriate educational approaches including verbal instruction, written materials, demonstration, visual aids, or technology-based tools based on patient learning preferences and capabilities. Material development creates or selects resources matching patient needs, employing appropriate language level, cultural relevance, and format accessibility rather than generic medication information.

IMPLEMENTATION

Recommendation communication employs structured formats including SBAR (Situation-Background-Assessment-Recommendation) to present findings, supporting evidence, and specific suggestions efficiently and persuasively. Collaborative discussion addresses prescriber questions, concerns, and alternative perspectives through collegial dialogue focused on patient benefit rather than professional authority. Implementation negotiation determines specific responsibilities, timeframes, and follow-up mechanisms ensuring clear accountability for agreed-upon interventions.

Direct Patient Care Activities

Medication therapy initiation implements agreed-upon treatment plans through appropriate prescribing, therapy scheduling, and initial dosing based on patient-specific factors. Administration technique instruction demonstrates proper medication use including inhaler technique, injection administration, transdermal application, or other specialized delivery methods requiring more than verbal direction. Self-monitoring training teaches patients appropriate techniques for home-based assessment including blood pressure measurement, blood glucose monitoring, symptom tracking, or other relevant parameters supporting therapy management.

Addressing Barriers to Implementation

Financial obstacle management navigates coverage issues, patient assistance programs, therapeutic alternatives, and discount options to overcome cost-related adherence barriers. Health literacy challenges addresses through plain language communication, teachback verification, focused information prioritization, and literacy-appropriate written materials rather than comprehensive but overwhelming education. Practical support coordination connects patients with medication management tools including pill organizers, reminder systems, administration aids, and technology support appropriate to individual needs and capabilities.

Table 2.4: Implementation Strategies for Pharmaceutical Care Plans

Implementation Type	Approaches	Documentation Elements	Outcome Measures
Direct Patient Care Activities	Medication counseling, adherence interventions, self-monitoring instruction	Content delivered, patient understanding assessment, materials provided	Knowledge assessment, skill demonstration, patient confidence
Provider Interventions	Drug therapy recommendations, collaborative medication management, consult responses	Clinical recommendations, supporting evidence, provider response	Recommendation acceptance rate, therapy changes, time to implementation
Health System Interventions	Protocol development, order set creation, formulary recommendations	System changes, implementation timeline, affected populations	Compliance rates, system utilization, process improvement metrics
Care Coordination	Transitions of care interventions, referrals, interprofessional collaboration	Hand-off information, referral details, team communication	Successful transitions, medication continuity, team awareness
Technology Implementation	Electronic alerts, decision support tools, telehealth services	Technology description, user training, workflow integration	Utilization rates, alert response, technology acceptance

Coordination with Healthcare Team

Care transition management ensures treatment plan implementation across settings including hospital discharge, post-acute care, and transitions between providers through active information transfer and coordination. Interprofessional communication shares implementation plans, responsibilities, and follow-up expectations with relevant team members including physicians, nurses, case managers, and other providers involved in patient care. Support service integration connects pharmaceutical care with related services including nutrition counseling, physical therapy, social work, and community support programs through appropriate referrals and information sharing.

Patient Engagement Strategies

Shared decision-making involves patients as active participants in implementation decisions, discussing options, preferences, and responsibilities rather than presenting fixed treatment directives. Motivational approaches employ techniques including importance and confidence scaling, value exploration, and discrepancy development to enhance patient commitment to agreed-upon treatment plans. Self-management support develops patient capabilities for independent medication management through gradually increasing responsibility, problem-solving skill development, and appropriate autonomy based on individual capacity.

MONITORING AND FOLLOW-UP

Parameter selection identifies appropriate indicators for tracking therapeutic response, adverse effects, and overall medication effectiveness based on pharmacological effects, individual risk factors, and treatment goals. Measurement frequency establishes appropriate intervals for reassessment based on medication characteristics, condition stability, and risk level, ranging from daily monitoring for high-risk therapies to quarterly or annual evaluation for stable chronic treatments. Threshold determination defines specific values or findings that would trigger intervention, including both insufficient therapeutic response and development of adverse effects requiring modification.

Clinical Outcome Evaluation

Effectiveness assessment compares current status against established therapeutic goals using objective measures including laboratory values, physical findings, or validated symptom scores appropriate to the condition. Adverse effect monitoring systematically evaluates for known or potential medication-related problems through targeted questioning, physical assessment, laboratory testing, or other appropriate surveillance methods. Unexpected outcome investigation explores unanticipated findings including lack of expected benefit, unusual reactions, or unexpected improvements to determine relationship to medication therapy versus other factors.

Adherence Monitoring

Refill pattern analysis examines prescription refill timing to calculate measures including proportion of days covered, medication possession ratio, or gaps in therapy revealing potential adherence issues before clinical deterioration. Self-reported adherence assessment employs structured questions or validated instruments during follow-up visits to identify emerging adherence challenges or persistent difficulties despite previous interventions. Therapeutic response correlation examines the relationship between adherence patterns and clinical outcomes, distinguishing between treatment failures due to non-adherence versus pharmacological ineffectiveness requiring different intervention approaches.

Therapy Modification

Dose adjustment implements changes based on monitoring findings, including titration for insufficient effect, reduction for adverse effects, or modification based on changing patient factors including weight, organ function, or drug interactions. Medication addition or discontinuation responds to monitoring results indicating need for supplemental therapy, alternative approaches, or cessation of medications providing inadequate benefit or unnecessary risk. Administration modification alters timing, frequency, or method of administration to address issues identified during monitoring including adverse effects, convenience barriers, or interaction management.

Long-term Follow-up Systems

Scheduled reassessment establishes systematic intervals for comprehensive medication review beyond condition-specific monitoring, ensuring continued appropriateness of all therapies as patient circumstances evolve. Care coordination maintains communication with other providers regarding medication changes, monitoring findings, and emerging concerns through appropriate documentation and direct communication. Proactive surveillance implements systematic approaches to identifying potential problems between scheduled visits through pharmacy system alerts, patient-reported outcome collection, or strategic interim contact for high-risk patients or therapies

DOCUMENTATION

Patient assessment findings record subjective and objective information gathered during evaluation, including medication history, clinical data, reported symptoms, and identified medication-related problems. Clinical interventions document specific actions taken including therapy recommendations, education provided, referrals made, and communications with other healthcare providers. Monitoring parameters specify indicators being tracked, measurement schedule, responsibility assignment, and action thresholds for future reference and continuity of care.

Table 2.5: Documentation Systems and Components for Clinical Pharmacy Services

Documentation Type	Purpose	Essential Elements	Format Examples
SOAP Note	Comprehensive clinical assessment and plan	Subjective, objective, assessment, plan sections	Electronic health record progress note, structured template
Pharmacy Consult Response	Focused response to specific clinical question	Question addressed, literature review, specific recommendation	Consult note, e-communication response
Medication Reconciliation	Document and resolve medication discrepancies	Prior to admission list, current list, discharge list with changes	Medication reconciliation form, transition document
Medication Therapy Management Note	Document comprehensive medication review	Medication-related problems, interventions, monitoring plan	MTM platform documentation, SNOMED coded entries
Intervention Documentation	Record specific clinical interventions	Problem identified, action taken, outcome	Pharmacy intervention database, billing documentation
Patient Education Record	Document patient teaching	Content covered, understanding assessment, materials provided	Education checklist, teach-back documentation

Documentation Standards

Problem-oriented format organizes information using standardized structures including subjective information, objective data, assessment, and plan (SOAP) or similar frameworks ensuring comprehensive and logical documentation. Terminology standardization employs consistent, precise language for describing medication therapy problems, interventions, and outcomes rather than variable or ambiguous terminology subject to interpretation. Evidence linkage connects recommendations and decisions to specific findings, literature, guidelines, or clinical reasoning supporting the chosen approach.

Documentation Systems

Electronic health record integration incorporates pharmacy documentation within shared patient records accessible to all team members rather than isolated pharmacy-specific systems. Structured templates implement standardized formats for common documentation scenarios including comprehensive medication reviews, targeted interventions, or follow-up assessments ensuring consistency and completeness. Interoperability considerations ensure critical medication information transfers appropriately between different healthcare systems, preventing information loss during care transitions.

Quality Documentation Practices

Temporal accuracy records the timing of assessments, interventions, and communications with date and time specificity, particularly for time-sensitive clinical situations. Objective recording distinguishes between directly observed information, patient-reported data, and provider assessment or interpretation rather than presenting all information as equivalent. Intervention tracking documents the complete sequence from identification through resolution for medication therapy problems, including intermediate steps, patient response, and final outcomes rather than isolated recommendations.

Documentation for Different Purposes

Clinical care documentation focuses on information supporting ongoing patient management, emphasizing actionable findings, specific plans, and follow-up requirements for care continuity. Billing documentation includes elements required for service reimbursement, ensuring appropriate coding, time specification, complexity assessment, and other factors supporting payment requirements. Quality measurement reporting captures data elements required for performance metrics, quality improvement initiatives, and regulatory requirements without disrupting clinical documentation flow.

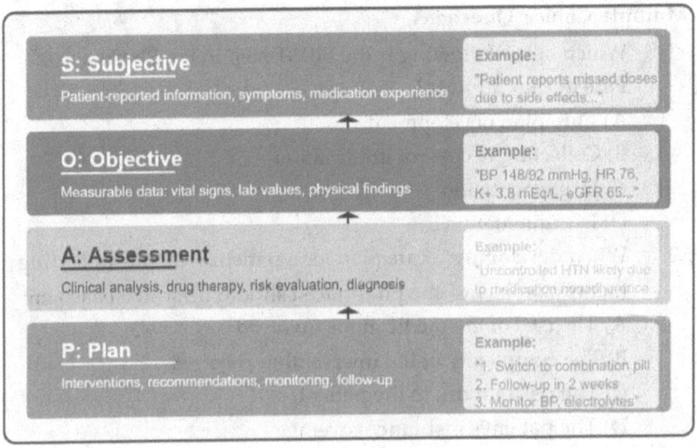

Figure 2.4: SOAP Documentation

Summary

- Comprehensive patient assessment involves gathering subjective and objective information through interviews, physical assessment, and review of medical records and laboratory data.

- Care planning requires identifying drug therapy problems, establishing therapeutic goals, and selecting appropriate interventions based on patient-specific factors.

- Implementation includes initiating, modifying, or discontinuing medication therapy with appropriate patient education and addressing potential barriers to adherence.

- Continuous monitoring evaluates therapeutic outcomes, adverse effects, and patient adherence using laboratory parameters, physical findings, and patient-reported outcomes.

- Documentation must be clear, concise, problem-oriented, and follow structured formats such as SOAP (Subjective, Objective, Assessment, Plan) to ensure continuity of care.

- Patient-centered care emphasizes shared decision-making, respect for patient preferences, and individualization of therapy based on unique patient needs.

- Effective communication with patients and healthcare providers is essential for successful implementation of the care plan and achievement of therapeutic goals.

Multiple Choice Questions

1. Which of the following is the FIRST step in the Pharmacists' Patient Care Process?
   A) Care plan development
   B) Collecting necessary information
   C) Implementation
   D) Documentation
2. When developing a care plan for a patient with multiple drug therapy problems, the pharmacist should prioritize based on:
   A) The cost of the medications involved
   B) The complexity of the intervention required
   C) The risk of harm to the patient
   D) The patient's insurance coverage
3. Which of the following assessment techniques would be MOST appropriate for evaluating a patient's medication adherence?
   A) Conducting a physical assessment
   B) Reviewing laboratory values
   C) Analyzing prescription refill history
   D) Performing a point-of-care test
4. A pharmacist is providing care to a patient with diabetes who has not reached their A1C goal. When implementing a medication adjustment, which of the following is the MOST important consideration?
   A) The cost of the new medication
   B) The patient's understanding and agreement with the plan
   C) The pharmacy's inventory of the medication
   D) The prescriber's preferred medication
5. Which documentation component includes the pharmacist's evaluation of collected data and identification of drug therapy problems?
   A) Subjective
   B) Objective
   C) Assessment
   D) Plan
6. When establishing monitoring parameters for a newly initiated antihypertensive medication, the pharmacist should:
   A) Focus exclusively on blood pressure measurements
   B) Establish parameters for both efficacy and adverse effects
   C) Rely solely on patient-reported outcomes
   D) Plan for one follow-up visit after therapy initiation

7. The MOST effective approach to follow-up for a patient started on warfarin therapy is:
   A) Instructing the patient to contact the pharmacist if they experience bleeding
   B) Scheduling regular INR monitoring with specific target ranges
   C) Recommending annual comprehensive medication reviews
   D) Advising the patient to follow up with their physician as needed
8. Which of the following best exemplifies the "Collect" phase of the Pharmacists' Patient Care Process?
   A) Documenting interventions in the patient's medical record
   B) Performing a comprehensive medication history
   C) Developing goals of therapy with the patient
   D) Communicating recommendations to other healthcare providers
9. A pharmacist has identified that a patient is experiencing an adverse drug reaction. The NEXT step in the patient care process should be to:
   A) Document the adverse drug reaction in the patient's record
   B) Develop a plan to address the adverse drug reaction
   C) Assess the severity and causality of the reaction
   D) Report the reaction to the FDA MedWatch program
10. Which of the following is an essential component of implementation in the patient care process?
    A) Identifying drug therapy problems
    B) Establishing goals of therapy
    C) Taking actions to achieve care plan goals
    D) Evaluating effectiveness of the care plan

Self-Assessment Questions

1. Describe the five components of the Pharmacists' Patient Care Process and explain how they form a continuous cycle of care.
2. Explain three assessment techniques a clinical pharmacist should use when gathering patient-specific information, and why each is important.
3. Identify the essential components of a comprehensive care plan and explain why each element is necessary.
4. Compare and contrast objective and subjective assessment data, providing examples of each and explaining their relative importance in clinical decision-making.
5. Describe three strategies for prioritizing drug therapy problems in a complex patient case with multiple medical conditions.
6. Explain how a clinical pharmacist should approach monitoring for both efficacy and safety when implementing a new medication therapy.
7. Discuss the importance of patient engagement in the care planning process and strategies to enhance patient participation.
8. Describe the key components of a well-documented SOAP note and explain why standardized documentation is important for clinical pharmacy practice.
9. Explain how pharmacists should establish appropriate follow-up parameters, including timing and methods, for different types of medication interventions.
10. Discuss how documentation of clinical pharmacy services contributes to quality improvement, research, and justification of pharmacy services.

Bibliography

1. Joint Commission of Pharmacy Practitioners. Pharmacists' patient care process. 2014. Available from: https://jcpp.net/wp-content/uploads/2016/03/PatientCareProcess-with-supporting-organizations.pdf
2. Tietze KJ. Clinical skills for pharmacists: a patient-focused approach. 3rd ed. St. Louis: Mosby Elsevier; 2012.
3. Strand LM, Cipolle RJ, Morley PC, Frakes MJ. The impact of pharmaceutical care practice on the practitioner and the patient in the ambulatory practice setting: twenty-five years of experience. Curr Pharm Des. 2004;10(31):3987-4001.
4. Cipolle RJ, Strand LM, Morley PC. Pharmaceutical care practice: the patient-centered approach to medication management. 3rd ed. New York: McGraw-Hill Medical; 2012.
5. Weed LL. Medical records that guide and teach. N Engl J Med. 1968;278(11):593-600.
6. Ramalho de Oliveira D, Brummel AR, Miller DB. Medication therapy management: 10 years of experience in a large integrated health care system. J Manag Care Pharm. 2010;16(3):185-195.
7. Rovers JP, Currie JD. A practical guide to pharmaceutical care. 3rd ed. Washington DC: American Pharmacists Association; 2007.
8. Hammond RW, Schwartz AH, Campbell MJ, Remington TL, Chuck S, Blair MM, et al. Collaborative drug therapy management by pharmacists—2003. Pharmacotherapy. 2003;23(9):1210-1225.
9. Hazen ACM, de Bont AA, Boelman L, Zwart DLM, de Gier JJ, de Wit NJ, et al. The degree of integration of non-dispensing pharmacists in primary care practice and the impact on health outcomes: a systematic review. Res Social Adm Pharm. 2018;14(3):228-240.
10. Barnett MJ, Frank J, Wehring H, Newland B, VonMuenster S, Kumbera P, et al. Analysis of pharmacist-provided medication therapy management (MTM) services in community pharmacies over 7 years. J Manag Care Pharm. 2009;15(1):18-31.

CHAPTER 3

EVIDENCE-BASED PRACTICE

Author

Mr. Srihari Krishna Indurti, PharmD Intern, Department of Pharmacy Practice, East Point College of Pharmacy, Benguluru, Karnataka, India

Abstract

Evidence-based pharmacy practice integrates best research evidence with clinical expertise and patient values to optimize medication therapy decisions. Literature evaluation skills include searching biomedical databases efficiently, understanding study designs, and interpreting statistical analyses to assess clinical significance beyond statistical significance. Clinical guideline interpretation requires evaluating recommendation strength, evidence quality, and applicability to specific patient populations while recognizing limitations and conflicts. Critical appraisal employs structured frameworks to evaluate literature validity, importance, and applicability through systematic assessment of methodology, bias risk, and result interpretation. Practical application involves integrating evidence with patient-specific factors including preferences, comorbidities, and social determinants through shared decision-making. This approach enables pharmacists to navigate information overload, resolve conflicting recommendations, address evidence gaps, and translate complex research into practical therapeutic decisions that balance scientific evidence with individualized patient care, ultimately improving medication therapy outcomes through rigorous, systematic application of best available evidence.

Keywords: *Clinical Literature Evaluation, Critical Appraisal, Guideline Implementation, Evidence Hierarchy, Therapeutic Decision-Making*

Learning Objectives

After completion of the chapter, the learners should be able to:

- Formulate answerable clinical questions using the PICO framework to guide effective literature searches.
- Evaluate primary literature for validity, reliability, and applicability to specific patient care scenarios.
- Interpret clinical practice guidelines including strength of recommendations and quality of evidence to inform therapeutic decision-making.
- Apply critical appraisal skills to different study designs including randomized controlled trials, observational studies, and systematic reviews.
- Integrate best research evidence with clinical expertise and patient values to optimize therapeutic decisions.
- Communicate evidence-based recommendations effectively to patients, caregivers, and healthcare professionals.

LITERATURE EVALUATION

Primary literature encompasses original research published in peer-reviewed journals, providing the most detailed methodology and results but requiring significant evaluation skills to assess quality and applicability. Secondary resources include systematic reviews and meta-analyses that synthesize multiple primary studies, offering higher-level evidence through systematic methodology and statistical pooling of results. Tertiary references provide summarized, pre-evaluated information including clinical databases (Micromedex, Lexicomp), evidence-based compendia (UpToDate, DynaMed), and pharmacy-specific resources (Pharmacist's Letter, APhA's Handbook of Nonprescription Drugs) that balance accessibility against potential publication delays and filtering bias. Point-of-care tools deliver concise, actionable information designed for clinical decision support at the time of patient care, sacrificing comprehensive detail for immediate utility in practice settings.

Search Strategy Development

Question formulation structures clinical uncertainties into searchable queries using frameworks such as PICO (Patient/Problem, Intervention, Comparison, Outcome) or PICOT (adding Time) to clarify search parameters and ensure relevant results. Database selection matches information needs with appropriate resources, distinguishing between comprehensive bibliographic databases (PubMed/MEDLINE,

Embase), subject-specific collections (PsycINFO, International Pharmaceutical Abstracts), and full-text aggregators (Ovid, EBSCO) based on topic, depth requirements, and access availability. Search technique optimization employs advanced features including controlled vocabulary (MeSH terms), field-specific searching, Boolean operators, truncation, and limits to balance search sensitivity (finding all relevant studies) against specificity (excluding irrelevant results) for efficient literature retrieval.

Study Design Recognition

Experimental designs include randomized controlled trials providing the strongest evidence for intervention effects through randomization and control group comparison, with variations including parallel group, crossover, factorial, and adaptive designs offering different advantages for specific research questions. Observational studies encompass cohort studies (following exposed and unexposed groups forward in time), case-control studies (comparing those with and without outcomes retrospectively), cross-sectional analyses (examining exposures and outcomes simultaneously), and case series/reports (describing individual patient experiences without comparison groups). Qualitative research employs methodologies including phenomenology, grounded theory, and ethnography to explore subjective experiences and perspectives through systematic non-numerical data collection and analysis, providing insights into patient preferences, experiences, and decision-making processes essential for patient-centered care.

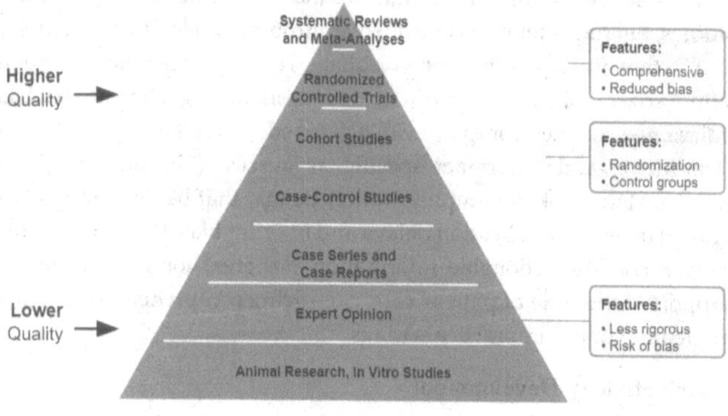

Figure 3.1: Hierarchy of Evidence

Statistical Concepts in Research

Significance testing evaluates whether observed differences likely represent true effects rather than chance findings, with p-values indicating probability of results occurring randomly and confidence intervals showing the range of plausible true values. Effect size measures quantify the magnitude of findings using metrics appropriate to the outcome type, including absolute risk reduction, relative risk, odds ratios, hazard ratios, mean differences, and number needed to treat, with clinical significance often requiring judgment beyond statistical significance alone. Methodological considerations including sample size adequacy, power calculations, multiple comparison adjustments, and intention-to-treat versus per-protocol analyses impact result interpretation and reliability, requiring assessment beyond headline findings to evaluate substantive meaning.

Table 3.1: Hierarchy of Evidence in Clinical Decision Making

Evidence Level	Study Types	Strengths	Limitations	Application Examples
Level I	Systematic reviews, meta-analyses of RCTs	Comprehensive analysis, reduced bias, statistical power	Heterogeneity between studies, publication bias	Treatment guidelines, formulary decisions
Level II	Well-designed RCTs	Control for confounding, randomization reduces bias	Limited generalizability, may not reflect real-world use	Drug efficacy determination, comparative effectiveness
Level III	Non-randomized controlled trials, cohort studies	Larger populations, longer follow-up, real-world settings	Selection bias, confounding variables	Safety surveillance, rare adverse effects
Level IV	Case-control studies, case series	Useful for rare conditions, hypothesis generation	Cannot establish causality, recall bias	Adverse event signals, unusual presentations
Level V	Expert opinion, mechanism-based reasoning	Provides guidance when higher evidence lacking	Subject to individual bias, lacks systematic evaluation	New therapies, rare conditions without research

Information Evaluation Frameworks

Validity assessment examines internal factors determining whether results represent true effects, including randomization quality, blinding, allocation concealment, follow-up completeness, and appropriate analysis methods. Importance evaluation considers effect magnitude, precision (confidence interval width), clinical significance thresholds, and relevance to patient-oriented rather than surrogate outcomes. Applicability analysis determines whether study populations, interventions, comparators, and settings reasonably translate to specific patient care scenarios, recognizing that methodologically strong studies may still have limited relevance to particular clinical situations. Synthesis approaches integrate findings across multiple studies with consideration of consistency, direction of effect, heterogeneity, and overall evidence quality rather than relying on isolated studies regardless of apparent quality.

CLINICAL GUIDELINES

Evidence collection systematically identifies, evaluates, and synthesizes relevant research through comprehensive literature searches, explicit inclusion criteria, and structured quality assessment. Recommendation formulation translates evidence into specific guidance through expert interpretation, considering both research findings and practical implementation factors, ideally using formalized consensus methods to minimize individual bias. Strength grading assigns levels to recommendations reflecting both evidence quality (from high-quality randomized trials to expert opinion) and benefit-risk assessment (from clear benefit-risk advantage to uncertain trade-offs), providing clinicians with transparency about recommendation foundations.

Quality Assessment Tools

AGREE II (Appraisal of Guidelines for Research and Evaluation) provides a validated framework evaluating guideline quality across six domains: scope and purpose, stakeholder involvement, development rigor, clarity of presentation, applicability, and editorial independence. GRADE (Grading of Recommendations Assessment, Development and Evaluation) offers a systematic approach to rating evidence quality and recommendation strength, explicitly considering study limitations, inconsistency, indirectness, imprecision, and publication bias. RIGHT (Reporting Items for Practice Guidelines in Healthcare) checklist ensures comprehensive reporting of guideline development processes, evidence foundations, and implementation considerations for transparency and usability.

Guideline Limitations and Considerations

Evidence gaps frequently necessitate recommendations based on lower-quality research or expert consensus when high-quality studies are unavailable for important clinical questions, requiring transparent acknowledgment of limitations. Applicability constraints arise from study populations that differ from diverse practice populations, particularly regarding age extremes, pregnancy, lactation, multimorbidity, and racial/ethnic diversity often underrepresented in research. Competing guidelines from different organizations sometimes provide conflicting recommendations for identical clinical questions due to different evidence interpretation, expert composition, or development methodologies, requiring comparative evaluation rather than arbitrary selection.

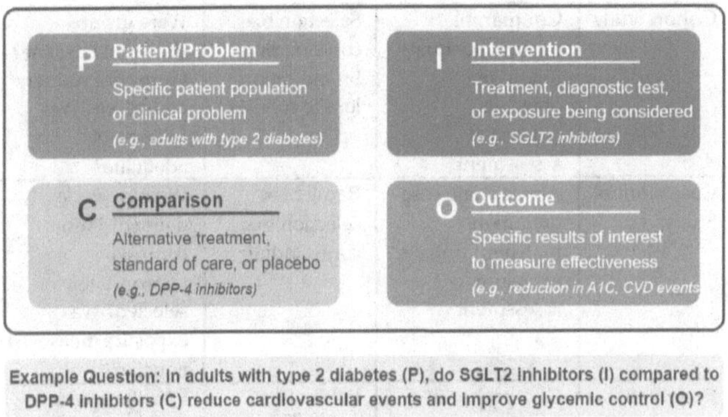

Figure 3.2: PICO Framework for Clinical Questions

Implementation

Adaptation to local context modifies guideline recommendations based on specific practice setting factors including population characteristics, resource availability, formulary constraints, and existing workflows rather than wholesale adoption without consideration of practical application barriers. Algorithm and protocol development translates guideline recommendations into operational workflows, order sets, and decision support tools facilitating consistent application across practitioners and settings. Measurement strategy identifies key performance indicators aligned with guideline recommendations, establishing baseline assessment, tracking mechanisms, and feedback systems to evaluate implementation success and areas requiring additional support.

Table 3.2: Critical Appraisal Elements for Common Study Designs

Study Design	Quality Indicators	Potential Biases	Validity Assessment Questions
Randomized Controlled Trial	Randomization method, allocation concealment, blinding, intention-to-treat analysis	Selection bias, performance bias, attrition bias, detection bias	Was randomization appropriate? Was blinding maintained? Were all participants accounted for?
Cohort Study	Comparable groups, adequate follow-up, objective outcomes assessment	Selection bias, confounding by indication, loss to follow-up	Were groups similar at baseline? Were confounders addressed? Was follow-up adequate?
Case-Control Study	Appropriate case definition, matched controls, exposure assessment	Recall bias, selection bias, confounding	Were cases clearly defined? Were controls appropriately selected? Was exposure measured equally?
Systematic Review	Comprehensive search, quality assessment, appropriate synthesis	Publication bias, study selection bias, heterogeneity	Was the search comprehensive? Were inclusion criteria appropriate? Was quality assessment conducted?
Clinical Practice Guideline	Systematic development, evidence grading, stakeholder involvement	Sponsor bias, expert bias, evidence selection bias	Was development systematic? Were conflicts disclosed? Is evidence grading transparent?

Guideline Evolution and Currency

Update processes maintain guideline relevance through scheduled comprehensive reviews (typically every 3-5 years) and interim updates for significant new evidence potentially changing recommendations. Living guidelines represent an emerging approach with continuous evidence surveillance and rapid recommendation modification as new research emerges, particularly valuable for rapidly evolving therapeutic areas. Harmonization efforts address proliferation and inconsistency through collaborative development across multiple organizations, adoption of common methodology standards, and explicit consideration of existing guidelines during development to minimize unexplained variations.

Table 3.3: Evaluation of Clinical Guidelines

Evaluation Domain	Assessment Elements	Quality Indicators	Red Flags
Development Methodology	Systematic literature review, evidence grading system, update frequency	AGREE II criteria compliance, transparent methods	Unclear development process, no systematic review
Stakeholder Involvement	Multidisciplinary panel, patient representation, external review	Diverse representation, transparent selection	Single specialty authorship, no patient perspective
Evidence Quality	Systematic evidence evaluation, strength of recommendation grading	GRADE approach, evidence tables	Missing evidence grades, selected citations
Recommendation Clarity	Specific actionable recommendations, implementation considerations	Clear directives, practical guidance	Vague recommendations, conflicting advice
Applicability	Resource implications, barriers assessment, monitoring criteria	Implementation tools, cost considerations	No implementation guidance, unrealistic recommendations
Editorial Independence	Funding sources, conflict of interest management	Transparent disclosures, conflict management	Undisclosed conflicts, industry funding without safeguards

CRITICAL APPRAISAL

Randomization evaluation assesses the process for allocation sequence generation and concealment to ensure true randomization rather than predictable or manipulable assignment potentially introducing selection bias. Blinding assessment examines measures to prevent knowledge of treatment assignment from influencing participants, clinicians, outcome assessors, and analysts, recognizing that different outcomes vary in susceptibility to expectation effects. Follow-up completeness examines attrition rates, reasons for withdrawal, and handling of missing data, with differential dropout between treatment arms or incomplete outcome data potentially biasing results regardless of initial randomization quality.

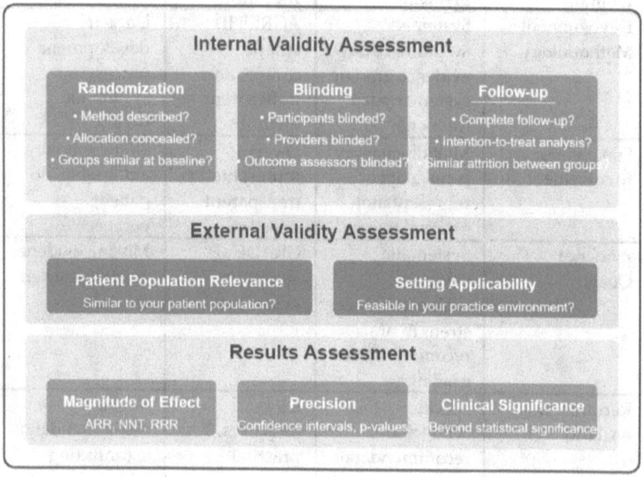

Figure 3.3: Critical Appraisal of Randomized Controlled Trials

Observational Study Evaluation

Selection bias assessment examines how study groups were assembled and whether systematic differences between comparison groups might explain observed outcomes independently of the intervention being studied. Confounding variable management evaluates techniques including restriction, matching, stratification, multivariable adjustment, and propensity scoring used to address known and measured potential confounders. Information bias examination considers whether data collection methods differed between comparison groups or over time, potentially creating artificial differences unrelated to true effects. Temporal relationship clarity ensures exposure preceded outcomes for causal inference, particularly important in case-control studies where retrospective design can create ambiguity about sequence.

Systematic Review and Meta-Analysis Assessment

Search comprehensiveness evaluates whether review methodology captured all relevant studies through appropriate database selection, search term development, inclusion of unpublished data sources, and language considerations. Study selection and extraction examines processes including duplicate independent screening, clear eligibility criteria, and standardized data collection to minimize bias during review construction. Heterogeneity management assesses approaches to study variability, including statistical testing (I^2 statistic, Cochran's Q), subgroup analyses, meta-regression, and appropriate model selection (fixed vs. random effects) based on diversity among included studies. Publication bias evaluation examines whether missing studies (typically negative results) might distort pooled conclusions, using funnel plots, statistical tests, and search strategies specifically addressing unpublished data.

Table 3.4: Applying Evidence to Patient Care Decision-Making

Decision Step	Considerations	Tools and Resources	Examples
Formulate Clinical Question	Patient-specific factors, therapeutic alternatives, outcomes of interest	PICO framework, clinical pathways	"In adults with type 2 diabetes and CKD (P), does an SGLT2 inhibitor (I) compared to standard therapy (C) reduce progression of kidney disease (O)?"
Locate Best Evidence	Appropriate information sources, search strategy, evidence hierarchy	PubMed Clinical Queries, Cochrane Library, guideline repositories	Systematic search of PubMed using MeSH terms "Sodium-Glucose Transporter 2 Inhibitors," "Diabetic Nephropathies," and "Disease Progression"
Critical Appraisal	Study validity, magnitude of effect, precision of results, applicability	Critical appraisal worksheets, evidence summary tools	Evaluation of CREDENCE trial using RCT appraisal checklist
Apply to Patient	Patient characteristics vs. study population, benefit-risk assessment, patient preferences	Shared decision-making tools, risk calculators, benefit-harm visualization	Assess patient's eGFR, albuminuria, comorbidities, and medication tolerance compared to study inclusion criteria
Evaluate Outcome	Therapeutic goals achievement, adverse effects, patient experience	Monitoring plans, outcome assessment tools	Track changes in eGFR, albuminuria, hospitalizations, and quality of life after implementing therapy

Pharmaceutical Industry-Sponsored Research

Design consideration examines whether study methodology favors the sponsor's product through comparator selection (placebo rather than active alternatives, inappropriate dosing of competitors), endpoint choice (surrogate markers, composite outcomes, post-hoc analyses), or participant selection (narrow criteria excluding challenging patients). Reporting completeness assesses whether all pre-specified outcomes appear in publications, as selective outcome reporting frequently favors statistically significant findings while omitting negative or neutral results. Disclosure transparency evaluates whether funding sources, author relationships with sponsors, data access, and analytical independence are fully declared and whether independent verification of findings was permitted.

Statistical vs. Clinical Significance

Absolute vs. relative effect distinction differentiates between percentage reductions (relative effects often appearing more impressive) and actual risk differences (absolute effects directly showing impact magnitude), with number needed to treat providing practical clinical context. Surrogate endpoint evaluation considers the validation strength between intermediate markers (laboratory values, imaging findings) and patient-oriented outcomes (mortality, symptoms, function, quality of life) determining whether statistical changes translate to meaningful benefits. Subgroup analysis scrutiny examines whether population segment findings represent pre-specified hypotheses with adequate statistical power or post-hoc observations at high risk for false positive findings due to multiple comparisons without appropriate adjustment.

Table 3.5: Common Statistical Concepts in Evidence Evaluation

Statistical Concept	Definition	Interpretation Considerations	Clinical Application
Absolute Risk Reduction (ARR)	Actual difference in event rates between treatment and control groups	Provides actual magnitude of effect	"Treatment reduced MI by 2% (from 5% to 3%)"
Number Needed to Treat (NNT)	Number of patients who need treatment to prevent one additional bad outcome	Lower values indicate more effective treatments	"NNT of 50 means 50 patients need treatment to prevent 1 event"

Statistical Concept	Definition	Interpretation Considerations	Clinical Application
Relative Risk Reduction (RRR)	Proportional reduction in risk between treatment and control groups	Can magnify small absolute differences	"Treatment reduced MI risk by 40% (from 5% to 3%)"
Confidence Interval (CI)	Range of values within which the true value likely lies	Width indicates precision, crossing null indicates non-significance	"95% CI of 0.8-1.2 crosses 1.0, suggesting non-significant result"
p-value	Probability of obtaining results at least as extreme if null hypothesis is true	Arbitrary significance thresholds, not a measure of effect size	"p<0.05 indicates statistical significance but not necessarily clinical importance"
Hazard Ratio (HR)	Ratio of hazards between treatment groups in time-to-event analysis	Time-dependent relative risk measure	"HR of 0.75 indicates 25% reduction in event rate at any given time"

APPLICATION TO PRACTICE

Evidence hierarchies establish frameworks for weighing different study types, traditionally placing systematic reviews and randomized trials above observational studies and expert opinion, though evolving models recognize that methodology quality within study types and question appropriateness sometimes outweigh rigid hierarchical placement. GRADE framework application systematically evaluates evidence quality (high, moderate, low, very low) and recommendation strength (strong or conditional/weak) based on balance of effects, certainty of evidence, resource considerations, and preference variability, providing structured guidance for evidence application. Shared decision-making integration combines best evidence with patient values and preferences through explicit discussion of benefits, harms, uncertainties, and alternatives rather than unilateral application of even high-quality evidence without patient engagement.

Clinical Expertise Integration

Knowledge gaps navigation addresses the frequent absence of perfect evidence for specific clinical scenarios through structured approaches including analogous population extrapolation, first principles application, risk-benefit modeling, and explicit uncertainty acknowledgment rather than abandoning evidence-based approaches entirely. Therapy individualization adapts population-based evidence to specific patients through consideration of pharmacokinetic/ pharmacodynamic factors, comorbidities, concurrent medications, genetic variations, and individual values not addressed in research populations. Conflicting evidence resolution approaches contradictory findings through consideration of methodology quality, population similarity to the current patient, recency, consistency with related evidence, and biological plausibility rather than selective citation supporting preconceived conclusions.

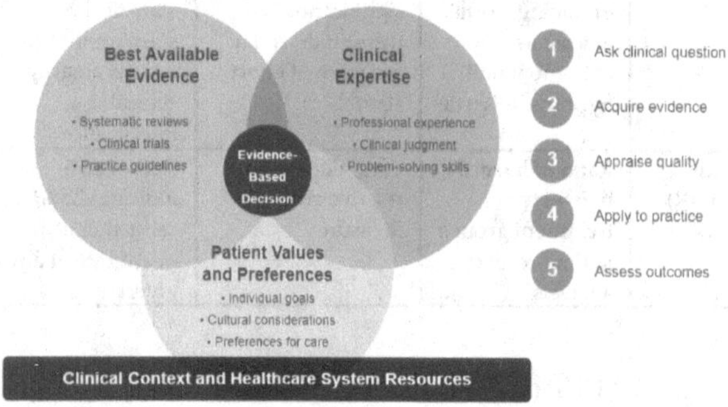

Figure 3.4: Evidence-Based Practice Model

Practice-Based Research Participation

Quality improvement integration embeds systematic data collection, intervention testing, and outcome evaluation into routine practice through methodologies including Plan-Do-Study-Act cycles, audit and feedback systems, and benchmarking against best practices or comparable organizations. Research network engagement connects individual practitioners with larger collaborative structures supporting multi-site investigations, data pooling, and standardized protocols addressing questions arising from practice that might otherwise remain unanswerable by individual clinicians. Practice-based evidence generation complements traditional research by systematically documenting real-world effectiveness, safety, and implementation considerations through structured data collection during routine care, particularly valuable for populations and interventions underrepresented in traditional clinical trials.

Technology-Enabled Evidence Application

Point-of-care tools integrate evidence into workflow through electronic clinical decision support delivering filtered, actionable information at the time and location of decision-making, balancing comprehensiveness against usability constraints. Mobile applications provide immediate access to drug information, calculators, guidelines, and primary literature through smartphones and tablets, enabling evidence retrieval in diverse practice settings without fixed computer access. Artificial intelligence applications emerging in literature surveillance, pattern recognition, risk prediction, and treatment recommendation generation offer potential to manage information volume exceeding human cognitive capacity, though requiring careful validation and appropriate practitioner oversight.

Continuing Professional Development

Self-assessment approaches identify personal knowledge gaps through structured reflection, practice audits, assessment tools, and peer feedback rather than pursuing continuing education based solely on interest or convenience. Targeted learning strategies address identified needs through appropriate educational methods including case-based learning, simulation, academic detailing, and spaced education rather than passive information exposure. Implementation planning moves beyond knowledge acquisition to skill development, behavior change, and practice integration through goal setting, barrier identification, and follow-up assessment focused on application rather than mere information retention.

Summary

- Comprehensive patient assessment involves gathering subjective and objective information through interviews, physical assessment, and review of medical records and laboratory data.

- Care planning requires identifying drug therapy problems, establishing therapeutic goals, and selecting appropriate interventions based on patient-specific factors.

- Implementation includes initiating, modifying, or discontinuing medication therapy with appropriate patient education and addressing potential barriers to adherence.

- Continuous monitoring evaluates therapeutic outcomes, adverse effects, and patient adherence using laboratory parameters, physical findings, and patient-reported outcomes.

- Documentation must be clear, concise, problem-oriented, and follow structured formats such as SOAP (Subjective, Objective, Assessment, Plan) to ensure continuity of care.

- Patient-centered care emphasizes shared decision-making, respect for patient preferences, and individualization of therapy based on unique patient needs.

- Effective communication with patients and healthcare providers is essential for successful implementation of the care plan and achievement of therapeutic goals.

Multiple Choice Questions

1. Which of the following represents the HIGHEST level of evidence in the evidence hierarchy?
   A) Expert opinion
   B) Case series
   C) Cohort study
   D) Systematic review of randomized controlled trials
2. When formulating a clinical question using the PICO framework, the letter "C" stands for:
   A) Clinical outcome
   B) Comparison or control
   C) Chronic condition
   D) Cost-effectiveness
3. A study reports that a new medication reduces the risk of stroke by 30% compared to standard therapy. The absolute risk reduction is 3% (from 10% to 7%). Which of the following represents the number needed to treat (NNT)?
   A) 3
   B) 10
   C) 30
   D) 33
4. Which of the following is the MOST appropriate approach when applying clinical practice guidelines to an elderly patient with multiple comorbidities?
   A) Strictly follow guideline recommendations regardless of patient factors
   B) Adapt recommendations based on patient-specific factors and preferences
   C) Ignore guidelines completely and rely on clinical experience
   D) Apply only the recommendations supported by randomized controlled trials
5. When evaluating a randomized controlled trial, which of the following would MOST significantly threaten its internal validity?
   A) Small sample size
   B) Single-center design
   C) Failure to maintain blinding
   D) Industry funding
6. A pharmacist is evaluating literature on a new medication for heart failure. Which of the following outcomes would provide

the STRONGEST evidence of clinical benefit?

A) Improvement in a surrogate marker like brain natriuretic peptide

B) Patient-reported improvement in symptoms

C) Reduction in hospitalization and mortality

D) Improvement in ejection fraction

7. When reviewing a meta-analysis, which of the following is the MOST important factor to consider when determining its quality?

   A) The number of included studies

   B) The journal's impact factor

   C) The heterogeneity among included studies

   D) The country where the analysis was conducted

8. Which statement best describes the appropriate use of clinical practice guidelines?

   A) Guidelines represent rules that must be followed in all clinical situations

   B) Guidelines replace clinical judgment in complex patient cases

   C) Guidelines provide recommendations based on evidence that must be contextualized

   D) Guidelines are primarily useful for research purposes, not clinical practice

9. When evaluating a study's statistical significance, which of the following statements is MOST accurate?

   A) A p-value <0.05 always indicates clinical importance

   B) Statistical significance does not necessarily imply clinical significance

   C) Confidence intervals are less informative than p-values

   D) Studies with p-values >0.05 provide no useful information

10. A pharmacist is applying evidence to a clinical decision for an individual patient. Which of the following should be considered ALONG WITH the evidence?

    A) Only the patient's medical conditions

    B) Only the medication's cost and accessibility

    C) Patient preferences, clinical context, and available resources

    D) Only the strength of the available evidence

Self-Assessment Questions

1. Explain the hierarchy of evidence in clinical decision-making, ranking different study types from strongest to weakest and explaining why they are ranked in this order.
2. Describe the PICO framework and explain how it helps formulate answerable clinical questions for evidence-based practice.
3. Identify three key components to evaluate when critically appraising a randomized controlled trial, and explain why each is important.
4. Explain the difference between absolute risk reduction (ARR) and relative risk reduction (RRR), including how each might influence clinical decision-making.
5. Describe three limitations of clinical practice guidelines and how pharmacists should account for these limitations when applying guidelines to individual patients.
6. Explain how confidence intervals help interpret the results of a clinical study and their advantage over p-values alone.
7. Discuss how pharmacists should approach situations where high-quality evidence is lacking but clinical decisions must still be made.
8. Describe the process of applying evidence-based medicine to an individual patient, including considerations beyond the evidence itself.
9. Explain the concept of number needed to treat (NNT) and how it can be used to compare different therapeutic interventions.
10. Discuss three strategies pharmacists can use to stay current with rapidly evolving medical literature and evidence.

Bibliography

1. Sackett DL, Rosenberg WM, Gray JA, Haynes RB, Richardson WS. Evidence based medicine: what it is and what it isn't. BMJ. 1996;312(7023):71-72.
2. Guyatt G, Rennie D, Meade MO, Cook DJ. Users' guides to the medical literature: a manual for evidence-based clinical practice. 3rd ed. New York: McGraw-Hill Education; 2015.
3. Straus SE, Glasziou P, Richardson WS, Haynes RB. Evidence-based medicine: how to practice and teach EBM. 5th ed. Edinburgh: Elsevier; 2019.
4. Schardt C, Adams MB, Owens T, Keitz S, Fontelo P. Utilization of the PICO framework to improve searching PubMed for clinical questions. BMC Med Inform Decis Mak. 2007;7:16.
5. Shaughnessy AF, Slawson DC, Bennett JH. Becoming an information master: a guidebook to the medical information jungle. J Fam Pract. 1994;39(5):489-499.
6. Institute of Medicine (US) Committee on Standards for Developing Trustworthy Clinical Practice Guidelines; Graham R, Mancher M, Miller Wolman D, Greenfield S, Steinberg E, editors. Clinical practice guidelines we can trust. Washington (DC): National Academies Press (US); 2011.
7. Higgins JPT, Thomas J, Chandler J, Cumpston M, Li T, Page MJ, Welch VA (editors). Cochrane handbook for systematic reviews of interventions version 6.3. Cochrane, 2022. Available from: www.training.cochrane.org/handbook
8. Shea BJ, Reeves BC, Wells G, Thuku M, Hamel C, Moran J, et al. AMSTAR 2: a critical appraisal tool for systematic reviews that include randomised or non-randomised studies of healthcare interventions, or both. BMJ. 2017;358:j4008.
9. Oxman AD, Guyatt GH. The science of reviewing research. Ann N Y Acad Sci. 1993;703:125-133.
10. Greenhalgh T, Howick J, Maskrey N; Evidence Based Medicine Renaissance Group. Evidence based medicine: a movement in crisis? BMJ. 2014;348:g3725.

CHAPTER 4

PATIENT INTERVIEW AND ASSESSMENT

Author

Dr. Usha Sri Pammi, Assistant Professor, Department of Pharmacy Practice, Sir C.R. Reddy College of Pharmaceutical Sciences, Eluru, Andhra Pradesh, India

Abstract

Effective patient interview and assessment techniques form the foundation of comprehensive medication management, beginning with advanced communication skills incorporating active listening, open-ended questioning, and empathetic response. Medical history gathering employs structured approaches to medication reconciliation, allergy assessment, and symptom evaluation while navigating challenges with recall accuracy and health literacy. Physical assessment includes targeted examination techniques relevant to medication therapy monitoring, focusing on vital signs, cardiopulmonary assessment, and organ-specific evaluations indicating drug efficacy or toxicity. Clinical documentation practices capture pertinent findings through standardized formats ensuring comprehensive, objective recording of subjective and objective data supporting clinical decisions. Cultural competency integrates awareness of diverse health beliefs, communication preferences, and medication practices across different populations, addressing language barriers, health disparities, and culturally-specific concerns. These integrated skills enable pharmacists to gather accurate, comprehensive patient information essential for identifying medication-related problems, developing appropriate interventions, and establishing therapeutic relationships founded on trust and mutual understanding.

Keywords: *Medication History Taking, Patient-Centered Communication, Therapeutic Relationship, Health Literacy, Culturally-Competent Care*

Learning Objectives

After completion of the chapter, the learners should be able to:

- Demonstrate effective patient-centered communication techniques including active listening, empathy, and appropriate questioning strategies.
- Conduct comprehensive medication history interviews that accurately capture prescription medications, over-the-counter products, supplements, and adherence patterns.
- Perform targeted physical assessment techniques relevant to medication therapy monitoring and evaluation.
- Document patient encounters comprehensively using standardized formats that support clinical decision-making and interprofessional communication.
- Apply principles of cultural competency to address diverse health beliefs, communication styles, and medication practices.
- Evaluate and address barriers to effective communication including health literacy limitations, language differences, and cognitive impairments.

COMMUNICATION SKILLS

Initial approach creates a positive first impression through appropriate introduction, professional appearance, and attention to environmental factors including privacy, seating arrangement, and minimization of barriers such as desks or computer screens. Non-verbal communication employs body language including eye contact, forward lean, and open posture demonstrating engagement, while facial expressions and gestures convey empathy and understanding beyond verbal content. Relationship development establishes trust through demonstrated respect for patient autonomy, recognition of expertise in their own experience, and authentic interest in their perspective rather than purely transactional interaction focused exclusively on information gathering.

Active Listening Techniques

Attentive presence demonstrates full engagement through undivided attention, minimized distractions, and visible focus on the patient rather than electronic records or other tasks during communication. Reflective responses restate key points in different words to verify understanding, demonstrate listening, and encourage elaboration on important topics. Non-judgmental acknowledgment recognizes patient experiences, concerns, and emotions without expressing approval or disapproval, creating safe space for honest disclosure of potentially sensitive information including non-adherence, alternative therapy use, or lifestyle factors affecting health.

Table 4.1: Effective Communication Techniques in Patient Interviewing

Communication Technique	Description	Application Examples	Barriers to Avoid
Active Listening	Full attention to verbal and nonverbal cues with reflective responses	"I hear you saying the side effects are concerning..."	Interrupting, premature problem-solving
Open-Ended Questioning	Questions requiring more than yes/no responses	"Tell me about your experience with this medication"	Multiple questions at once, leading questions
Empathetic Responses	Acknowledging emotions without judgment	"That sounds really frustrating to deal with"	Dismissing concerns, false reassurance
Teach-Back Method	Having patients restate information in their own words	"To make sure I explained clearly, could you tell me how you'll take this medication?"	Asking "Do you understand?" which invites yes bias
Silence	Strategic pauses allowing patient reflection and response	3-5 second pause after asking about concerns	Filling silence with excessive talking
Chunking and Checking	Presenting information in small segments with comprehension checks	Explain one aspect of therapy, verify understanding, then continue	Information overload without verification
Body Language	Nonverbal cues showing engagement and openness	Eye contact, forward lean, open posture	Physical barriers, distracting behaviors
Summarizing	Concise restatement of key points	"So the main concerns are the cost and remembering to take it twice daily"	Omitting important details, misrepresenting concerns

Questioning Approaches

Open-ended inquiry employs questions that cannot be answered with simple yes/no responses, beginning with broad prompts such as "What concerns brought you here today?" or "Tell me about your experience with this medication" before narrowing to specific details. Closed questioning strategically obtains precise information when required, including timing, frequency, or specific symptom characteristics after establishing broader context through open approaches. Funnel technique progresses systematically from general to specific information, beginning with patient-directed narrative before focusing on details necessary for clinical decision-making, balancing efficiency with patient-centered communication.

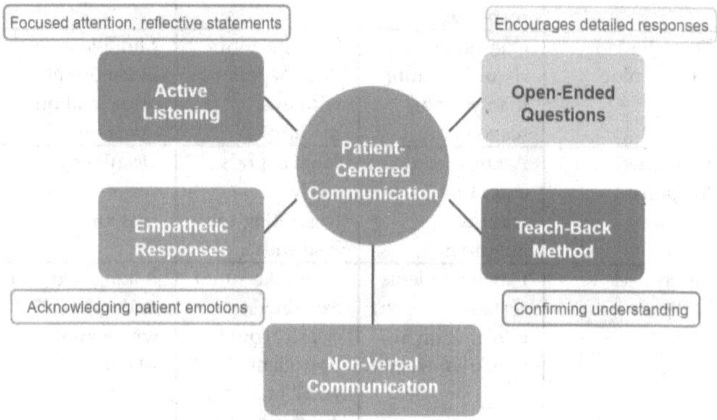

Figure 4.1: Effective Communication Techniques

Patient Education Principles

Health literacy adaptation matches communication complexity to individual comprehension capabilities, using plain language (approximately 6th-8th grade level for most patients), defining medical terminology when necessary, and confirming understanding through teach-back techniques. Chunking and pacing divides information into manageable segments presented at appropriate speed with opportunities for questions between segments, preventing cognitive overload that impairs retention and understanding. Visual reinforcement supplements verbal information with written materials, diagrams, models, or demonstrations enhancing comprehension through multiple learning modalities, particularly important for conceptually complex or detailed instructions.

Challenging Communication Scenarios

Emotion management responds constructively to patient distress, anger, or anxiety through acknowledgment, legitimization, and appropriate empathic responses rather than defensive reactions or premature reassurance that may inhibit expression of legitimate concerns. Health belief navigation addresses perspectives that differ from conventional medical understanding through respectful exploration rather than confrontation, identifying underlying concerns driving seemingly irrational positions and finding common ground for shared decision-making. Language barrier management employs professional interpreters (preferably trained medical interpreters rather than family members) for limited English proficiency, utilizing best practices including first-person speech, manageable information segments, and direct patient engagement rather than speaking to the interpreter.

MEDICAL HISTORY TAKING

Current medication profile documents all active treatments including prescription medications, over-the-counter products, dietary supplements, and complementary/alternative therapies with specific details on drug name, strength, dose, frequency, timing, and duration of use. Administration assessment explores how patients actually take medications versus prescribed directions, identifying intentional modifications, administration challenges, or misunderstandings requiring clarification or regimen adjustment. Medication experience evaluation examines perceived effectiveness, side effects (both confirmed and suspected), and overall satisfaction with current and previous therapies, providing crucial context for treatment decisions beyond objective clinical parameters.

Table 4.2: Components of Medication History

History Component	Information to Obtain	Suggested Questions	Documentation Elements
Current Prescription Medications	Name, dose, frequency, duration, indication	"What prescription medications are you currently taking? What is each one for?"	Complete list with strength, route, frequency, duration, prescriber
Over-the-Counter Products	Name, dose, frequency,	"What medications do	Complete list with patterns of

History Component	Information to Obtain	Suggested Questions	Documentation Elements
	reason for use	you buy without a prescription? How often do you take them?"	use and self-treatment purposes
Dietary Supplements/Herbals	Name, formulation, dose, reason for use	"Do you take any vitamins, minerals, or herbal supplements?"	Product details, formulation, brands, self-reported benefits
Medication Allergies	Specific agent, reaction type, timing, severity	"Have you ever had an allergic reaction to a medication? What happened?"	Specific agent, reaction description, temporal relationship, interventions required
Medication Efficacy	Perceived benefit, symptom control, therapeutic goals	"How well do you feel your blood pressure medicine is working?"	Patient-reported efficacy, objective measures if available
Adverse Effects	Current or previous side effects, management strategies	"Have you noticed any unwanted effects from your medications?"	Specific effects, severity, timing, management approaches
Adherence Patterns	Missed doses, modified regimens, adherence barriers	"How often do you miss taking your medications? What makes it difficult?"	Self-reported adherence, specific barriers, modification patterns
Medication Storage	Storage locations, organization systems	"Where and how do you store your medications?"	Storage conditions, organization methods, potential safety issues
Administration Techniques	Device use, timing, with/without food	"Can you show me how you use your inhaler?"	Technique assessment, timing relative to meals, administration challenges

Medication Allergy Assessment

Reaction characterization distinguishes between true allergies (immunologic reactions including IgE-mediated anaphylaxis or delayed hypersensitivity) and intolerances (predictable side effects including gastrointestinal distress or headache) through detailed description of specific symptoms, timing, and severity. Cross-reactivity evaluation identifies potential risks across related medications based on chemical structure and documented patterns, preventing unnecessary avoidance of entire drug classes when isolated agents are problematic. Documentation standards record specific reaction details rather than vague labels like "allergy," enabling accurate risk assessment for future prescribing decisions based on reaction type, severity, and certainty of causation rather than overgeneralized precautions.

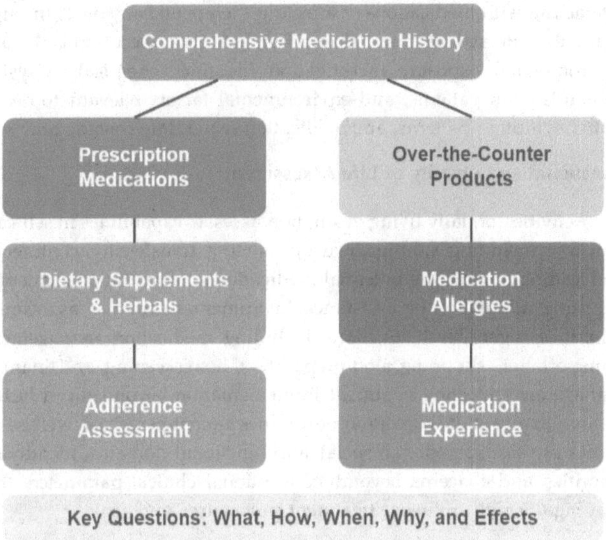

Figure 4.2: Components of Comprehensive Medication History

Medical History Domains

Disease state inventory comprehensively documents acute and chronic conditions including diagnosis dates, treatment history, current status, and relationship to medication therapy, extending beyond primary concerns to seemingly unrelated conditions potentially affecting medication selection or response. Surgical and procedural history records relevant interventions including dates, complications, and resulting anatomical changes potentially affecting medication absorption or administration, such as gastric bypass, ostomy placement, or vascular access devices. Family history identifies hereditary conditions and treatment responses among first-degree relatives providing context for current health risks and potential medication effectiveness or adverse effect patterns suggested by genetic relationships.

Social and Lifestyle Assessment

Substance use evaluation systematically assesses tobacco, alcohol, caffeine, and illicit substance consumption including amount, frequency, duration, and attempts at cessation, recognizing significant implications for medication metabolism, interactions, and treatment adherence. Dietary patterns examination explores typical intake, restrictions, cultural practices, and nutritional supplements potentially interacting with medications or affecting therapeutic outcomes through nutrient interactions or absorption effects. Occupational and environmental exposure investigation identifies chemicals, physical demands, shift patterns, and environmental factors relevant to health status, symptom patterns, and medication scheduling considerations.

Functional and Quality of Life Assessment

Activities of daily living evaluation assesses capabilities in self-care functions including bathing, dressing, toileting, transferring, continence, and feeding, identifying potential medication administration challenges requiring adaptation or assistance. Instrumental activities assessment examines higher-level functions including medication management, transportation, shopping, food preparation, housekeeping, and financial management affecting treatment implementation beyond direct health status. Quality of life exploration examines patient-perceived well-being across physical, emotional, social, and functional domains, identifying priorities and concerns beyond conventional clinical parameters that may significantly influence treatment preferences and goals.

PHYSICAL ASSESSMENT

Blood pressure measurement employs proper technique including appropriate cuff size, patient positioning, resting period, and repeated measurements when indicated, with recognition of factors affecting readings including white coat effect, recent activity, or time relative to medication administration. Heart rate and respiratory assessment evaluates rate, rhythm, depth, and effort, noting relationship to exertion, medication effects, or underlying conditions beyond simple numerical documentation. Body composition evaluation includes weight, height, body mass index, and when

Table 4.3: Physical Assessment Parameters for Medication Monitoring

Body System	Assessment Components	Medication Monitoring Applications	Documentation
Cardiovascular	Blood pressure, heart rate, rhythm, edema	Antihypertensives, heart failure therapy, anticoagulants	Vital signs with position, cardiac exam findings, edema grading
Respiratory	Respiratory rate, oxygen saturation, breath sounds, inhaler technique	Bronchodilators, inhaled corticosteroids, oxygen therapy	Respiratory parameters, auscultation findings, inhaler technique assessment
Neurological	Mental status, coordination, gait, reflexes	Anticonvulsants, antipsychotics, Parkinson's medications	Standardized assessment scales, specific neurological findings
Dermatological	Skin integrity, rashes, injection sites, wounds	Topical medications, biologics, anticoagulants	Description, location, size, appearance with photo documentation if applicable
Gastrointestinal	Abdominal examination, bowel patterns, liver assessment	Laxatives, antidiarrheals, hepatotoxic medications	Abdominal findings, stool characteristics, hepatic assessment
Musculoskeletal	Range of motion, strength, gait assessment	Pain medications, muscle relaxants, osteoporosis therapy	Functional assessments, pain scales, mobility measures
Endocrine	Weight, body mass index, glucose monitoring	Diabetes medications, thyroid therapy, corticosteroids	Weight trends, glycemic patterns, metabolic parameters
Sensory	Vision, hearing, taste alterations	Ototoxic medications, ophthalmics, taste-altering drugs	Sensory changes, functional impact, screening test results

relevant, waist circumference or more detailed composition assessment, with interpretation considering trends over time rather than isolated measurements.

Systems-Focused Examination

Cardiovascular assessment includes heart sound evaluation, jugular venous pressure estimation, extremity examination for edema, pulses, and perfusion status, with findings interpreted in context of medication effects including volume status changes, rate/rhythm alterations, or peripheral circulation effects. Respiratory examination evaluates breathing pattern, breath sounds, cough characteristics, and signs of respiratory distress, particularly relevant for medications affecting respiratory function or used to treat pulmonary conditions. Neurological screening assesses relevant functions including mental status, coordination, gait, and reflexes as appropriate to medication regimens with potential neurological effects or for conditions where neurological function affects medication use capability.

Medication-Specific Physical Findings

Adverse effect manifestations identifies physical signs of medication-related problems including rashes, edema, tremor, drowsiness, dry mouth, or specific patterns associated with particular drug classes, distinguishing between expected, tolerable effects and those requiring intervention. Efficacy indicators evaluates physical findings reflecting treatment response including blood pressure control, heart failure symptoms, respiratory function, pain behaviors, or other observable markers of therapeutic effect or failure. Monitoring parameter assessment collects physical findings required for ongoing therapy management including weight for heart failure patients, respiratory rate for opioid recipients, or neurological status for seizure medication management.

Point-of-Care Testing

Glucose monitoring employs appropriate technique and timing relative to meals and medications, with interpretation considering patterns rather than isolated readings for therapy adjustment decisions. International normalized ratio (INR) testing provides immediate warfarin effect assessment allowing real-time dosage adjustment and shorter follow-up intervals when outside therapeutic range. Respiratory function measurement including peak flow or spirometry offers objective assessment of airway obstruction response to therapy and guides treatment intensification or maintenance decisions for respiratory conditions.

Technology-Enhanced Assessment

Remote monitoring integration incorporates data from patient-used devices including home blood pressure monitors, continuous glucose monitoring systems, or activity trackers into clinical assessment, extending evaluation beyond episodic clinic measurements. Digital health applications employ smartphone-based or wearable technology collecting relevant physiological parameters, symptom reports, or functional measures providing longitudinal data between visits. Telehealth examination adapts physical assessment techniques to virtual platforms through structured protocols, patient self-examination guidance, and appropriate technology utilization while recognizing inherent limitations requiring mitigation or in-person follow-up when indicated.

CLINICAL DOCUMENTATION

Care continuity documentation ensures critical information transfers effectively between providers and settings, highlighting active problems, current medication regimens, recent changes, planned monitoring, and follow-up requirements essential for seamless transitions. Quality measurement reporting captures elements required for quality initiatives, performance metrics, and population health management without compromising narrative clarity or clinical utility. Legal protection documentation creates defensible records demonstrating appropriate assessment, decision-making processes, interventions, patient education, and follow-up planning that would withstand scrutiny in potential liability situations.

Documentation Formats

SOAP format organizes information into Subjective (patient-reported symptoms, experiences, and concerns), Objective (measured findings, examination results, and test data), Assessment (clinical interpretation and problem evaluation), and Plan (treatment decisions, monitoring strategy, and follow-up arrangements) providing comprehensive, logical structure. Problem-oriented medical record establishes separate documentation for each active issue with corresponding assessment and plan rather than undifferentiated narratives combining multiple problems. Progress note structures document interval changes, intervention responses, and plan modifications between comprehensive evaluations, focusing on relevant developments rather than repeating stable information.

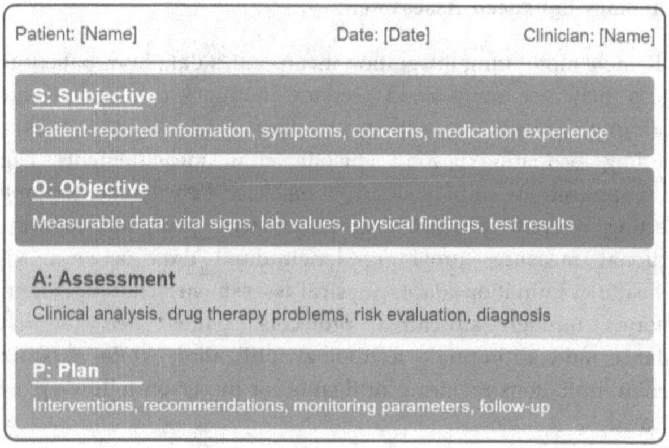

Figure 4.3: SOAP Documentation Format

Documentation Content Elements

Patient demographics records essential identifying information, contact details, insurance coverage, preferred language, and other administrative data supporting care delivery and appropriate communication. Encounter specifics document visit type, reason for encounter, setting, individuals present, and time parameters establishing context for the documented interaction. Information sources clearly identify whether reported history came directly from the patient, family members, caregivers, previous records, or other providers, establishing data reliability context for clinical decision-making.

Quality Documentation Principles

Objectivity distinguishes between observed facts and provider interpretation through clear language choices, quotation of patient statements rather than characterization, and explicit reasoning connecting findings to conclusions. Specificity employs precise descriptions including quantification where possible (e.g., "edema extending 4cm above medial malleolus" rather than "significant edema") and exact timing rather than vague temporal references. Relevance focuses content on information influencing clinical decision-making, patient care, or required reporting rather than extraneous details diluting important findings or creating unnecessarily lengthy documents.

Table 4.4: SOAP Documentation for Patient Assessment

SOAP Component	Content Elements	Documentation Examples	Common Pitfalls
Subjective	Patient-reported symptoms, medication experiences, concerns	"Patient reports 'feeling dizzy' for 3 days after starting new blood pressure medication. Describes lightheadedness when standing quickly."	Mixing objective data into subjective, omitting patient's own words
Objective	Measured parameters, observable findings, laboratory data	"BP 118/64 mmHg seated, 98/52 mmHg standing. HR increases from 72 to 95 bpm with position change. Recent labs: K+ 3.3 mEq/L (↓ from 3.8 last month)."	Incomplete data, undated laboratory values, missing relevant metrics
Assessment	Clinical interpretation, drug therapy problems identified	"Orthostatic hypotension likely due to hydrochlorothiazide initiated 1 week ago, possibly exacerbated by hypokalemia. Patient at increased fall risk."	Unsupported conclusions, failure to connect findings to medications
Plan	Specific interventions, monitoring approach, follow-up	"1. Reduce HCTZ from 25mg to 12.5mg daily. 2. Add potassium supplement 20mEq daily. 3. Instruct on slow position changes. 4. Recheck BP and K+ in 1 week."	Vague recommendations, unspecified monitoring parameters, no timeline

Electronic Documentation Considerations

Template customization adapts standard formats to specific practice needs, patient populations, or visit types while maintaining structural consistency and required elements across encounters. Copy-forward functionality employs appropriate technology capabilities for efficiency while avoiding perpetuation of outdated information, clearly distinguishing between historical and current data, and updating all relevant sections rather than isolated elements. Alert and decision support integration incorporates system-generated recommendations, warnings, or reminders within documentation while maintaining narrative coherence and professional assessment rather than uncritical acceptance of automated suggestions.

CULTURAL COMPETENCY

Self-reflection examines personal beliefs, biases, and assumptions about different cultural groups that may unconsciously influence patient interactions, including recognition of one's own cultural perspectives rather than viewing them as neutral or universal standards. Knowledge acquisition builds understanding of health beliefs, practices, and communication styles among commonly encountered cultural groups while avoiding stereotyping through recognition of individual variation within cultural communities. Skill-building develops practical abilities for cross-cultural communication including appropriate greeting customs, eye contact norms, personal space considerations, and communication styles varying across cultural contexts.

Cross-Cultural Communication

Language adaptation addresses both linguistic translation needs and communication style preferences, including directness versus indirectness, emotional expressiveness norms, and formality expectations varying across cultures. Family involvement navigates different expectations regarding decision-making roles, information sharing, and appointment participation while balancing patient autonomy with cultural norms about family engagement. Non-verbal sensitivity recognizes cultural variations in gesture meaning, touch appropriateness, silence interpretation, and other non-verbal elements that may significantly affect rapport and understanding across cultural boundaries.

Health Belief Systems

Explanatory model elicitation explores how patients understand their health conditions including perceived causes, expected timeline, treatment expectations, and feared consequences, which may differ significantly from biomedical frameworks depending on cultural background. Traditional healing integration acknowledges complementary approaches including traditional medicine practitioners, herbal remedies, spiritual practices, or healing rituals that patients may utilize alongside conventional treatments, requiring respectful exploration rather than dismissal.

Table 4.5: Cultural Considerations in Medication Assessment

Cultural Domain	Assessment	Adaptation Strategies	Documentation
Health Beliefs	Traditional healing practices, causation beliefs	Explore health perspectives, integrate traditional approaches	"Patient incorporates traditional herbal tea alongside prescribed medications; reports no interference"
Language and Communication	Primary language, health literacy, communication preferences	Use professional interpreters, adapted materials, teach-back verification	"Assessment conducted with certified Spanish interpreter. Pictogram medication schedule provided."
Family Involvement	Decision-making roles, caregiver involvement, privacy expectations	Include appropriate family members	"Patient's daughter (primary caregiver) included in medication counseling at patient's request"
Dietary Practices	Cultural food preferences, fasting practices, dietary restrictions	Adapt medication timing to accommodate practices, food interactions	"Medication schedule adjusted to accommodate Ramadan fasting; daily doses consolidated to post-sunset"
Complementary Therapies	Traditional medicines, herbal remedies, alternative practitioners	Non-judgmental inquiry, assess potential interactions	"Currently taking ginseng root preparation (2g daily) alongside prescribed medications; potential interaction with warfarin discussed"
Time Orientation	Attitudes toward preventive care, appointment keeping	Align recommendations with cultural time perspectives	"Preventive statin therapy framed in context of maintaining family role responsibilities"
Trust and Relationships	Authority perceptions, historical healthcare experiences, trust development	Build relationship before recommendations, acknowledge historical context	"Initial visit focused on relationship building; medication review deferred to follow-up at patient's request"

Religious considerations addresses how faith traditions influence health decisions including medication components of animal origin, fasting practices affecting administration timing, or beliefs about suffering, healing, and medical intervention requiring accommodation within treatment plans.

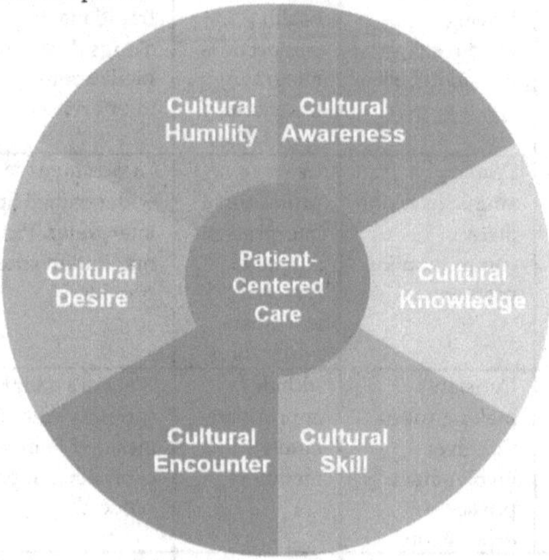

Figure 4.4: Cultural Competency

Social Determinants Recognition

Access barrier identification recognizes challenges including transportation limitations, insurance restrictions, work scheduling conflicts, and financial constraints disproportionately affecting certain cultural communities and requiring practical solutions beyond clinical recommendations alone. Discrimination experience awareness acknowledges how previous negative healthcare encounters involving prejudice, stereotyping, or cultural insensitivity may affect current interactions through heightened vigilance, communication hesitancy, or institutional distrust requiring intentional relationship building. Social support assessment examines available resources within family systems, community networks, and cultural institutions that may significantly influence treatment implementation, adherence capacity, and overall health outcomes beyond individual factors.

Culturally Responsive Care

Treatment adaptation modifies standard approaches to accommodate cultural preferences while maintaining clinical effectiveness, including medication selection considering dietary restrictions, formulation choices respecting cultural beliefs, or administration timing coordinated with religious practices. Educational approach customization develops information delivery methods aligned with cultural learning preferences, health literacy levels, and community norms regarding health communication. Interpreter collaboration employs professional language services effectively through appropriate pre-session briefing, direct patient engagement rather than interpreter focus, manageable information segments, and awareness of potential cultural mediation beyond literal translation occurring during interpreted encounters.

Summary

- Evidence-based practice integrates the best available research evidence with clinical expertise and patient values to guide clinical decision-making.

- Literature evaluation involves assessing study design, methodology, statistical analysis, and clinical relevance to determine applicability to patient care.

- Critical appraisal skills allow pharmacists to evaluate research validity, results reliability, and potential biases that might influence study conclusions.

- Clinical practice guidelines provide standardized recommendations but must be applied with consideration of individual patient circumstances and preferences.

- Implementing evidence into practice requires balancing research findings with patient-specific factors, clinical judgment, and practical constraints of the healthcare setting.

- The hierarchy of evidence ranges from expert opinion (lowest level) to systematic reviews and meta-analyses of randomized controlled trials (highest level).

- Practical application of evidence-based practice includes formulating clinical questions, efficiently searching literature resources, and translating findings into patient care recommendations.

Multiple Choice Questions

1. Which communication technique is MOST effective for encouraging patients to share detailed information about their medication experience?
   A) Using yes/no questions
   B) Maintaining uninterrupted eye contact
   C) Using open-ended questions
   D) Providing written questionnaires
2. A patient tells a pharmacist, "I don't take that blood pressure pill because it makes me dizzy." The MOST appropriate response would be:
   A) "You should speak with your doctor about that."
   B) "You shouldn't stop taking prescribed medications."
   C) "Tell me more about the dizziness you experienced."
   D) "Would you like to try a different medication instead?"
3. Which of the following is the MOST important component to include when documenting an adverse drug reaction?
   A) The brand name of the medication
   B) The specific symptoms, timing, and relationship to medication use
   C) The prescriber's contact information
   D) The pharmacy where the medication was dispensed
4. When conducting a focused physical assessment for a patient on furosemide therapy, which of the following would be MOST important to evaluate?
   A) Heart rate and rhythm
   B) Respiratory rate
   C) Lower extremity edema
   D) Pupillary response
5. A pharmacist is interviewing a patient from a cultural background different from their own. The MOST appropriate approach is to:
   A) Assume cultural practices based on the patient's apparent ethnicity
   B) Avoid discussing cultural influences on medication use
   C) Ask respectful questions about how cultural factors may influence medication use
   D) Provide the same medication counseling used for all patients
6. When obtaining a medication history, which of the following would provide the MOST accurate information about a

patient's actual medication use?

A) Reviewing the patient's electronic health record

B) Asking the patient to bring in all medications and reviewing them together

C) Calling the patient's pharmacy for a medication list

D) Reviewing the medication list from the patient's last hospitalization

7. Which of the following is an example of the subjective component of a SOAP note?

A) "Blood pressure 142/88 mmHg"

B) "Patient reports taking medication 'only when needed'"

C) "Lisinopril 10 mg daily"

D) "Potassium 3.8 mEq/L"

8. A pharmacist is assessing a patient's understanding of their new medication regimen. The MOST effective method would be to:

A) Ask the patient if they have any questions

B) Provide written instructions and confirm the patient can read

C) Ask the patient to demonstrate how they will take their medications

D) Have the patient sign a form acknowledging receipt of counseling

9. When interviewing an elderly patient with hearing impairment, which approach is MOST appropriate?

A) Speaking much louder than normal

B) Facing the patient, speaking clearly at a moderate pace, and reducing background noise

C) Writing all questions and information on paper

D) Directing questions to the patient's caregiver instead

10. Which of the following best demonstrates cultural competency in pharmacy practice?

A) Using the same approach for all patients regardless of background

B) Memorizing cultural practices of different ethnic groups

C) Acknowledging one's own cultural biases and adapting care to individual patient needs

D) Avoiding discussions about cultural beliefs related to medications

Self-Assessment Questions

1. Describe three active listening techniques that clinical pharmacists can use during patient interviews and how each improves information gathering.
2. Explain the difference between open-ended and closed-ended questions, providing examples of each and when each type is most appropriate during a patient interview.
3. Outline the key components of a comprehensive medication history and explain why each component is important for clinical decision-making.
4. Describe three physical assessment skills that are particularly relevant for pharmacists to master, and explain how each relates to medication therapy evaluation.
5. Explain the teach-back method, including how to implement it effectively and why it's superior to simply asking "Do you understand?"
6. Describe the components of a SOAP note and explain why this documentation format is valuable for clinical pharmacy practice.
7. Explain how cultural factors might influence medication-taking behaviors and how pharmacists should address these factors during patient assessment.
8. Discuss three strategies pharmacists can use to effectively communicate with patients who have low health literacy.
9. Explain how nonverbal communication affects the patient interview process and provide examples of positive nonverbal behaviors pharmacists should demonstrate.
10. Describe how a pharmacist should approach sensitive topics (e.g., medication adherence, substance use) during a patient interview to maximize honest disclosure

Bibliography

1. Berger BA. Communication skills for pharmacists: building relationships, improving patient care. 3rd ed. Washington DC: American Pharmacists Association; 2009.
2. Smith RC, Fortin AH, Dwamena F, Frankel RM. An evidence-based patient-centered method makes the biopsychosocial model scientific. Patient Educ Couns. 2013;91(3):265-270.
3. Tully MP. Articulating the value of the clinical pharmacist: implications for pharmacy education. Pharmacy. 2018;6(3):58.
4. Bickley LS, Szilagyi PG. Bates' guide to physical examination and history taking. 12th ed. Philadelphia: Wolters Kluwer; 2017.
5. Ha JF, Longnecker N. Doctor-patient communication: a review. Ochsner J. 2010;10(1):38-43.
6. Weed LL. Medical records that guide and teach. N Engl J Med. 1968;278(12):652-657.
7. Kleinman A, Benson P. Anthropology in the clinic: the problem of cultural competency and how to fix it. PLoS Med. 2006;3(10):e294.
8. Schwartzman E, Hsu DI, Law AV, Chung EP. Assessment of patient communication skills during OSCE: examining effectiveness of a training program in minimizing inter-grader variability. Patient Educ Couns. 2011;83(3):472-477.
9. Naughton CA. Patient-centered communication. Pharmacy. 2018;6(1):18.
10. Campinha-Bacote J. The process of cultural competence in the delivery of healthcare services: a model of care. J Transcult Nurs. 2002;13(3):181-184.

CHAPTER 5

CLINICAL SKILLS AND TOOLS

Author

Mr. Gourab Saha, Associate Professor, Department of Pharmaceutics, College of Pharmaceutical Sciences, Berhampur, Mohada, Odisha, India

Abstract

Clinical laboratory interpretation and diagnostic testing represent essential components of comprehensive medication management. Common laboratory tests provide critical insights into organ function, disease progression, and medication effects, requiring pharmacists to understand indications, limitations, and interference factors affecting result interpretation. Therapeutic drug monitoring optimizes medications with narrow therapeutic indices through appropriate timing, sampling techniques, and clinical decision-making based on pharmacokinetic principles. Point-of-care testing enables rapid clinical decisions through immediately available results for anticoagulation management, glycemic control, and infectious disease screening. Clinical significance assessment distinguishes between statistical variations and meaningful changes requiring intervention, considering patient-specific factors and trending results over time. Reference range interpretation addresses population variations, methodology differences, and condition-specific targets beyond standard laboratory norms. These integrated skills enable pharmacists to effectively monitor medication therapy, identify drug-related problems, recommend appropriate interventions, and collaborate with healthcare teams using objective data to optimize patient outcomes through evidence-based medication management.

Keywords: *Laboratory Monitoring, Therapeutic Range, Pharmacokinetic Assessment, Clinical Interpretation, Diagnostic Testing*

Learning Objectives

After completion of the chapter, the learners should be able to:

- Interpret common laboratory tests relevant to medication therapy including renal function, hepatic function, hematology, and therapeutic drug levels.
- Apply principles of therapeutic drug monitoring including appropriate timing, sampling techniques, and target range interpretation for narrow therapeutic index medications.
- Utilize point-of-care testing technologies for immediate clinical decision-making in areas including anticoagulation, diabetes, and infectious disease management.
- Differentiate between statistically significant and clinically significant laboratory values requiring intervention.
- Analyze laboratory data in the context of patient-specific factors including age, gender, comorbidities, and ethnicity that affect reference ranges.
- Develop monitoring plans incorporating appropriate laboratory tests, frequencies, and parameters based on medication therapy and patient characteristics.

COMMON LABORATORY TESTS

Hemoglobin and hematocrit evaluation assesses oxygen-carrying capacity, identifying anemia potentially caused by medications (chemotherapy, anticonvulsants, NSAIDs), exacerbated by drug therapy (proton pump inhibitors reducing iron absorption), or requiring medication dosage adjustments (erythropoietin-stimulating agents). White blood cell analysis examines total count and differential percentages, detecting neutropenia from myelosuppressive drugs (antineoplastics, carbamazepine, clozapine), infections potentially requiring antimicrobial therapy, or inflammatory conditions affecting medication response. Platelet assessment identifies thrombocytopenia from medications (heparin, chemotherapy, valproic acid) potentially requiring dose adjustment, discontinuation, or alternative therapy selection, while also guiding antiplatelet and anticoagulant management decisions.

Electrolyte Panel Assessment

Sodium interpretation evaluates hyponatremia potentially caused by medications (diuretics, SSRIs, carbamazepine) or hypernatremia from sodium-containing formulations (IV antibiotics, sodium polystyrene sulfonate), with both abnormalities potentially requiring therapy modification. Potassium analysis identifies hyperkalemia from medications (ACE inhibitors, ARBs, potassium-sparing diuretics, potassium supplements) or hypokalemia from diuretics (thiazides, loop diuretics), insulin, or beta-agonists, requiring either intervention or preventive management. Calcium examination detects hypercalcemia potentially exacerbated by thiazide diuretics or caused by vitamin D toxicity, versus hypocalcemia from medications (bisphosphonates, denosumab, phenytoin) potentially requiring supplementation or drug modification.

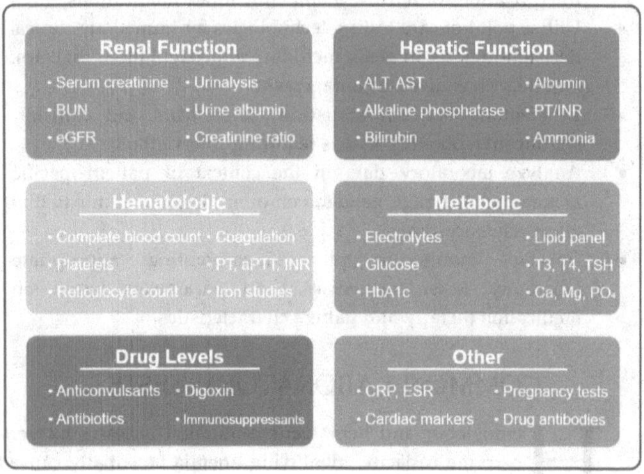

Figure 5.1: Common Laboratory Tests for Medication Monitoring

Renal Function Evaluation

Serum creatinine assessment estimates kidney function, recognizing limitations including delayed response to acute kidney injury, muscle mass dependence affecting interpretation in elderly or cachectic patients, and medication interference (trimethoprim, cimetidine). Estimated glomerular filtration rate calculation applies formulas including Cockcroft-Gault (historically used for drug dosing), MDRD, or CKD-EPI equations, with appropriate selection based on intended use and patient characteristics. Blood urea nitrogen examination provides complementary renal function assessment, with elevations potentially indicating prerenal causes (dehydration, heart failure) versus intrinsic renal injury, influencing medication selection and dosing decisions.

Table 5.1: Common Laboratory Tests for Medication Monitoring

Test Category	Specific Tests	Medication Monitoring Applications	Critical Values/Action Thresholds
Renal Function	Serum creatinine, BUN, eGFR, urinalysis	Renally eliminated medications, nephrotoxic agents, dosage adjustments	SCr increase ≥0.3 mg/dL in 48 hours, eGFR <30 mL/min requiring dose adjustment
Hepatic Function	ALT, AST, alkaline phosphatase, bilirubin, albumin	Hepatically metabolized drugs, hepatotoxic agents, protein binding assessment	ALT/AST >3x ULN, bilirubin >2x ULN requiring therapy discontinuation
Hematologic	CBC with differential, platelets, INR, aPTT	Anticoagulants, myelosuppressive agents, hematologic toxicities	Platelets <50,000/mm³, ANC <1,000/mm³, INR >4.0 without bleeding
Metabolic	Electrolytes, glucose, HbA1c, lipid panel	Diuretics, diabetes medications, cardiovascular agents	K+ <3.0 or >5.5 mEq/L, Na+ <125 or >150 mEq/L, glucose <70 or >400 mg/dL
Cardiac	Troponin, BNP, CK, digoxin level	Cardiovascular medications, cardiotoxic agents, heart failure therapy	Troponin elevation, BNP >500 pg/mL with symptoms, digoxin >2.0 ng/mL
Endocrine	TSH, free T4, cortisol, testosterone	Thyroid medications, hormone therapy, adrenal suppressants	TSH <0.1 or >10 mIU/L, critically low cortisol with symptoms
Inflammatory	ESR, CRP, procalcitonin	Anti-inflammatory agents, infection assessment, autoimmune therapies	CRP >100 mg/L, procalcitonin >0.5 ng/mL suggesting bacterial infection

Test Category	Specific Tests	Medication Monitoring Applications	Critical Values/Action Thresholds
Therapeutic Drug Levels	Anticonvulsant levels, antimicrobial levels, immunosuppressant levels	Narrow therapeutic index drugs, individualized dosing	Drug-specific toxic thresholds (e.g., vancomycin trough >20 mcg/mL)

Hepatic Function Tests

Transaminase evaluation (ALT, AST) detects hepatocellular injury potentially caused by medications (statins, acetaminophen, isoniazid), requiring risk-benefit assessment for continuation, dose adjustment, or discontinuation. Alkaline phosphatase and gamma-glutamyl transferase assessment identifies cholestatic patterns potentially indicating drug-induced injury (amoxicillin-clavulanate, oral contraceptives, anabolic steroids) with different management implications than hepatocellular damage. Bilirubin analysis distinguishes between direct (conjugated) and indirect (unconjugated) elevations, with patterns helping differentiate medication effects on various hepatic processes including uptake, conjugation, and excretion.

Metabolic Assessment

Glucose measurement evaluates hyperglycemia potentially caused or exacerbated by medications (corticosteroids, atypical antipsychotics, protease inhibitors) or hypoglycemia from excessive antidiabetic therapy, requiring dose adjustment or regimen modification. Hemoglobin A1C assessment provides longer-term glycemic control evaluation, guiding diabetes medication selection, dosage titration, and regimen intensification decisions based on target attainment. Lipid panel analysis guides cardiovascular risk management through statin selection and dosing, identifies secondary dyslipidemia from medications (thiazides, beta-blockers, antiretrovirals), and monitors for adverse effects of lipid-lowering therapies.

THERAPEUTIC DRUG MONITORING

Narrow therapeutic index identifies medications where small concentration differences significantly affect safety and efficacy, requiring individualized dosing beyond standardized regimens to maintain optimal range. Pharmacokinetic variability addresses medications with unpredictable absorption, distribution, metabolism, or elimination across individuals due to genetic polymorphisms, organ dysfunction, drug interactions, or physiological differences requiring direct concentration measurement rather than dose-based estimation. Clinical response correlation assesses situations where therapeutic effects or toxicity signs poorly correspond with dosing, including cases of suspected non-adherence, malabsorption, drug interactions, or altered protein binding affecting active drug fraction.

Table 5.2: Therapeutic Drug Monitoring Parameters

Drug Category	Specific Agents	Sampling	Target Ranges	Monitoring
Anticonvulsants	Phenytoin, carbamazepine, valproic acid, lamotrigine	Trough levels, steady state (≥5 half-lives), consistent timing	Phenytoin: 10-20 mcg/mL, Carbamazepine: 4-12 mcg/mL, Valproic acid: 50-100 mcg/mL	Initially monthly, then every 3-6 months or with regimen changes
Antimicrobials	Vancomycin, aminoglycosides, voriconazole	Vancomycin: trough before 4th dose, Aminoglycosides: peak 30 min after infusion, trough before next dose	Vancomycin trough: 10-15 mcg/mL (uncomplicated), 15-20 mcg/mL (severe), Gentamicin peak: 5-10 mcg/mL, trough <2 mcg/mL	Vancomycin: weekly, Aminoglycosides: after 3rd dose, then 2-3 times weekly
Immunosuppressants	Tacrolimus, cyclosporine, sirolimus, mycophenolate	Trough levels, consistent timing relative to dose,	Tacrolimus: 5-15 ng/mL, Cyclosporine: 100-400 ng/mL	Initially 2-3 times weekly, then weekly for 1 month

Drug Category	Specific Agents	Sampling	Target Ranges	Monitoring
Antiarrhythmics	Digoxin, amiodarone, procainamide	Digoxin: sample ≥6-8 hours post-dose, Amiodarone: trough level	Digoxin: 0.8-2.0 ng/mL, Amiodarone: 1.0-2.5 mcg/mL	Digoxin: after 7-10 days, then every 3-6 months, Amiodarone: every 6-12 months
Antipsychotics	Clozapine, haloperidol, risperidone	Trough levels, steady state, consistent timing	Clozapine: 350-600 ng/mL, Haloperidol: 5-15 ng/mL	Initially monthly, then every 3-6 months or with regimen changes
Mood Stabilizers	Lithium	12-hour post-dose, consistent timing, hydration status	Lithium: 0.6-1.2 mEq/L (indication-dependent)	Weekly until stable, then every 3-6 months or with regimen changes
Bronchodilators	Theophylline	Peak: 2 hours post-dose, Trough: before next dose	Theophylline: 10-20 mcg/mL	After 3-5 days, then every 6-12 months or with regimen changes
Anti-rejection	Mycophenolic acid	12-hour trough, 2-hour post-dose (AUC estimation)	Trough >1.3 mcg/mL, AUC 30-60 mg.h/L	Weekly x 1 month, then monthly x 3 months, then every 3-6 months

Anticonvulsant Monitoring

Phenytoin assessment addresses highly variable metabolism, non-linear pharmacokinetics, and numerous drug interactions, typically targeting total concentrations of 10-20 mcg/mL with free fraction monitoring (1-2 mcg/mL) when protein binding alterations exist. Carbamazepine evaluation considers autoinduction requiring dose titration, active metabolite contribution, and interaction potential, generally targeting 4-12 mcg/mL with sampling timing considerations for extended-release formulations. Valproic acid monitoring guides therapy with concentration targets varying by indication (50-100 mcg/mL for epilepsy, sometimes lower for psychiatric indications), with particular attention to protein binding changes affecting interpretation of total concentrations.

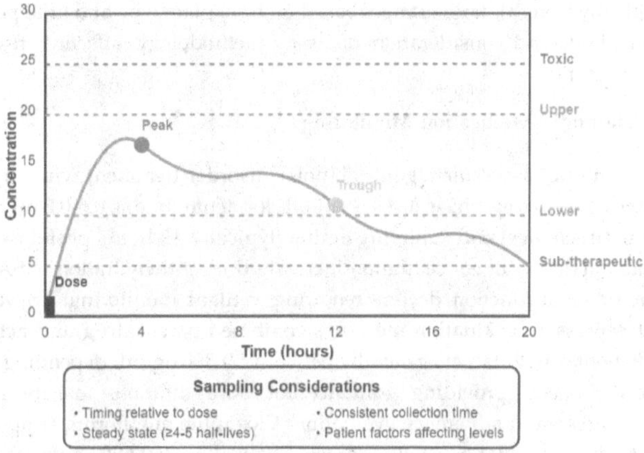

Figure 5.2: Therapeutic Drug Monitoring Parameters

Antimicrobial Monitoring

Vancomycin assessment optimizes therapy through trough monitoring (traditionally 10-20 mcg/mL based on infection site, now often using AUC/MIC ratio targeting 400-600 mg•hr/L) with timing precision critical for accurate interpretation. Aminoglycoside evaluation employs either peak/trough combinations or extended-interval (Hartford) regimen monitoring with appropriate sampling times based on dosing strategy, considering both efficacy (peak concentrations) and toxicity risk (trough or total exposure). Voriconazole monitoring addresses significant inter-individual pharmacokinetic variability from CYP2C19 polymorphisms and numerous drug interactions, targeting 1-5.5 mcg/mL (higher end for central nervous system infections) to balance efficacy against concentration-dependent adverse effects.

Cardiovascular Drug Monitoring

Digoxin assessment targets concentrations generally between 0.5-0.9 ng/mL for heart failure (lower than historical ranges) or up to 2.0 ng/mL for rate control in atrial fibrillation, with sampling at least 6-8 hours post-dose and consideration of factors affecting interpretation including renal function, electrolyte status, and thyroid function. Antiarrhythmic monitoring includes agents such as lidocaine (1.5-5.0 mcg/mL), procainamide (4-10 mcg/mL, with N-acetylprocainamide metabolite), and amiodarone (0.5-2.5 mcg/mL), each requiring specific timing, therapeutic range, and interpretation considerations. Immunosuppressant evaluation guides therapy with agents including cyclosporine, tacrolimus, and sirolimus, each requiring specific timing (typically trough), target ranges based on transplant type and time post-transplant, and consideration of assay methodology affecting result interpretation.

Psychotropic Medication Monitoring

Lithium assessment guides bipolar disorder treatment with target ranges varying by phase (0.8-1.2 mEq/L for acute mania, 0.6-0.8 mEq/L for maintenance) and sampling timing (typically 12 hours post-dose at steady state), with concentration increases during dehydration, NSAID use, or renal function decline requiring vigilant monitoring. Tricyclic antidepressant evaluation measures combined parent drug and active metabolites with targets generally between 50-300 ng/mL depending on specific agent, providing guidance for dose titration, toxicity risk assessment, and adherence evaluation. Clozapine monitoring supports therapy optimization with targets typically 350-600 ng/mL for schizophrenia response, potentially lower for other indications, while also monitoring norclozapine metabolite and clozapine/norclozapine ratio providing metabolism assessment.

Monitoring Implementation

Sampling time optimization ensures collection at appropriate intervals relative to dose administration based on specific drug characteristics, typically trough (pre-dose) for many agents, but peak or specific post-dose timing for others depending on pharmacokinetic properties and clinical question being addressed. Steady state consideration recognizes that accurate interpretation generally requires sampling after approximately 4-5 half-lives of consistent dosing, with premature measurement potentially misleading unless intentionally measuring peak effects during loading dose strategies. Documentation standards record essential contextual information including sampling time relative to last dose, current dosing regimen duration, concomitant medications affecting interpretation, and relevant clinical parameters such as renal function, hepatic status, and albumin levels when applicable.

POINT-OF-CARE TESTING

Self-monitoring implementation establishes appropriate testing frequency based on diabetes type, medication regimen (particularly for insulin or sulfonylureas), glycemic control stability, and presence of hypoglycemia unawareness, with structured recording of results. Accuracy verification ensures proper technique, unexpired strips/sensors, appropriate coding when required, and periodic comparison with laboratory values to detect systematic errors or device malfunction. Pattern recognition analyzes results across different contexts (fasting, pre-meal, post-meal, bedtime) to identify specific problem times requiring targeted intervention rather than global medication adjustments based on isolated readings or A1C alone.

Table 5.3: Point-of-Care Testing Applications in Pharmacy Practice

Test Type	Testing Parameters	Clinical Applications
Blood Glucose	Capillary blood glucose, continuous glucose monitoring	Diabetes management, hypoglycemia assessment, medication adjustment
Coagulation	INR, PT	Warfarin management, anticoagulation clinic services
Lipid Panel	Total cholesterol, HDL, LDL, triglycerides	Cardiovascular risk assessment, statin therapy monitoring
A1C	Glycated hemoglobin	Diabetes monitoring, therapy evaluation, screening
Infectious Disease	Influenza, Group A Strep, COVID-19	Diagnostic screening, treatment decisions, public health
Kidney Function	Albumin/creatinine ratio, eGFR calculation	Chronic kidney disease monitoring, medication dosing
Liver Function	ALT, bilirubin	Hepatotoxicity monitoring, jaundice assessment
Therapeutic Levels	Phenytoin, lithium, digoxin	Dose adjustment, toxicity assessment
Pregnancy	hCG	Medication safety assessment, teratogenic exposure
Drug Screening	Various drugs of abuse	Medication adherence, substance use monitoring

Anticoagulation Monitoring

International Normalized Ratio (INR) testing utilizes portable devices measuring prothrombin time with conversion to standardized INR values, allowing warfarin management through immediate dose adjustment rather than delayed laboratory-based decisions. Quality control implementation ensures accurate results through appropriate device maintenance, control testing, and periodic comparison with laboratory values, particularly when therapeutic decisions diverge from clinical expectations. Algorithm-based management employs standardized protocols for dose adjustment based on current INR, target range, previous stability, and intervening factors (diet changes, medication additions/discontinuations, illness) potentially affecting anticoagulation status.

Lipid Testing

Cholesterol screening provides rapid total cholesterol and often HDL measurement allowing preliminary cardiovascular risk assessment and therapy initiation in settings where laboratory testing creates barriers to care initiation. Follow-up protocols establish appropriate confirmation of point-of-care results with laboratory testing before long-term therapy decisions, particularly when values are borderline or inconsistent with clinical context. Patient engagement utilization leverages immediate result availability for enhanced education regarding cardiovascular risk, lifestyle modification importance, and medication benefit demonstration through visual representation of current status compared to targets.

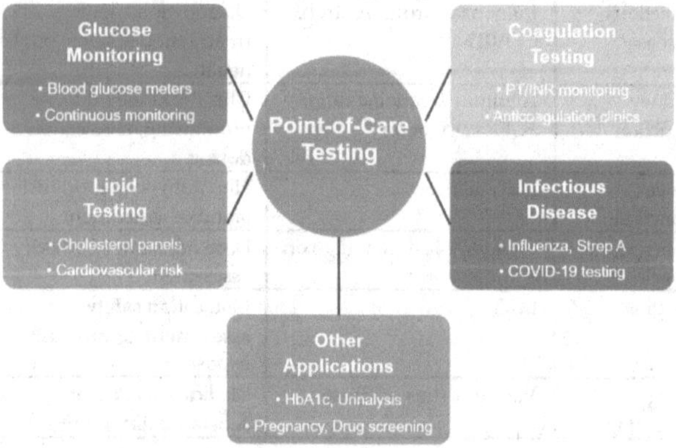

Figure 5.3: Applications of Point-of-Care Testing

Hemoglobin A1C Assessment

Diabetes diagnosis application implements screening in accordance with guidelines defining diabetes (≥6.5%) and prediabetes (5.7-6.4%) thresholds, with appropriate confirmation for values near diagnostic cut-points. Therapy adjustment utilizes results to guide medication selection, dosage titration, and regimen intensification based on target achievement relative to individualized goals. Limitations recognition addresses potential result distortion in conditions affecting red blood cell lifespan (hemolytic anemia, recent transfusion, hemoglobinopathies) or specific hemoglobin variants, requiring alternative monitoring approaches when these factors are present.

Infectious Disease Testing

Influenza diagnosis employs rapid antigen or molecular tests with result interpretation considering prevalence, test characteristics (sensitivity/specificity), and clinical presentation to guide appropriate antiviral therapy initiation. Streptococcal pharyngitis detection utilizes rapid antigen tests with understanding of negative result limitations potentially requiring culture confirmation based on clinical suspicion and patient characteristics. HIV screening implements rapid antibody testing in diverse settings, with appropriate protocols for confirmatory testing, linkage to care, and immediate counseling based on preliminary results.

CLINICAL SIGNIFICANCE

Interpreting Clinical Relevance

Magnitude assessment evaluates whether statistically significant laboratory changes represent clinically meaningful differences requiring intervention versus minor fluctuations within expected biological variation despite crossing reference range boundaries. Trend analysis examines sequential results over time rather than isolated values, identifying directional changes potentially requiring intervention before conventional reference ranges are exceeded. Context integration considers laboratory findings within the complete clinical picture including symptoms, other test results, medication effects, and pre-existing conditions rather than isolated interpretation of individual values.

Laboratory Error Identification

Pre-analytical factor assessment evaluates collection conditions potentially affecting results including timing relative to meals or medications, tourniquet duration, patient posture, sample hemolysis, or improper specimen handling. Analytical error recognition identifies patterns suggesting laboratory processing issues including implausible values, inconsistency between related parameters, or sudden changes without clinical explanation. Confirmation strategies implement appropriate verification approaches for unexpected results through repeat testing, alternative methodologies, or different specimen types depending on the specific test and clinical urgency.

Table 5.4: Interpreting Clinical Significance of Laboratory Abnormalities

Assessment Factor	Evaluation Approach	Examples of Significant Changes
Magnitude of Change	Percent change from baseline, absolute value change	SCr increase >50% from baseline, K+ change >1.0 mEq/L in 24 hours
Rate of Change	Time course analysis, trend direction	Platelet count decreasing 50,000/day, steadily rising aminotransferases
Relationship to Reference Range	Distance from normal range, crossing critical thresholds	Mild elevation (1-2x ULN) vs. severe (>3x ULN) for liver enzymes
Clinical Context	Patient symptoms, disease state, expected medication effects	Asymptomatic vs. symptomatic hyponatremia, expected vs. unexpected neutropenia
Pattern Recognition	Characteristic patterns indicating specific problems	Cholestatic vs. hepatocellular injury pattern, high anion gap vs. normal anion gap acidosis
Multiple Related Parameters	Constellation of findings suggesting syndrome	Combined hyperkalemia, metabolic acidosis, and rising creatinine suggesting acute kidney injury
Temporal Relationship to Therapy	Timing relative to medication initiation, dose changes	Thrombocytopenia beginning 7-14 days after heparin initiation suggesting HIT
Reversibility	Response to intervention, discontinuation effect	Improvement in renal function after drug discontinuation suggesting drug-induced nephrotoxicity

Screening vs. Diagnostic Interpretation

Sensitivity and specificity application considers the purpose of testing, recognizing that screening tests typically prioritize sensitivity (minimizing false negatives) while diagnostic confirmation often emphasizes specificity (minimizing false positives). Predictive value assessment interprets results considering disease prevalence in the specific population, recognizing that positive predictive value decreases significantly for positive results in low-prevalence situations despite unchanged test characteristics. Sequential testing interpretation applies principles of pre-test and post-test probability, using initial results to refine the likelihood of disease before applying subsequent test interpretation rather than viewing each test in isolation.

Age and Population Considerations

Pediatric parameter adjustment interprets results against age-appropriate references rather than adult ranges, recognizing developmental changes in laboratory values throughout childhood and adolescence affecting clinical significance. Geriatric interpretation considers age-related physiological changes potentially altering reference ranges while distinguishing between "normal aging" and pathological processes requiring intervention despite age-adjusted expectations. Pregnancy-specific ranges applies trimester-specific reference intervals for parameters significantly affected by normal pregnancy physiology including thyroid function, glucose tolerance, and hematologic values to prevent misclassification of normal changes as pathological.

Intervention Thresholds

Treatment initiation targets identifies laboratory values warranting new therapy introduction, such as LDL cholesterol levels for statin initiation based on cardiovascular risk category or HbA1c thresholds for antihyperglycemic therapy according to current guidelines. Dose adjustment parameters establishes values indicating need for medication dosage modification, including renal function thresholds for renally-eliminated drugs or neutrophil count cut-offs for myelosuppressive agent management. Emergency intervention levels recognizes critical values requiring immediate clinical action, such as critical potassium abnormalities, extreme glucose deviations, or dangerous drug concentrations necessitating urgent notification and intervention protocols

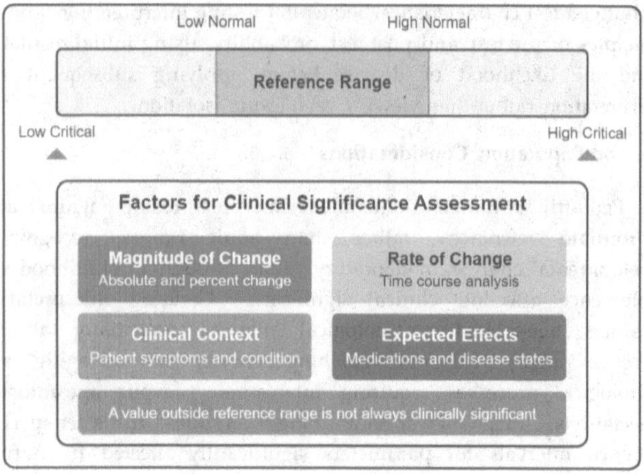

Figure 5.4: Clinical Significance of Laboratory Results

REFERENCE RANGES

Establishment methodology understands how reference ranges are typically derived from measurements in presumably healthy populations, usually encompassing the central 95% of values (±2 standard deviations from the mean) rather than representing absolute limits of normality. Population specificity recognizes that reference intervals may vary based on factors including the laboratory's specific measurement methods, equipment calibration, and reference population characteristics potentially differing from local patient demographics. Biological variation consideration acknowledges that many analytes fluctuate within individuals over time due to circadian rhythms, seasonal variations, or physiological cycles, affecting interpretation of values near reference boundaries.

Specialized Reference Considerations

Sex-specific ranges applies gender-appropriate intervals for parameters with significant biological differences between males and females, including hemoglobin, creatinine, liver enzymes, and certain hormones to prevent misclassification based on inappropriate comparisons. Ethnic and racial variations recognizes potential differences in laboratory parameters across population groups, including hemoglobin A1C interpretation, estimated GFR calculations, and bone mineral density assessment requiring appropriate reference selection. Geographic adjustments considers regional variations in "normal" values for certain parameters including vitamin D levels, thyroid function in iodine-deficient regions, or liver function in areas with high hepatitis prevalence.

Table 5.5: Laboratory Reference Range Considerations

Consideration Factor	Impact on Interpretation	Examples	Adjustment
Age-Specific Variations	Different normal ranges based on age groups	Alkaline phosphatase higher in children/adolescents, creatinine lower in elderly	Use age-adjusted reference ranges, formulas (e.g., pediatric GFR)
Sex Differences	Physiological differences between males and females	Hemoglobin (M: 13.5-17.5 g/dL, F: 12.0-16.0 g/dL), Creatinine typically lower in females	Apply sex-specific reference ranges and formulas
Pregnancy-Related Changes	Physiological adaptations during pregnancy	Decreased albumin, increased alkaline phosphatase, expanded plasma volume affecting concentrations	Use pregnancy-specific reference ranges by trimester
Racial/Ethnic Considerations	Genetic variations affecting normal values	Lower eGFR with same creatinine in Black patients, hemoglobin variants in different ethnic groups	Apply race-specific adjustment factors when validated
Laboratory Methodology	Different techniques producing different results	Immunoassay vs. chromatographic drug levels, different creatinine assays	Know methodology used, ensure consistent testing method
Diurnal Variations	Normal fluctuations throughout the day	Cortisol (highest in morning), iron (highest in morning), testosterone	Time-specific reference ranges, consistent sampling times
Fasting vs. Non-fasting	Food effects on certain parameters	Glucose, triglycerides, certain drug levels affected by food	Note fasting status, use appropriate reference ranges

Consideration Factor	Impact on Interpretation	Examples	Adjustment
Acute Phase Response	Inflammatory conditions affecting baseline values	Decreased albumin, increased ferritin during inflammation	Consider inflammatory markers when interpreting affected tests
Analytical Interference	Substances affecting test accuracy	Hemolysis affecting potassium, biotin supplementation affecting immunoassays	Note potential interferents, consider repeat testing
Disease-Specific Targets	Therapeutic goals different from normal ranges	Lower LDL targets in high cardiovascular risk, higher hemoglobin targets in certain conditions	Apply condition-specific target ranges rather than normal ranges

Laboratory Method Variations

Methodology differences recognizes that various analytical techniques for measuring the same parameter may yield systematically different results, requiring method-specific reference ranges rather than universal standards, particularly relevant when comparing results across different facilities. Standardization initiatives implements programs harmonizing results across different platforms through reference materials, calculation adjustments, or reporting conventions, as seen with hemoglobin A1C, lipid measurements, and certain hormone assays. Unit conversion applies appropriate mathematical transformations when comparing results reported in different units (conventional versus SI) while recognizing that simple conversion may not account for methodological differences beyond unit systems.

Therapeutic Targets vs. Reference Ranges

Treatment goal distinction differentiates between population reference ranges and clinical targets established for specific conditions, recognizing that optimal management often aims for values outside typical reference intervals based on evidence from intervention trials. Risk-based targets implements individualized goals based on comprehensive risk assessment rather than fixed cut-points, as seen in blood pressure management, lipid targets, or glycemic control where appropriate values vary based on comorbidities, age, and overall risk profile. Suboptimal range identification recognizes values that while technically within reference limits may still represent suboptimal status warranting intervention, such as "normal" but insufficient vitamin D levels or borderline-high cardiovascular risk factors in high-risk individuals.

Reporting Format Interpretation

Flagging systems understands laboratory highlighting methods for abnormal results, distinguishing between different levels of deviation (mildly abnormal versus critical) while recognizing that flagging reflects statistical boundaries rather than clinical significance judgments. Numerical precision considers the appropriate number of decimal places for clinical decision-making, avoiding over-precision suggesting greater accuracy than methodologically justified or under-precision obscuring clinically meaningful differences. Directional indicators interprets symbols (↑,↓) or terms (elevated, decreased) correctly within the specific laboratory's reporting convention, particularly important for parameters where directionality may be ambiguous without clear indication

Summary

- Interpretation of common laboratory tests (CBC, metabolic panels, lipid profiles, liver and kidney function tests) is essential for monitoring medication efficacy and toxicity.
- Therapeutic drug monitoring requires understanding of pharmacokinetic principles, sampling timing, and therapeutic ranges for narrow therapeutic index drugs.
- Point-of-care testing provides immediate results for clinical decision-making in areas such as anticoagulation management, diabetes care, and infectious disease diagnosis.
- Clinical significance of laboratory values must be assessed in context of patient-specific factors, disease states, and medication regimens rather than in isolation.
- Reference ranges vary by laboratory, patient demographics, and clinical context, requiring careful interpretation of results that fall outside standard ranges.
- Monitoring parameters should be established for each medication, including baseline assessments, follow-up intervals, and specific laboratory or clinical markers.
- Recognition of drug-laboratory test interactions is crucial to avoid misinterpretation of results and inappropriate clinical decisions.

Multiple Choice Questions

1. A patient's serum creatinine has increased from 0.9 mg/dL to 1.3 mg/dL over three days after starting a new medication. Which of the following would be the MOST appropriate initial action?

   A) Immediately discontinue the medication

   B) Calculate the percent change and estimated GFR to assess clinical significance

   C) Assume it is laboratory error and ignore the result

   D) Order dialysis consultation

2. When monitoring vancomycin therapy for a patient with MRSA bacteremia, the MOST appropriate time to collect a trough level is:

   A) 30 minutes after the end of the infusion

   B) 2 hours after the end of the infusion

   C) Immediately before the fourth dose

   D) Midway between doses

3. Which of the following point-of-care tests provides the MOST valuable information for long-term diabetes management?

   A) Random blood glucose

   B) Hemoglobin A1C

   C) Fasting blood glucose

   D) Urine glucose

4. A patient's INR is 4.8 while on warfarin therapy with a target range of 2.0-3.0. The patient reports no bleeding symptoms. Which of the following is the MOST appropriate assessment?

   A) This is not clinically significant as the patient has no symptoms

   B) This represents a critical value requiring immediate intervention

   C) This is an expected variation for patients on warfarin therapy

   D) This result is likely a laboratory error and should be repeated

5. Which laboratory parameter is MOST useful for distinguishing between acute and chronic kidney injury?

   A) Blood urea nitrogen (BUN)

   B) Serum creatinine

   C) Estimated glomerular filtration rate (eGFR)

   D) Presence of kidney damage markers like albuminuria

6. When interpreting aminoglycoside levels, which of the following statements is MOST accurate?
   A) Peak levels correlate with efficacy, while trough levels correlate with toxicity
   B) Only trough levels are necessary for monitoring
   C) Levels should be drawn at the same time daily regardless of dosing schedule
   D) Therapeutic ranges are the same for all indications
7. Which of the following represents the MOST appropriate use of point-of-care testing in pharmacy practice?
   A) Replacing comprehensive laboratory testing
   B) Screening and monitoring for specific conditions with immediate results
   C) Diagnosing complex medical conditions
   D) Reducing the need for physician visits
8. A patient's potassium level is reported as 5.7 mEq/L (reference range: 3.5-5.0 mEq/L). Which of the following factors is MOST important to consider when assessing this result?
   A) The patient's diet
   B) The collection technique and sample handling
   C) The patient's ethnic background
   D) The time of day the sample was collected
9. Which of the following best describes the clinical application of therapeutic drug monitoring for phenytoin?
   A) Samples should be drawn at the same time each day
   B) Free phenytoin levels are unnecessary when total levels are available
   C) Albumin levels should be considered when interpreting total phenytoin levels
   D) Phenytoin follows linear pharmacokinetics at all doses
10. When interpreting laboratory results for a geriatric patient, which of the following is MOST important to consider?
   A) Age-specific reference ranges may differ from those for younger adults
   B) Laboratory tests are generally more accurate in older adults
   C) Most medication dosing should be based on actual body weight
   D) Kidney function naturally improves with age

Self-Assessment Questions

1. Explain the difference between a screening test and a diagnostic test, and provide an example of each in the context of pharmacy practice.
2. Describe three factors that can cause variations in laboratory reference ranges and how these factors should be considered when interpreting test results.
3. Explain the concepts of sensitivity and specificity in laboratory testing and why they are important considerations when selecting and interpreting tests.
4. For a drug that requires therapeutic drug monitoring (e.g., vancomycin), explain the appropriate timing of sample collection and why this timing is critical.
5. Describe three point-of-care tests commonly performed in pharmacy settings and the clinical applications of each.
6. Explain how to determine if a change in a laboratory value represents a clinically significant finding versus a normal variation.
7. Describe how renal function tests should be interpreted and applied to medication dosing, including considerations for special populations.
8. Explain the concept of critical values for laboratory tests and the pharmacist's responsibility when encountering them.
9. Discuss how pharmacists should interpret drug levels for medications with active metabolites (e.g., digoxin), and how this affects clinical decision-making.
10. Explain how to correlate laboratory findings with clinical signs and symptoms when monitoring for medication efficacy and toxicity.

Bibliography

1. Lee M. Basic skills in interpreting laboratory data. 6th ed. Bethesda: American Society of Health-System Pharmacists; 2017.
2. Winter ME. Basic clinical pharmacokinetics. 5th ed. Philadelphia: Lippincott Williams & Wilkins; 2010.
3. Burtis CA, Bruns DE. Tietz fundamentals of clinical chemistry and molecular diagnostics. 7th ed. St. Louis: Elsevier Saunders; 2015.
4. Kang JS, Lee MH. Overview of therapeutic drug monitoring. Korean J Intern Med. 2009;24(1):1-10.
5. Nichols JH. Point-of-care testing: performance improvement and evidence-based outcomes. Clin Lab Med. 2007;27(4):723-748.
6. Murphy JE. Clinical pharmacokinetics. 6th ed. Bethesda: American Society of Health-System Pharmacists; 2017.
7. Horn JR, Hansten PD. Drug interactions: insights and observations. Pharmacy Times. 2013;79(3):80.
8. Dasgupta A. Therapeutic drug monitoring: newer drugs and biomarkers. 1st ed. London: Academic Press; 2012.
9. McPherson RA, Pincus MR. Henry's clinical diagnosis and management by laboratory methods. 23rd ed. St. Louis: Elsevier; 2017.
10. Soldin SJ, Soldin OP. Therapeutic drug monitoring in pediatrics. Ther Drug Monit. 2002;24(1):1-8.

CHAPTER 6

DRUG INFORMATION RESOURCES

Author

Mr. Sri Venkatesh Uriti, Associate Professor, Department of Pharmacology, Sri Sivani College of Pharmacy, Etcherla, Srikakulam, Andhra Pradesh, India

Abstract

Reviewing the complex and vast pharmaceutical information requires mastery of diverse resources and retrieval methodologies essential for evidence-based practice. Primary literature evaluation encompasses journal article analysis, preprint assessment, and clinical trial interpretation with emphasis on methodological quality, bias identification, and applicability determination. Secondary resources provide synthesized information through systematic reviews, meta-analyses, and evidence summaries offering comprehensive evaluations of therapeutic approaches with structured quality assessment. Electronic databases facilitate efficient information retrieval through specialized platforms including PubMed, Embase, and Cochrane Library, each requiring specific search strategies and controlled vocabulary mastery. Clinical decision support tools integrate patient-specific data with medication knowledge bases through computerized alerts, order sets, and interactive applications supporting point-of-care decisions. Information retrieval skills combine systematic search strategy development, resource selection based on question type, critical evaluation of conflicting information, and effective communication of complex findings to various audiences. This detailed approach enables pharmacists to address medication information needs with accuracy, efficiency, and clinical relevance while navigating information overload and evaluating source credibility.

Keywords: *Biomedical Literature, Information Retrieval, Evidence Synthesis, Clinical Databases, Knowledge Management*

Learning Objectives

After completion of the chapter, the learners should be able to:

- Evaluate primary literature sources including peer-reviewed journals, clinical trials, and pre-publication research for quality, relevance, and applicability.
- Utilize secondary drug information resources including systematic reviews, meta-analyses, and evidence summaries to inform clinical decision-making.
- Conduct efficient literature searches using electronic databases and appropriate search strategies to answer specific clinical questions.
- Apply clinical decision support tools appropriately to enhance medication safety, therapeutic selection, and patient-specific dosing.
- Develop systematic information retrieval skills including search strategy formulation, resource selection, and critical evaluation of conflicting information.
- Communicate complex pharmaceutical information effectively to diverse audiences including patients, healthcare providers, and administrators.

PRIMARY LITERATURE

Impact factor assessment evaluates journal quality through citation metrics while recognizing limitations including field-specific variation, potential manipulation, and the imperfect relationship between citation frequency and clinical relevance. Peer review process understanding recognizes different models including traditional blind review, open peer review, and post-publication evaluation, each with strengths and limitations affecting publication quality and reliability. Publication bias awareness acknowledges systematic distortion in the published literature, with positive studies more likely to be published than negative findings, particularly affecting meta-analyses and systematic reviews drawing primarily from published sources.

Study Design Recognition

Experimental designs include randomized controlled trials providing the strongest evidence for intervention effects through randomization and control group comparison, with variations including parallel group, crossover, factorial, and adaptive designs offering different advantages for specific research questions.

Table 6.1: Primary Literature Types and Evaluation

Study Type	Characteristics	Strengths	Limitations
Randomized Controlled Trials	Experimental design with randomized intervention assignment	Minimizes selection bias, controls for confounders, establishes causality	Limited external validity, short duration, selected populations
Observational Studies (Cohort)	Follows groups with/without exposure over time	Large populations, long-term outcomes, real-world setting	Selection bias, confounding variables, loss to follow-up
Observational Studies (Case-Control)	Compares cases with outcome to controls without	Efficient for rare outcomes, multiple exposure assessment	Recall bias, selection bias, temporal relationship challenges
Systematic Reviews/Meta-analyses	Comprehensive analysis of multiple studies	Increased statistical power, reduced bias, synthesized evidence	Heterogeneity between studies, publication bias
Case Reports/Series	Detailed reports of individual cases or small groups	Identifies rare adverse effects, generates hypotheses	Cannot establish causality or frequency, reporting bias
Pharmacokinetic/Pharmacodynamic Studies	Examines drug disposition and effects	Establishes dosing, identifies interactions, special populations	Small sample sizes, controlled conditions
Health Economics/Outcomes Research	Evaluates cost-effectiveness, quality of life	Real-world effectiveness, economic impact, patient-centered outcomes	Methodological complexity, generalizability concerns

Observational studies encompass cohort studies (following exposed and unexposed groups forward in time), case-control studies (comparing those with and without outcomes retrospectively), cross-sectional analyses (examining exposures and outcomes simultaneously), and case series/reports (describing individual patient experiences without comparison groups). Meta-analytic methodology combines results from multiple individual studies through statistical pooling, with understanding of heterogeneity assessment, publication bias evaluation, and statistical models essential for appropriate interpretation.

Critical Reading Strategies

Introduction assessment evaluates whether authors establish clear research questions, provide sufficient background justifying the study, and frame hypotheses appropriately within existing literature. Methods evaluation examines study design appropriateness for the research question, participant selection and characteristics, intervention details, outcome definition and measurement, and statistical approach adequacy. Results interpretation considers both statistical and clinical significance, appropriate presentation of findings, handling of missing data, and congruence between described methods and reported outcomes. Discussion analysis evaluates whether authors appropriately contextualize findings within existing literature, acknowledge limitations honestly, and draw conclusions justified by the actual results rather than overreaching claims.

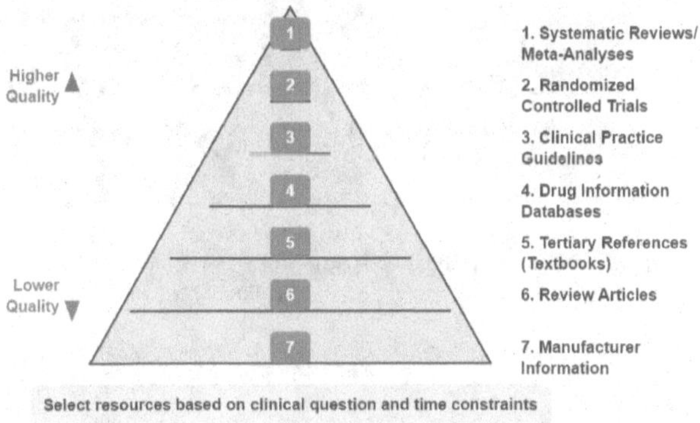

Figure 6.1: Hierarchy of Drug Information Resources

Industry-Sponsored Research Considerations

Financial relationship disclosure examines transparency regarding funding sources, author conflicts of interest, and potential commercial influences on study design, analysis, or reporting. Study design evaluation assesses whether methodology favors sponsor products through comparator selection (placebo rather than active alternatives, inappropriate dosing of competitors), endpoint choice (surrogate markers, composite outcomes, post-hoc analyses), or participant selection (narrow criteria excluding challenging patients). Publication planning awareness recognizes strategic approaches potentially fragmenting results across multiple publications ("salami slicing"), selective outcome reporting, or delayed/suppressed publication of unfavorable findings, requiring comprehensive literature search beyond individual articles.

Application to Practice

Patient applicability assessment evaluates whether study populations reasonably represent clinical practice populations through examination of inclusion/exclusion criteria, demographic characteristics, comorbidity profiles, and concurrent medication use. Clinical significance determination distinguishes between statistical significance and meaningful clinical impact through consideration of effect size, absolute versus relative differences, number needed to treat/harm, and patient-oriented versus surrogate outcomes. Practice change threshold establishes appropriate evidentiary standards for modifying clinical practice based on study quality, consistency with existing evidence, risk-benefit balance, and available alternatives rather than responding to individual publications in isolation.

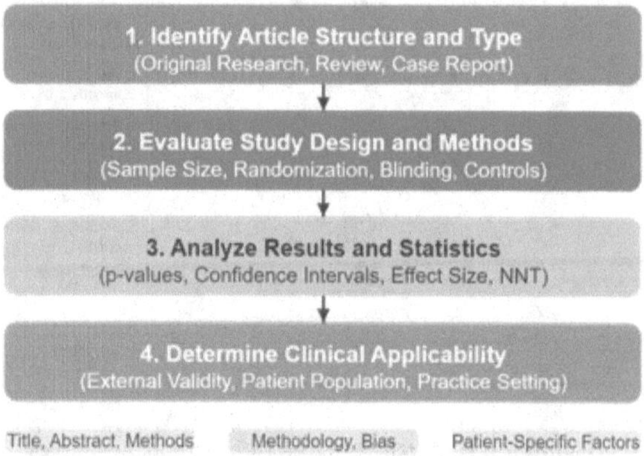

Figure 6.2: Primary Literature Evaluation Process

SECONDARY RESOURCES

Quality assessment employs tools such as AMSTAR-2 (Assessing the Methodological Quality of Systematic Reviews) examining search comprehensiveness, study selection methodology, quality evaluation of included studies, appropriate synthesis methods, and publication bias assessment. Forest plot interpretation analyzes graphical representations of meta-analysis results, including individual study findings, weighting, confidence intervals, heterogeneity assessment, and overall effect estimates with appropriate uncertainty measures. Cochrane Collaboration resources represent particularly rigorous systematic reviews following standardized methodology, comprehensive searching, and structured quality assessment, though covering limited topics and sometimes lacking practical implementation guidance despite methodological excellence.

Evidence-Based Summaries

Clinical Evidence (BMJ) provides systematic condition-based reviews categorizing interventions as beneficial, likely beneficial, trade-off between benefits and harms, unknown effectiveness, unlikely beneficial, or likely ineffective based on systematic literature evaluation. ACP Journal Club selects methodologically sound, clinically relevant studies from over 120 journals with structured abstracts and expert commentary highlighting practical implementation considerations beyond statistical findings. Essential Evidence Plus integrates evidence-based summaries with clinical decision support tools including calculators, guidelines, and patient information organized around clinical questions with strength of evidence ratings for recommendations.

Pharmacotherapy Textbooks

Comprehensive references including DiPiro's Pharmacotherapy: A Pathophysiologic Approach provide detailed disease-oriented chapters integrating pathophysiology, clinical presentation, and complete therapeutic management with extensive referencing supporting recommendations. Specialized textbooks address focused therapeutic areas with greater depth, including Koda-Kimble and Young's Applied Therapeutics (case-based approach), Casebook in Clinical Pharmacokinetics and Drug Dosing, and Pediatric Injectable Drugs (The Teddy Bear Book) for specialized practice areas. Currency limitations affect all print resources, with publication cycles of 2-5 years potentially outdating specific recommendations despite accurate foundational information, requiring supplementation with more frequently updated resources for rapidly evolving therapeutic areas.

Clinical Practice Guidelines

Developer evaluation assesses guideline source credibility through examination of sponsoring organization, panel composition, methodological rigor, evidence evaluation transparency, and conflict of interest management. Recommendation grading systems interpret strength designations including various frameworks (GRADE, USPSTF, ACC/AHA) connecting recommendation strength to evidence quality, benefit-risk assessment, and degree of consensus among experts. Implementation tools assessment examines whether guidelines include practical resources supporting application including algorithms, decision aids, order sets, and quality measures rather than solely providing conceptual recommendations without operational guidance.

Drug Information Compendia

American Hospital Formulary Service (AHFS) Drug Information provides comprehensive, evidence-based, independently written monographs organized by therapeutic class with extensive referencing, pharmacokinetic data, off-label uses, and dosing recommendations. Clinical Pharmacology powered by ClinicalKey offers electronic drug monographs with screening for interactions, duplicate therapy, allergies, and pregnancy/lactation considerations alongside IV compatibility information and patient education materials. Specialized references address specific information needs including Briggs' Drugs in Pregnancy and Lactation, Micromedex IV Compatibility, and Natural Medicines Comprehensive Database for complementary and alternative products.

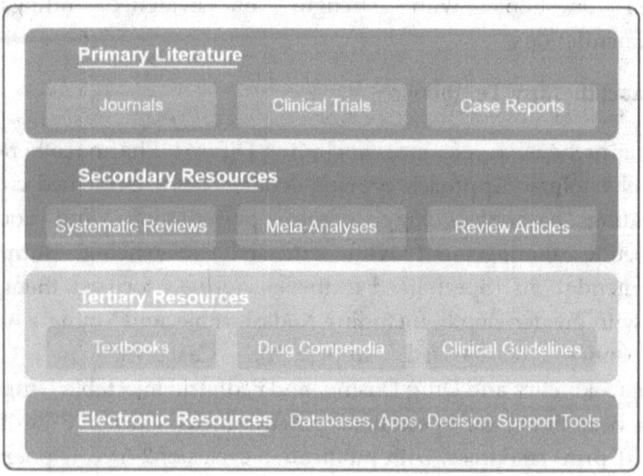

Figure 6.3: Types of Drug Information Resources

ELECTRONIC DATABASES

PubMed/MEDLINE search optimization employs advanced features including Medical Subject Heading (MeSH) terms, field-specific searching, filters, Boolean operators, and citation mapping to efficiently retrieve relevant literature from over 30 million biomedical citations. Embase utilization accesses European and international pharmaceutical literature with particular strengths in drug safety, pharmacovigilance, and regulatory information often not fully indexed in MEDLINE, with Emtree controlled vocabulary enhancing precision. International Pharmaceutical Abstracts provides specialized coverage of pharmacy-specific literature including pharmaceutical science, pharmacy practice, and pharmaceutical education journals alongside meeting abstracts not consistently included in broader biomedical databases.

Full-Text Aggregators

Ovid platform delivers integrated access to multiple resources including MEDLINE, Embase, and full-text journals with consistent interface, linking between databases, and specialized search tools including natural language processing. ClinicalKey consolidates full-text access to Elsevier journals, textbooks, clinical practice guidelines, drug information, and patient education materials with clinically-focused search capabilities and point-of-care organization. Access considerations include institutional subscription limitations, embargoes on recent content, and variable coverage across therapeutic areas requiring understanding of collection strengths and limitations for efficient information retrieval.

Table 6.2: Secondary Drug Information Resources

Resource Category	Examples	Characteristics	Applications	Limitations
Comprehensive Drug References	Micromedex, Lexicomp, Clinical Pharmacology	Detailed monographs, multiple content areas, regular updates	Complete drug information, off-label uses, detailed dosing	Subscription cost, information density, overwhelming detail
Pharmacotherapy Textbooks	DiPiro's Pharmacotherapy, Koda-Kimble and Young's	Disease-oriented chapters, evidence summaries,	Background knowledge, pathophysiology integration,	Publication lag time, rapid outdating for evolving therapies

Resource Category	Examples	Characteristics	Applications	Limitations
	Applied Therapeutics	clinical application	therapeutic approaches	
Clinical Practice Guidelines	ACC/AHA Heart Failure Guidelines, IDSA Antimicrobial Guidelines	Evidence-based recommendations, graded evidence quality	Standard of care determination, treatment algorithms	Potential conflicts of interest, update delays, generalizability issues
Systematic Reviews	Cochrane Database, Drug Effectiveness Review Project	Rigorous methodology, comprehensive search, evidence grading	Comparative effectiveness, therapy selection, formulary decisions	Limited scope, publication delays, varying methodological quality
Drug Handbooks	Sanford Guide to Antimicrobial Therapy, Pediatric Dosing Handbook	Concise, focused information, point-of-care format	Quick reference, common scenarios, standard dosing	Limited detail, simplified recommendations, narrow scope
Disease-Specific Resources	NCCN Guidelines, GOLD COPD Guidelines	Condition-specific recommendations, specialized content	Specialty practice, complex conditions, staging-based therapy	Narrow focus, specialty bias, limited medication detail
Drug Interaction References	Drug Interaction Facts, Stockley's Drug Interactions	Mechanism details, clinical significance ratings, management strategies	Interaction screening, polypharmacy assessment, risk management	Theoretical interactions, limited clinical context, evolving evidence
Adverse Reaction References	Meyler's Side Effects of Drugs, Drug-Induced Diseases	Comprehensive ADR listings, causality assessment, management approaches	ADR identification, differential diagnosis, preventive strategies	Reporting bias, causality uncertainty, prevalence limitations

Evidence-Based Medicine Resources

Cochrane Library provides access to high-quality systematic reviews, controlled trials registry, methodology resources, and health technology assessments with standardized methodology and minimal commercial influence. DynaMed synthesizes evidence into clinically-organized topics with explicit evidence grading, practice recommendations, and frequent updates (typically within 24 hours of major new evidence publication). UpToDate offers comprehensive, expert-authored topics organized around clinical questions with graded recommendations, extensive references, patient information, and drug interaction checking, though with potential expert opinion influence despite explicit evidence grading.

Medication-Specific Databases

Micromedex Solutions provides comprehensive drug information including FDA-approved and off-label uses, detailed dosing, adverse effects, interactions, IV compatibility, pregnancy/lactation data, and comparative efficacy information with explicit evidence ratings. Lexicomp delivers monographs with consistent organization, rapid navigation between sections, customizable interaction screening, extensive calculations, and integration with electronic health records in many institutions. Facts & Comparisons eAnswers offers detailed comparison charts, product identification tools, extensive patient counseling information, and formulary management features alongside core drug information monographs.

Specialized Electronic Resources

Drug interaction databases including Micromedex Drug Interactions, Drug Interaction Facts, and Lexi-Interact provide mechanistic explanations, clinical significance ratings, management recommendations, and primary literature citations beyond simple interaction identification. Pharmacogenomic resources such as PharmGKB, CPIC guidelines, and FDA Table of Pharmacogenomic Biomarkers connect genetic variations to medication response, dosing recommendations, and clinical implementation strategies for precision medicine applications. Adverse reaction databases including FDA Adverse Event Reporting System (FAERS), VigiBase (WHO), and EudraVigilance (EMA) provide post-marketing surveillance data on emerging safety concerns beyond clinical trial experience

Table 6.3: Electronic Database Characteristics and Search Strategies

Database	Content Coverage	Unique Features	Search Functionalities	Effective Search Strategies
PubMed/MEDLINE	Biomedical literature, >30 million citations	MeSH controlled vocabulary, clinical queries filters	Boolean operators, field tags, filters	Use MeSH terms, apply clinical queries filters, limit to publication types
Embase	Biomedical literature with European/ drug focus	Emtree thesaurus, drug and adverse event emphasis	Similar to MEDLINE plus drug searching	Use Emtree terms, drug subheadings, adverse event searching
Cochrane Library	Systematic reviews, controlled trials	Methodologically rigorous reviews, trials database	Topic browsing, intervention searching	Use MeSH terms, review vs. trials database selection, protocol access
Scopus/Web of Science	Citation databases across disciplines	Citation tracking, author searching, impact metrics	Citation analysis, journal metrics	Forward/backward citation searching, journal impact analysis
Clinical Trials Registries	Ongoing and completed clinical trials	Unpublished results, trial protocols	Condition, intervention, location searching	Use multiple terms for condition/intervention, status filters
FDA/EMA Databases	Regulatory submissions, approvals, safety alerts	Original submission data, regulatory decisions	Drug approval searching, safety alerts	Use both trade/generic names, application number searching
Google Scholar	Broad academic literature	Citation tracking, full-text searching	Simple interface, citation linking	Use quotation marks for phrases, author: and site: operators

CLINICAL DECISION SUPPORT TOOLS

Computerized provider order entry (CPOE) systems incorporate medication-specific safeguards including dose range checking, renal adjustment alerts, allergy screening, drug-drug interaction warnings, and pregnancy precautions at the point of prescribing. Clinical decision support rules deliver patient-specific, evidence-based recommendations triggered by specific clinical conditions, laboratory values, or medication combinations identified within electronic health records. Integration challenges include alert fatigue from excessive warnings, interoperability limitations between systems, and potential workflow disruptions requiring ongoing optimization balancing safety benefits against operational efficiency.

Point-of-Care Reference Applications

Mobile application selection evaluates factors including content quality, update frequency, offline functionality, interface usability, and integration capabilities across different clinical reference tools. Epocrates provides rapid drug information access including dosing, adverse effects, contraindications, drug interactions, pill identification, and clinical practice guidelines with particular strength in concise point-of-care information. Pharmacist's Letter/Prescriber's Letter delivers monthly updates on emerging evidence, new medications, safety concerns, and clinical controversies with concise recommendations, comparison charts, and patient education materials focused on practice-changing developments.

Drug Interaction Screening Tools

Significance classification systems categorize interaction severity using various frameworks including categorical ratings (minor/moderate/major), numeric scales, or descriptive classifications based on potential clinical consequences, quality of evidence, and management difficulty. Management recommendation evaluation assesses practical guidance including monitoring parameters, dosage adjustments, scheduling modifications, or alternative therapy suggestions beyond simply identifying potential interactions. Filter customization adapts alerting thresholds to specific practice settings, patient populations, or individual risk factors to balance comprehensive screening against alert volume management.

Table 6.4: Clinical Decision Support Tools

Tool Type	Examples	Functionalities	Implementation
Medication Alert Systems	Drug-drug interaction alerts, dose checking, allergy warnings	Real-time notifications, severity stratification, override tracking	Alert fatigue management, relevance thresholds, workflow integration
Dosing Calculators	Renal dosing, pediatric dosing, anticoagulation management	Patient-specific parameters, evidence-based algorithms, documentation	Validation against guidelines, interface design, calculation transparency
Treatment Pathways	Order sets, clinical pathways, protocol automation	Standardized approach, guideline alignment, decision trees	Customization capability, update processes, user acceptance
Mobile Applications	Epocrates, Micromedex, specialty-specific apps	Point-of-care information, offline access, quick reference	Evidence validation, update frequency, information source
Risk Calculators	CHA_2DS_2-VASc, ASCVD risk, Cockcroft-Gault	Evidence-based algorithms, patient-specific inputs, guidance integration	Algorithm validation, appropriate application
Therapeutic Monitoring Systems	Anticoagulation management, diabetes monitoring, pharmacokinetic services	Tracking parameters, trend analysis, intervention recommendations	Integration with laboratory data, alert thresholds, documentation
Pharmacogenomic Tools	Gene-drug interaction checkers, dosing guidance, interpretation	Genetic variant interpretation, clinical recommendations, reference information	Evidence quality, recommendation clarity, clinical integration
Prescription Writing Systems	E-prescribing, medication reconciliation tools, discharge prescribing	Safety checks, formulary integration, patient instructions	Interoperability, user interface, safety feature effectiveness

Calculation and Conversion Tools

Dosing calculators implement appropriate formulas for weight-based, body surface area, or organ function-adjusted medication dosing with verification mechanisms preventing mathematical errors during high-stress situations. Pharmacokinetic tools employ appropriate models for specialized dosing situations including aminoglycoside dosing (population-based or individualized), vancomycin dosing (trough-based or AUC-based), and anticoagulation management incorporating patient-specific factors. Conversion utilities facilitate accurate transformation between different measurement units, dosage forms, or equivalent dosing across therapeutic alternatives while maintaining clinical appropriateness beyond simple mathematical conversion.

Patient Education Resources

Health literacy appropriate materials provide medication information at suitable reading levels (typically 5th-6th grade), appropriate language translations, and visual aids supporting comprehension across diverse patient populations. Interactive tools engage patients through medication reminder applications, symptom tracking functionality, and two-way communication features enhancing adherence and self-management capabilities. Multimedia resources employ videos, animations, and graphics explaining complex medication concepts including mechanism of action, administration techniques, and self-monitoring expectations in accessible formats for diverse learning styles.

INFORMATION RETRIEVAL SKILLS

PICO framework structures information needs into answerable questions specifying Patient/Problem, Intervention, Comparison, and Outcome components to clarify search parameters and ensure relevance of retrieved information. Background versus foreground question distinction differentiates between general knowledge needs (typically addressed through textbooks or summaries) and specific clinical decisions (requiring more detailed primary literature or specialized resources). Searchable question conversion transforms clinical uncertainties into effective search terminology including appropriate synonyms, related concepts, and controlled vocabulary terms matching database indexing systems.

Search Strategy Development

Controlled vocabulary utilization employs database-specific thesaurus terms including Medical Subject Headings (MeSH) in

MEDLINE, Emtree terms in Embase, or similar structured terminology in other resources to improve search precision beyond keyword variations. Boolean operator application combines search concepts appropriately using AND (narrowing results by requiring multiple concepts), OR (broadening results by including synonyms or related terms), and NOT (excluding specific concepts with careful consideration of potential relevant exclusion). Limits and filters application refines results through appropriate restrictions including publication type, date ranges, study design, patient age groups, or language while avoiding overly restrictive parameters potentially excluding relevant information.

Table 6.5: Information Retrieval and Analysis Process

Process Step	Actions	Tools and Resources	Common Pitfalls
Question Formulation	Define PICO elements, determine question type, specify scope	PICO framework, background resources, clinical context assessment	Overly broad questions, missing critical elements, undefined scope
Resource Selection	Choose appropriate resources based on question type	Resource matrix, search strategies by question type, access considerations	Overreliance on familiar resources, ignoring specialized databases
Search Strategy Development	Construct logical search with appropriate terms and operators	Controlled vocabularies (MeSH, Emtree), Boolean operators, search filters	Too narrow/broad terms, missing synonyms, improper Boolean logic
Literature Retrieval	Execute search, save results, obtain full-text	Database interfaces, citation management software, document delivery	Inadequate documentation, poor organization, limited access methods
Critical Appraisal	Evaluate methodology, validity, applicability	Critical appraisal worksheets, validity assessment tools, bias evaluation frameworks	Accepting conclusions without methodology evaluation, confirmation bias

Process Step	Actions	Tools and Resources	Common Pitfalls
Information Synthesis	Integrate findings, resolve conflicts, develop recommendations	Evidence tables, grading frameworks, clinical context integration	Cherry-picking supportive evidence, ignoring conflicting data
Response Formulation	Tailor information to requestor needs, appropriate format and detail	Communication templates, clinical relevance frameworks, audience analysis	Information overload, inappropriate detail level, unclear recommendations
Documentation	Record question, resources, strategy, response	Standardized documentation forms, searchable database, quality metrics	Insufficient detail, missing search strategy, inadequate response rationale

Database Selection Logic

Information type matching selects appropriate resources based on specific needs including primary literature (bibliographic databases), synthesized evidence (systematic reviews, guidelines), drug-specific information (specialized compendia), or point-of-care guidance (decision support tools). Currency requirements consideration selects resources based on information time-sensitivity, ranging from constantly updated surveillance databases for emerging safety concerns to stable foundational knowledge where historical sources remain relevant. Access method evaluation considers institutional subscriptions, professional membership benefits, publicly available resources, and point-of-care availability in selecting practical information pathways for different practice settings.

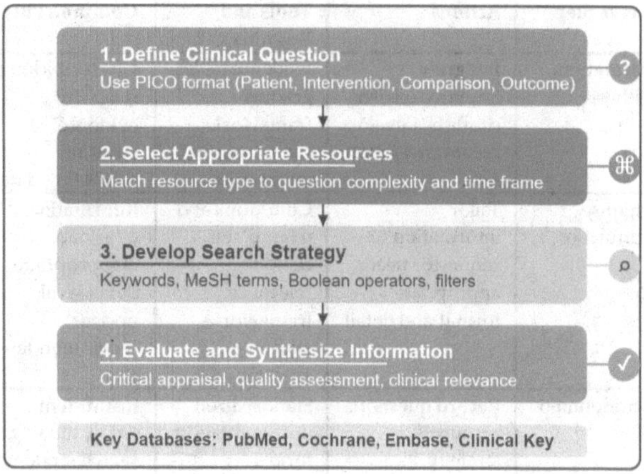

Figure 6.4: Systematic Information Retrieval

Efficient Search Execution

Advanced interface feature utilization employs database-specific capabilities including proximity operators, truncation, wildcard characters, phrase searching, and field-specific limitations to optimize retrieval precision. Citation pearl growing begins with a highly relevant source and expands through related articles functions, citation tracking (works citing the original source), and reference examination (works cited by the original source) to build comprehensive literature identification. Search documentation maintains records of search strategies, databases accessed, and filters applied to enable strategy refinement, reproducibility for similar questions, and methodological transparency for formal reviews.

Search Result Management

Relevance assessment evaluates retrieved information against the original clinical question through rapid title and abstract screening, distinguishing between directly applicable, potentially useful, and irrelevant results based on PICO element matching. Citation management employs software tools including EndNote, Zotero, or Mendeley to organize references, store full-text articles, annotate important findings, and generate properly formatted citations for formal writing. Knowledge organization systems develop personal or team-based structures for storing, categorizing, and retrieving information for future use through taxonomies, tagging systems, or specialized knowledge bases supporting cumulative expertise development.

Summary

- Primary literature includes original research published in peer-reviewed journals, representing the most current but also most complex source of drug information.

- Secondary resources such as review articles, textbooks, and compendia provide synthesized information that is more accessible but may not reflect the most recent evidence.

- Electronic databases (PubMed, Embase, Cochrane) allow efficient searching of medical literature using appropriate search strategies and MeSH terms.

- Clinical decision support tools include point-of-care resources that integrate drug information with patient-specific factors to guide therapeutic decisions.

- Information retrieval skills include formulating answerable clinical questions, selecting appropriate resources, and efficiently extracting relevant information.

- Critical evaluation of drug information resources requires assessment of authorship, publication date, methodology, potential bias, and applicability to specific patient scenarios.

- Communicating drug information effectively to patients and healthcare providers requires adapting complex information to the recipient's level of understanding and specific needs.

Multiple Choice Questions

1. Which of the following is the MOST appropriate resource for finding detailed information about a drug's pharmacokinetic properties?
   A) Hospital formulary
   B) Drug package insert
   C) Clinical practice guideline
   D) Pharmacy dispensing software
2. A physician asks about the efficacy of a new medication compared to standard therapy. Which resource would provide the HIGHEST level of evidence to answer this question?
   A) Pharmacology textbook
   B) Drug manufacturer's website
   C) Systematic review and meta-analysis
   D) Expert opinion paper
3. When using PubMed for a literature search, which of the following search strategies is MOST likely to yield focused, relevant results?
   A) Using very broad search terms to capture all possible articles
   B) Limiting the search to articles published within the last year
   C) Using MeSH terms combined with appropriate filters and Boolean operators
   D) Searching only for free full-text articles
4. A pharmacist needs to quickly determine an appropriate dose adjustment for a renally impaired patient. The MOST efficient reliable resource would be:
   A) Calling the drug manufacturer
   B) A specialized drug dosing handbook or database
   C) Conducting a comprehensive literature search
   D) Consulting with a nephrologist
5. Which of the following is the MOST important limitation of secondary drug information resources?
   A) They typically require subscription access
   B) Information may be outdated depending on publication date
   C) They present information without critical analysis
   D) They contain only FDA-approved information

6. When evaluating drug information from a pharmaceutical company's medical information department, the pharmacist should be MOST concerned about:
   A) Potential bias in how information is presented
   B) Delays in receiving a response
   C) Complex scientific language
   D) Limited historical information
7. Which of the following is the BEST approach when drug information resources provide conflicting recommendations?
   A) Always follow the most recently published information
   B) Evaluate the quality and strength of evidence supporting each recommendation
   C) Follow the recommendation from the most prestigious journal
   D) Use the information that best confirms the pharmacist's initial impression
8. Clinical decision support tools are MOST valuable for:
   A) Replacing clinical judgment in complex cases
   B) Providing patient-specific recommendations based on individual factors
   C) Eliminating the need for drug information specialists
   D) Storing patient medication histories
9. When providing drug information in response to a clinical question, which of the following is MOST important to include?
   A) All available information on the topic
   B) Only information that supports the recommended action
   C) A response tailored to the specific question with appropriate clinical context
   D) Information from as many different sources as possible
10. Which of the following statements about clinical practice guidelines is MOST accurate?
    A) They should be followed without modification for all patients
    B) They represent consensus expert opinion but may not always reflect the strongest evidence
    C) They are updated continuously as new evidence emerges
    D) They are primarily useful for research purposes rather than clinical practice

Self-Assessment Questions

1. Compare and contrast primary, secondary, and tertiary drug information resources, providing examples of each and when each type would be most appropriate to use.
2. Explain the PICO framework for formulating clinical questions and how it guides effective information retrieval.
3. Describe three key elements to evaluate when assessing the quality and reliability of a drug information resource.
4. Explain the advantages and limitations of using electronic databases compared to print resources for drug information.
5. Describe the process for conducting a systematic literature search, including selection of appropriate databases and development of search strategies.
6. Discuss three factors that should be considered when evaluating the clinical applicability of information found in primary literature.
7. Explain how clinical decision support tools can enhance medication safety and provide examples of common tools used in pharmacy practice.
8. Describe strategies for efficiently evaluating a medication's safety profile when limited information is available about a newly approved drug.
9. Explain the concept of "information mastery" and how pharmacists can apply it to manage the volume of available drug information.
10. Discuss ethical considerations in using and communicating drug information, including managing conflicts of interest and addressing information gaps.

Bibliography

1. Malone PM, Kier KL, Stanovich JE, Malone MJ. Drug information: a guide for pharmacists. 6th ed. New York: McGraw-Hill Education; 2018.
2. Guyatt G, Rennie D, Meade MO, Cook DJ. Users' guides to the medical literature: a manual for evidence-based clinical practice. 3rd ed. New York: McGraw-Hill Education; 2015.
3. Koh EY, Chui WK. Use of information sources by cancer patients: results of a systematic review of the research literature. Inf Res. 2016;21(4):paper 727.
4. MacLure K, Paudyal V, Stewart D. Reviewing the literature, how systematic is systematic? Int J Clin Pharm. 2016;38(3):685-694.
5. Walker E, Rew K, Hawkins L. Developing a drug information service for a university hospital-based drug information centre. Health Info Libr J. 2006;23(2):102-108.
6. Perrier L, Farrell A, Ayala AP, Lightfoot D, Kenny T, Aaronson E, et al. Effects of librarian-provided services in healthcare settings: a systematic review. J Am Med Inform Assoc. 2014;21(6):1118-1124.
7. Kupferberg N, Protus BM. Accuracy and completeness of drug information in Wikipedia: an assessment. J Med Libr Assoc. 2011;99(4):310-313.
8. Shebl NA, Franklin BD, Barber N. Clinical decision support systems and antibiotic use. Pharm World Sci. 2007;29(4):342-349.
9. Bright TJ, Wong A, Dhurjati R, Bristow E, Bastian L, Coeytaux RR, et al. Effect of clinical decision-support systems: a systematic review. Ann Intern Med. 2012;157(1):29-43.
10. Kawamoto K, Houlihan CA, Balas EA, Lobach DF. Improving clinical practice using clinical decision support systems: a systematic review of trials to identify features critical to success. BMJ. 2005;330(7494):765.

CHAPTER 7

MEDICATION THERAPY MANAGEMENT

Author

Dr. Hema Arya, Assistant Professor, Department of Pharmaceutical Chemistry, School of Pharmacy, Sharda University, Greater Noida, Uttar Pradesh, India

Abstract

Medication therapy management (MTM) provides a systematic framework for optimizing therapeutic outcomes through comprehensive medication review, problem identification, and targeted interventions. Comprehensive medication reviews systematically evaluate all medications including prescription, non-prescription, supplements, and complementary therapies through structured assessment of indication, effectiveness, safety, and adherence. Drug therapy problem identification employs standardized taxonomies categorizing issues including unnecessary therapy, suboptimal dosing, adverse effects, interactions, and adherence barriers requiring resolution. Intervention strategies encompass prescriber collaboration, medication regimen optimization, patient education, care coordination, and documentation with appropriate follow-up planning. Evaluation methodologies assess clinical, economic, and humanistic outcomes through both objective measures and patient-reported experiences using validated instruments and systematic data collection. Quality metrics demonstrate MTM impact through standardized measures addressing medication appropriateness, adherence rates, adverse event reduction, and therapeutic goal achievement. This patient-centered approach improves medication use through personalized interventions addressing specific medication-related needs while reducing healthcare costs, preventing adverse events, and enhancing quality of life through optimized pharmacotherapy.

Keywords: *Comprehensive Medication Review, Pharmaceutical Care, Drug-Related Problems, Therapeutic Optimization, Outcome Assessment*

Learning Objectives

After completion of the chapter, the learners should be able to:

- Conduct comprehensive medication reviews systematically assessing indication, effectiveness, safety, and adherence for all medications.
- Identify and categorize drug therapy problems using standardized taxonomies addressing unnecessary therapy, dosing issues, adverse effects, interactions, and adherence barriers.
- Implement targeted intervention strategies addressing identified medication-related problems through prescriber collaboration, regimen optimization, and patient education.
- Design appropriate follow-up evaluation plans to assess intervention outcomes, therapeutic goal achievement, and resolution of identified problems.
- Apply quality metrics and performance measures to demonstrate the impact of medication therapy management services on patient outcomes.
- Develop systematic approaches for prioritizing patients who would benefit most from comprehensive medication management services.

MEDICATION REVIEW

Medication inventory compilation documents all active treatments including prescription medications, over-the-counter products, supplements, and alternative therapies through multiple source verification including patient interviews, prescription records, previous medical records, and caregiver reports. Indication assessment evaluates each medication against documented medical conditions, identifying both untreated conditions requiring therapy and medications without clear indications for potential discontinuation. Regimen analysis examines the complete medication profile for therapeutic duplication, potential interactions, inappropriate combinations, and cumulative anticholinergic or sedative burden beyond evaluation of individual medications in isolation.

Table 7.1: Medication Review Components

Review Component	Assessment Elements	Clinical Tools
Medication Reconciliation	Prescription medications, OTCs, supplements, sample medications	Brown bag review, patient interview guide, EHR medication history
Indication Assessment	FDA-approved uses, evidence-based off-label uses, therapeutic duplication	Clinical guidelines, formulary criteria, diagnosis-medication matching tools
Effectiveness Evaluation	Therapeutic goal achievement, symptom control, disease markers	Disease-specific monitoring parameters, patient-reported outcomes
Safety Analysis	Adverse effects, contraindications, high-risk medications, drug interactions	Beers Criteria, STOPP/START, interaction checkers, adverse effect scales
Adherence Assessment	Refill patterns, self-reported adherence, barriers to adherence	Morisky scale, refill records, pill counts, adherence barrier questionnaires
Medication Costs	Out-of-pocket expenses, insurance coverage, financial burden	Pricing tools, assistance program eligibility, therapeutic alternatives
Patient Understanding	Knowledge of purpose, directions, monitoring, precautions	Teach-back assessment, medication knowledge questionnaires
Care Coordination	Communication with providers, care transitions, fragmentation issues	Care team roster, SBAR communication, transition documentation

Targeted Medication Review Focus

High-risk medication identification prioritizes review for medications with elevated safety concerns including those on Beers Criteria for older adults, ISMP high-alert medications, narrow therapeutic index drugs, or those requiring specialized monitoring parameters. Disease-specific evaluation addresses medication appropriateness for specific conditions including heart failure, diabetes, chronic kidney disease, or behavioral health disorders through condition-focused review against current treatment guidelines and quality measures. Care transition assessment specifically examines medication changes during transfers between settings including hospital discharge, long-term care placement, or provider changes to identify unintentional discrepancies, inappropriate continuations, or communication gaps.

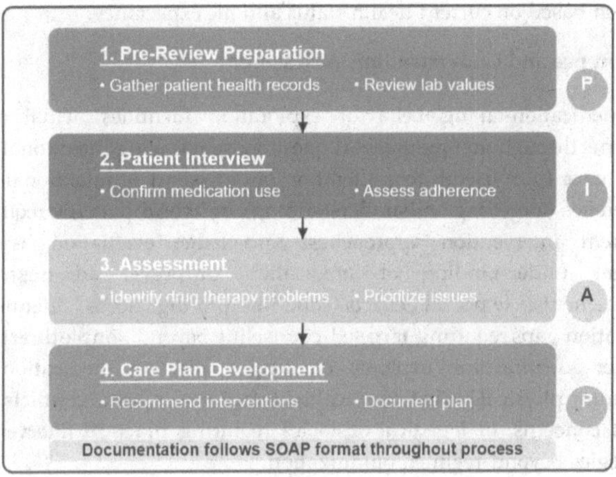

Figure 7.1: Medication Review Process

Patient-Specific Appropriateness Evaluation

Dosage optimization assesses medication quantities, frequencies, and timing against patient-specific factors including age, weight, organ function, genetics, and comorbidities to identify potential adjustments beyond standard dosing recommendations. Administration practicality evaluates whether prescribed regimens align with patient capabilities including physical limitations, swallowing difficulties, cognitive status, and daily routines that may impair proper medication use despite appropriate selection. Cost consideration examines financial impact of medication regimens including insurance coverage, copayment burden, and availability of more affordable alternatives with similar efficacy to address economic barriers to adherence.

Evidence Application to Individual Patients

Guideline individualization adapts standardized recommendations to specific patient circumstances, recognizing when guideline-recommended therapy requires modification based on comorbidities, patient preferences, prognosis, or competing health priorities. Benefit-risk assessment weighs potential therapeutic advantages against possible harms for each medication within the specific patient context rather than population-averaged expectations, particularly important for preventive therapies in elderly or multi-morbid patients. Deprescribing consideration systematically evaluates opportunities to discontinue medications with unfavorable risk-benefit profiles, questionable ongoing need, or minimal benefit relative to treatment burden based on current health status and life expectancy.

Adherence and Understanding Assessment

Medication-taking behavior exploration identifies actual usage patterns through non-judgmental questioning revealing intentional non-adherence (purposeful dose alteration or omission), unintentional non-adherence (forgetting, misunderstanding), or hybrid patterns requiring different intervention approaches. Knowledge evaluation assesses patient understanding of medication purposes, administration requirements, expected effects, and monitoring needs, identifying education gaps requiring targeted counseling beyond simple directions. Barrier identification explores challenges affecting medication use including physical limitations, health literacy issues, belief conflicts, side effect concerns, or logistical obstacles requiring practical intervention strategies beyond regimen optimization.

DRUG THERAPY PROBLEMS

Hepler and Strand classification categorizes medication-related problems into seven categories: unnecessary therapy, need for additional therapy, ineffective drug, dosage too low, adverse drug reaction, dosage too high, and non-compliance—providing a comprehensive framework addressing both clinical and behavioral aspects of medication management. PCNE (Pharmaceutical Care Network Europe) taxonomy employs a multi-dimensional approach categorizing problems, causes, interventions, and outcomes with hierarchical sub-classifications allowing detailed documentation of pharmaceutical care activities. VA MedSAFE classification system addresses medication safety specifically through categories including prescribing problems, dispensing issues, administration errors, monitoring failures, and patient-related factors contributing to adverse drug events.

Indication-Related Problems

Unnecessary medication identification recognizes therapies without current indications including those prescribed for self-limited conditions that resolved, prophylactic treatments no longer needed, or medications continued through clinical inertia despite lack of ongoing benefit. Untreated condition recognition identifies documented diagnoses without appropriate pharmacotherapy, including both completely untreated conditions and partially treated conditions requiring additional therapy for comprehensive management. Inappropriate drug selection addresses medications unsuitable for specific patient conditions based on contraindications, precautions, or availability of more effective alternatives for the documented indication.

Table 7.2: Drug Therapy Problem Classification and Assessment

Problem Category	Definition	Assessment Indicators	Resolution Approaches
Unnecessary Drug Therapy	Medication without valid indication	No current diagnosis matching medication, duplicate therapy, therapy duration exceeded	Discontinuation, tapering plan, therapeutic substitution
Need for Additional Therapy	Untreated condition requiring medication	Untreated diagnosis, suboptimal prophylaxis, preventive therapy indicated	Therapy initiation, preventive medication addition, adjunctive therapy
Ineffective Drug	Wrong drug for condition	Lack of response, disease progression despite therapy, inappropriate drug selection	Therapeutic substitution, augmentation strategy, alternate drug class
Dosage Too Low	Subtherapeutic dose	Inadequate response, subtherapeutic levels, underdosed for indication	Dose increase, frequency adjustment, formulation change
Adverse Drug Reaction	Undesirable effect	Symptoms of ADR, laboratory evidence of toxicity, intolerable side effects	Dose reduction, scheduling change, therapeutic alternative, adjunctive therapy
Dosage Too High	Excessive dose	Toxicity symptoms, supratherapeutic levels, inappropriate for patient factors	Dose reduction, frequency adjustment, extended-release conversion
Nonadherence	Failure to take medication as prescribed	Missed doses, improper administration,	Simplification, adherence aids, cost reduction

Problem Category	Definition	Assessment Indicators	Resolution Approaches
Drug Interactions	Medication combinations causing undesirable effects	Potential or actual drug-drug, drug-food, drug-disease interactions	Spacing doses, alternative agent, monitoring plan, dose adjustment
Inappropriate Selection	Medication not optimal for patient	More effective, safer, or cost-effective alternatives available	Therapeutic substitution, guideline-directed alternatives
Medication Access	Barriers to obtaining medications	Insurance issues, availability problems, cost barriers	Prior authorization, assistance programs, therapeutic substitution

Effectiveness Problems

Suboptimal response identification recognizes inadequate therapeutic outcomes despite medication adherence, potentially requiring dosage adjustment, regimen intensification, or alternative therapy selection. Inappropriate drug selection for efficacy addresses medications unlikely to achieve desired outcomes based on patient-specific factors including genetic variations affecting response, disease severity exceeding medication capabilities, or past treatment failures with similar agents. Dosage insufficiency identifies underdosing relative to therapeutic needs including doses below evidence-based recommendations, failure to titrate to effect, or inappropriate intervals allowing breakthrough symptoms between doses.

Safety Problems

Adverse drug reactions include both predictable side effects (dose-dependent, pharmacologically expected) and idiosyncratic reactions (immunologic, unpredictable) requiring different management approaches including dosage reduction, alternative therapy selection, or supportive management. Drug-drug interactions occur through various mechanisms including pharmacokinetic effects (altered absorption, distribution, metabolism, or elimination) and pharmacodynamic effects (synergistic or antagonistic activity at receptors or physiological systems) with clinical significance varying from theoretical concerns to life-threatening consequences. Drug-disease interactions represent situations where medications adversely affect coexisting conditions including beta-blockers exacerbating asthma, NSAIDs worsening heart failure, or anticholinergics complicating narrow-angle glaucoma, requiring alternative therapy selection or careful risk-benefit assessment.

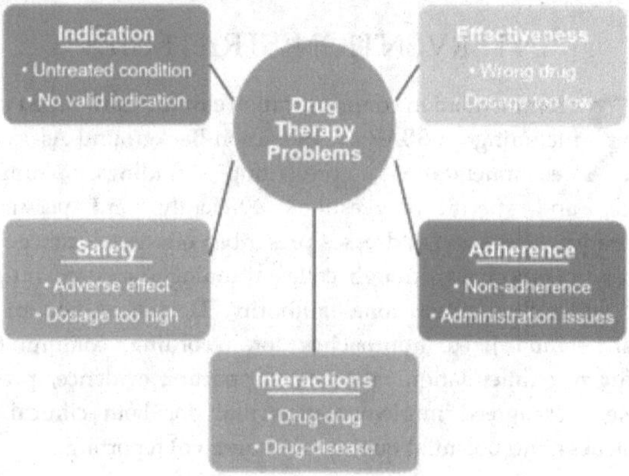

Figure 7.2: Common Drug Therapy Problems

Practical Use Problems

Administration difficulties encompass challenges with proper medication use including physical inability to manipulate packaging, swallowing difficulties with solid dosage forms, complexity of administration techniques for specialized formulations, or timing challenges with frequent daily dosing. Financial barriers include cost-related non-adherence due to high copayments, coverage limitations, or formulary restrictions, requiring therapy adjustments balancing clinical appropriateness against economic accessibility. Knowledge deficits involve insufficient understanding of proper use including misconceptions about administration timing, uncertainty about managing missed doses, or lack of awareness regarding important monitoring parameters or potential interactions requiring education intervention.

Monitoring-Related Problems

Inadequate monitoring identifies situations where essential laboratory or clinical parameters remain unevaluated despite being necessary for therapy management, including therapeutic drug levels, organ function assessment, or specific efficacy/toxicity markers. Inappropriate parameter selection addresses monitoring of irrelevant markers or incorrect test timing providing misleading information for therapy decisions, such as random rather than trough drug levels or non-fasting lipid assessment. Failure to respond to monitoring results involves situations where appropriate testing occurred but results indicating necessary therapy modifications were not implemented, representing an action gap rather than information deficit.

INTERVENTION STRATEGIES

Recommendation communication employs structured formats including SBAR (Situation-Background-Assessment-Recommendation) presenting findings, supporting evidence, and specific suggestions efficiently and persuasively. Collaborative discussion addresses prescriber questions, concerns, and alternative perspectives through collegial dialogue focused on patient benefit rather than professional authority. Documentation protocols establish standardized approaches for recording communications including recommendation rationale, supporting evidence, prescriber response, and agreed implementation plan for both clinical record completeness and potential quality measurement reporting.

Patient-Directed Interventions

Education enhancement employs targeted approaches addressing specific knowledge deficits identified during assessment, using appropriate health literacy level, preferred learning style, and focused content prioritization rather than comprehensive but overwhelming information. Administration simplification implements practical strategies reducing regimen complexity including consolidated administration times, extended-release formulations when appropriate, combination products, or calendar-based packaging reducing cognitive burden. Adherence tool selection matches appropriate support mechanisms to specific adherence barriers including pill organizers for forgetfulness, reminder systems for complex schedules, administration aids for physical limitations, or cost reduction strategies for financial barriers.

Regimen Optimization Strategies

Therapeutic substitution recommends alternative medications within the same class offering advantages in safety, efficacy, convenience, or cost while maintaining therapeutic intent for the original indication. Dosage adjustment implements changes based on patient-specific factors including organ function, drug interactions, genetic variations, age-related changes, or observed response and tolerance beyond standard dosing recommendations. Administration timing modification reorganizes medication schedules to enhance effectiveness (coordinating with meals, circadian variations, or symptom patterns), minimize adverse effects (separating interacting medications), or improve adherence (aligning with established daily routines).

Table 7.3: MTM Intervention Strategies and Implementation

Intervention Type	Implementation Approaches	Documentation Elements	Follow-up Requirements
Medication Changes	Discontinuation, dose adjustment, therapeutic substitution, initiation	Specific recommendation, rationale, evidence basis, prescriber response	Verify implementation, assess impact, monitor for withdrawal
Adherence Interventions	Simplification, reminder systems, packaging changes, cost reduction	Identified barriers, specific solutions, patient acceptance	Adherence reassessment, refinement of strategy, reinforcement
Educational Interventions	Counseling, written materials, demonstration, teach-back	Content covered, understanding assessment, reinforcement plan	Knowledge reassessment, behavior change evaluation, reinforcement needs
Monitoring Plans	Laboratory tests, self-monitoring, symptom tracking, follow-up schedule	Parameters, target values, frequency, responsibility, alert thresholds	Results review, plan adjustments, adherence to monitoring
Care Coordination	Provider communication, specialist referral, care transition planning	Communication method, information shared, response received	Closed-loop communication, integration of recommendations
Self-Management Support	Goal setting, action planning, problem-solving strategies	Patient goals, action steps, barriers addressed, support resources	Progress toward goals, barrier resolution, skill development
Regimen Optimization	Timing adjustments, administration route changes, formulation changes	Current issues, specific changes, implementation instructions	Feasibility assessment, practical challenges, effectiveness
Cost Interventions	Generic substitution, therapeutic alternatives	Cost before/after, program details, application status	Application completion, benefit verification, sustainability

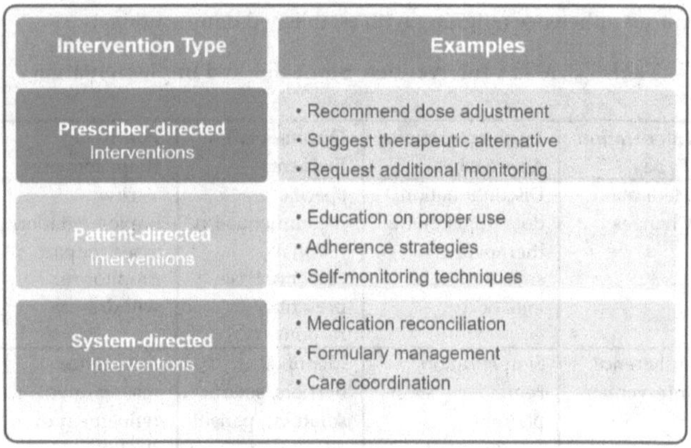

Figure 7.3: MTM Interventions

Formulary and Insurance Navigation

Prior authorization management develops supporting documentation addressing coverage criteria including diagnosis confirmation, previous therapy trials, contraindications to preferred alternatives, and clinical justification for non-formulary medications requiring special approval. Therapeutic alternative identification selects clinically appropriate options within insurance coverage parameters, balancing medical necessity against financial access considerations. Patient assistance program utilization connects eligible patients with pharmaceutical manufacturer programs, copayment assistance foundations, or medication discount services reducing financial barriers for essential therapies with limited insurance coverage.

Coordination with Healthcare Team

Care transition communication ensures critical medication information transfers effectively between settings through standardized formats including reconciliation documentation, therapy change rationale, monitoring requirements, and follow-up plans. Specialist consultation facilitates appropriate referrals for complex medication issues requiring additional expertise including nephrology for complex renal dosing, psychiatry for challenging psychotropic management, or pain management for complex analgesic regimens. Ancillary service coordination connects medication management with related supports including home health for administration assistance, nutrition services for diet-medication interactions, or social work for financial resource identification

FOLLOW-UP EVALUATION

Clinical parameter monitoring evaluates objective measures of medication effectiveness including physiological markers (blood pressure, blood glucose, lipid levels), symptom scales (pain scores, depression inventories), or functional assessments (activity tolerance, sleep quality) comparing baseline to post-intervention status. Patient-reported outcome collection systematically gathers subjective experiences including symptom improvement, quality of life changes, satisfaction with therapy, and perceived benefit beyond clinician-measured parameters. Medication-specific monitoring implements appropriate surveillance for individual agents including therapeutic drug levels for narrow-index medications, laboratory testing for potential toxicities, or physical assessment for specific adverse effects requiring early detection.

Table 7.4: MTM Outcome Evaluation Framework

Outcome	Evaluation Methods	Measurement Tools	Documentation
Clinical Outcomes	Disease marker monitoring, symptom assessment, event tracking	Laboratory values, validated symptom scales, event counts	Baseline and follow-up values, goal achievement, trending
Humanistic Outcomes	Quality of life assessment, satisfaction measurement, functional status	SF-36, treatment satisfaction questionnaires, functional scales	Standardized scores, comparative analysis, patient-reported changes
Economic Outcomes	Cost analysis, healthcare utilization tracking, work productivity	Medication costs, hospitalization/ED visits, work absence days	Pre/post comparison, cost avoidance calculations, ROI analysis
Process Measures	Intervention completion rates, recommendation acceptance, monitoring adherence	Chart review, tracking systems, patient follow-up	Percentage completion, acceptance rates, adherence rates
Medication-Specific Outcomes	Adverse event resolution, therapeutic goal achievement, adherence improvement	Side effect scales, therapeutic targets, adherence measures	Specific medication outcomes, resolution documentation

Outcome	Evaluation Methods	Measurement Tools	Documentation
Patient Engagement	Knowledge improvement, self-efficacy enhancement, behavior change	Knowledge assessments, self-efficacy scales, behavior tracking	Pre/post comparisons, qualitative assessments, engagement metrics
Care Coordination	Communication effectiveness, care transition success, fragmentation reduction	Provider feedback, transition measure tools, care coordination scales	Communication completion, transition success rates, fragmentation metrics
Patient-Centered Goals	Goal achievement, patient priority alignment, personalized outcomes	Goal attainment scaling, personalized outcome measures	Goal progress documentation, patient satisfaction with goal achievement

Follow-up Timing Considerations

Risk-based scheduling establishes follow-up intervals proportional to potential harm, with high-risk situations (narrow therapeutic index drugs, recent significant changes, complex regimens in vulnerable patients) requiring more frequent assessment than stable, low-risk therapy. Pharmacokinetic timing aligns reassessment with expected steady-state achievement, typically after 4-5 half-lives of consistent dosing for most medications, but potentially requiring extended observation for drugs with active metabolites or delayed effects. Condition-specific protocols implement disease-appropriate monitoring schedules including weekly INR for new warfarin users, monthly monitoring during antidepressant initiation, or quarterly assessment for stable chronic disease management.

Non-Response Management

Adherence verification distinguishes between treatment failure despite proper medication use versus inadequate therapy implementation through prescription refill review, direct observation, therapeutic drug monitoring, or structured patient interviewing. Dosage titration implements systematic increases within safety parameters for medications requiring individualized adjustment to effect, particularly common with antihypertensives, diabetes medications, and pain management. Alternative therapy progression follows structured approaches for sequential medication trials when initial selections prove inadequate, maintaining therapeutic class changes, combination strategies, or mechanism switches depending on specific condition treatment algorithms.

Adverse Effect Management

Causality assessment evaluates the relationship between suspected adverse effects and medications using structured approaches including temporal relationship, dechallenge/rechallenge response, alternative explanations, and known reaction patterns to distinguish medication effects from disease progression or coincidental symptoms. Expectedness evaluation determines whether observed effects represent known, anticipated reactions manageable through supportive care versus unexpected or severe reactions requiring therapy modification or discontinuation. Management strategy selection implements appropriate approaches including dosage reduction, administration modification, prophylactic treatment of side effects, or therapy discontinuation based on reaction severity, therapeutic importance, and available alternatives.

Long-Term Monitoring Systems

Systematic follow-up scheduling establishes structured approaches to ongoing monitoring including visit frequency, responsibility assignment, and specific parameter evaluation for chronic medication therapy beyond initial intervention periods. Technology-enabled monitoring employs remote assessment tools including home monitoring devices, smartphone applications, or telehealth connections maintaining surveillance between in-person visits particularly valuable for patients with geographic access limitations. Alert system implementation establishes automatic notifications for significant laboratory changes, missed follow-up appointments, or refill lapses identifying potential problems requiring intervention before clinical deterioration

QUALITY METRICS

Comprehensive medication review completion tracks the percentage of eligible patients receiving structured evaluation of complete medication regimens, typically targeting high-risk populations including those with multiple chronic conditions, polypharmacy, recent hospitalizations, or high-risk medication use. Medication reconciliation performance measures documentation of systematic comparison between medication lists during care transitions including hospital admission, discharge, and transfers between care settings with resolution of identified discrepancies. Drug therapy problem resolution monitors identification and addressment of medication-related problems with tracking of problem types, intervention strategies, and resolution rates to identify common issues and successful approaches.

Outcome Measure Development

Clinical goal attainment tracks achievement of condition-specific targets including blood pressure control (<130/80 mmHg), diabetes management (HbA1c <7% for most adults), or lipid management (LDL reduction appropriate to risk category) following medication therapy interventions. Adverse event reduction monitors medication-related complications including hypoglycemic episodes, fall incidents, or preventable adverse drug reactions before and after medication management service implementation. Healthcare utilization impact assesses changes in emergency department visits, hospitalizations, or unplanned care related to medication issues following comprehensive medication management implementation.

Table 7.5: MTM Quality Metrics and Program Evaluation

Metric Category	Specific Measures	Calculation Method	Benchmarking Considerations
Operational Metrics	Number of MTM cases, completion rates, time per encounter	Count, percentage, average time calculation	Compare to organization standards, national averages, historical trends
Intervention Metrics	Problems identified per patient, recommendations per patient, acceptance rates	Ratio calculation, percentage accepted	Complexity-adjusted comparisons, prescriber-specific analysis
Clinical Outcome Metrics	Clinical goal achievement, disease control rates, event prevention	Percentage at goal, event rates, NNT calculations	Risk-adjusted outcomes, comparable patient populations
Economic Metrics	Cost avoidance, ROI, hospitalization reduction	Cost calculation methodologies, utilization reduction	Valid comparison groups, comprehensive cost capture
Patient-Reported Metrics	Satisfaction scores, quality of life improvement, medication experience	Survey tools, standardized instruments	Baseline comparisons, comparable service benchmarks

Metric Category	Specific Measures	Calculation Method	Benchmarking Considerations
Provider Impact Metrics	Prescriber satisfaction, collaboration rates, recommendation uptake	Provider surveys, collaboration measures	Provider-specific trending, comparable service standards
Adherence Impact Metrics	PDC/MPR improvement, persistence rates, self-reported adherence	Calculation from refill data, survey tools	Pre/post comparison, population norms
Population Health Metrics	Percentage of eligible patients served, high-risk patient reach, health disparities	Population-based calculations	Demographic analysis, disparity measures, population penetration

Star Rating and Performance Measures

Medicare Part D measures includes medication adherence metrics for diabetes medications, renin-angiotensin system antagonists, and statins (proportion of days covered ≥80%), along with high-risk medication avoidance in elderly patients significantly affecting plan quality ratings and payment. HEDIS measures encompasses numerous medication-related metrics including appropriate treatment for conditions like asthma and COPD, monitoring for patients on persistent medications, and potentially inappropriate medication use in older adults used by numerous quality reporting programs. PQA (Pharmacy Quality Alliance) measures provides standardized metrics addressing medication safety, adherence, and appropriate use adopted across multiple quality reporting programs and increasingly linked to value-based payment models.

Economic Impact Assessment

Direct cost evaluation quantifies changes in medication expenditures resulting from interventions including reduction in unnecessary medications, conversion to lower-cost alternatives, or prevention of adverse drug events requiring additional treatment. Indirect cost impact measures broader economic effects including reduced emergency visits, hospitalizations, or unplanned care attributable to improved medication management beyond direct medication cost considerations. Return on investment calculation compares program implementation costs (personnel time, technology, facilities) against total economic benefit demonstrating financial sustainability beyond clinical outcomes, typically finding $3-5 return for every $1 invested in comprehensive medication management services.

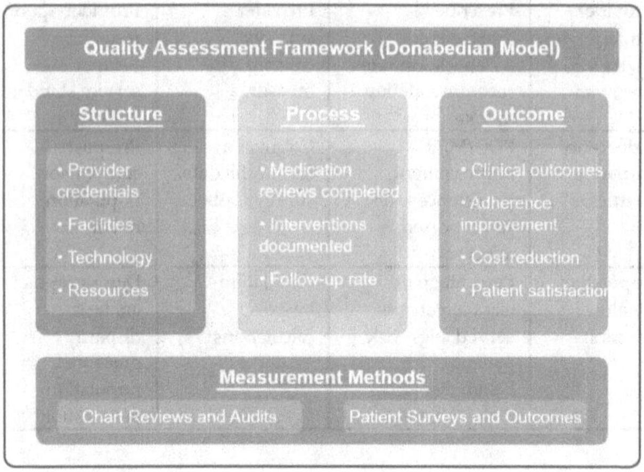

Figure 7.4: MTM Quality Metrics

Patient Experience Measurement

Satisfaction assessment employs validated instruments measuring patient perceptions of medication management services including perceived value, communication quality, problem resolution effectiveness, and likelihood to recommend services to others. Quality of life impact evaluates changes in patient-reported functional status, symptom burden, activity participation, and overall well-being following medication optimization beyond specific clinical parameters. Medication burden perception measures patient-experienced treatment complexity, regimen manageability, and confidence in medication self-management before and after intervention, recognizing that subjective burden often differs from objective regimen complexity.

Continuous Quality Improvement

Benchmark comparison evaluates performance against similar organizations, published standards, or historical baselines identifying relative strengths and improvement opportunities beyond isolated metric review. Root cause analysis examines underlying factors contributing to quality shortfalls, identifying systemic issues rather than individual performance gaps requiring process redesign rather than targeted interventions. Performance feedback loops provide regular metric review with frontline practitioners, identifying barriers to improvement, successful strategies, and necessary resource adjustments to continuously enhance service quality beyond initial implementation

Summary

• Comprehensive medication review involves systematically evaluating all medications a patient is taking to identify actual and potential drug therapy problems.

• Common drug therapy problems include unnecessary therapy, suboptimal dosing, adverse reactions, interactions, nonadherence, and untreated indications.

• Intervention strategies range from dose adjustments and medication changes to patient education, simplified regimens, and collaborative care planning.

• Follow-up evaluation is essential to assess the effectiveness of interventions, monitor for new problems, and make additional adjustments to the medication regimen.

• Quality metrics for MTM services include process measures (documentation, follow-up completion) and outcome measures (clinical endpoints, patient satisfaction, cost savings).

• Prioritization of drug therapy problems based on clinical significance, urgency, and potential for harm ensures efficient use of clinical resources.

• Interprofessional collaboration in MTM enhances patient outcomes through coordinated care approaches and comprehensive treatment planning.

Multiple Choice Questions

1. Which of the following is MOST essential to include in a comprehensive medication review?
   A) Insurance information for all medications
   B) Verification of adherence patterns and medication-taking behaviors
   C) Cost comparison between brand and generic medications
   D) Complete medication administration records from all hospitalizations
2. When prioritizing drug therapy problems for intervention, which of the following should receive the HIGHEST priority?
   A) A medication without a clear indication
   B) A medication that could be switched to a lower-cost alternative

C) A potentially serious drug interaction that poses immediate risk
D) A medication with suboptimal dosing frequency

3. Which of the following best describes a drug therapy problem classified as "needs additional therapy"?
A) Patient taking simvastatin 40 mg daily with an LDL of 150 mg/dL
B) Patient with hypertension not receiving any antihypertensive medication
C) Patient taking duplicate calcium channel blockers
D) Patient experiencing cough from lisinopril therapy

4. A key difference between MTM documentation and traditional pharmacy dispensing documentation is:
A) MTM documentation includes the prescription number
B) MTM documentation focuses on clinical assessment and interventions
C) MTM documentation is only required for billing purposes
D) MTM documentation is completed exclusively by technicians

5. Which of the following would be the MOST appropriate follow-up interval for a patient whose antihypertensive medication was changed during an MTM session?
A) One year
B) Six months
C) Two to four weeks
D) Next day

6. Which of the following quality metrics would BEST measure the clinical impact of MTM services?
A) Number of MTM sessions conducted per month
B) Average time spent per MTM encounter
C) Percentage of patients achieving therapeutic goals after MTM interventions
D) Revenue generated from MTM services

7. A pharmacist identifies that a patient is taking ibuprofen 800 mg three times daily along with warfarin. This drug therapy problem is BEST classified as:
A) Unnecessary drug therapy
B) Dosage too high
C) Adverse drug reaction
D) Drug interaction

8. Which of the following is the MOST appropriate approach when a drug therapy problem requires physician intervention?

   A) Tell the patient to discuss the issue with their physician

   B) Make a specific recommendation with supporting evidence to the physician

   C) Change the therapy and inform the physician afterward

   D) Suggest the patient discontinue the medication immediately

9. The BEST indicator of successful resolution of drug therapy problems identified during MTM is:

   A) Patient satisfaction with the service

   B) Number of recommendations accepted by prescribers

   C) Achievement of clinical goals and improved outcomes

   D) Reduced medication costs for the patient

10. Which of the following statements about MTM billing is MOST accurate?

    A) MTM services can only be billed under Medicare Part D

    B) Documentation requirements are the same for all payers

    C) Time spent is the only factor determining reimbursement

    D) Different billing codes exist based on the complexity and time of services

Self-Assessment Questions

1. Describe the key components of a comprehensive medication review (CMR) and explain how each component contributes to identifying drug therapy problems.
2. Explain the difference between a targeted medication review and a comprehensive medication review, including when each would be most appropriate.
3. Identify and describe the major categories of drug therapy problems with an example of each and potential resolution strategies.
4. Discuss three strategies for prioritizing interventions when multiple drug therapy problems are identified during an MTM session.
5. Explain how pharmacists should document MTM services to demonstrate clinical value and support billing requirements.
6. Describe three approaches to measuring the economic impact of MTM services and the advantages and limitations of each approach.
7. Explain the process for developing a personal medication record (PMR) and medication action plan (MAP) with patients, including key elements of each.
8. Discuss three common barriers to implementing MTM services in pharmacy practice and strategies to overcome them.
9. Explain how pharmacists should approach follow-up evaluation after implementing medication therapy changes, including timing and assessment parameters.
10. Describe how quality metrics can be used to evaluate and improve MTM services, providing examples of process and outcome measures.

Bibliography

1. Bluml BM. Definition of medication therapy management: development of profession-wide consensus. J Am Pharm Assoc. 2005;45(5):566-572.
2. Cipolle RJ, Strand LM, Morley PC. Pharmaceutical care practice: the patient-centered approach to medication management. 3rd ed. New York: McGraw-Hill Medical; 2012.
3. Isetts BJ, Schondelmeyer SW, Artz MB, Lenarz LA, Heaton AH, Wadd WB, et al. Clinical and economic outcomes of medication therapy management services: the Minnesota experience. J Am Pharm Assoc. 2008;48(2):203-211.
4. Viswanathan M, Kahwati LC, Golin CE, Blalock SJ, Coker-Schwimmer E, Posey R, et al. Medication therapy management interventions in outpatient settings: a systematic review and meta-analysis. JAMA Intern Med. 2015;175(1):76-87.
5. American Pharmacists Association, National Association of Chain Drug Stores Foundation. Medication therapy management in pharmacy practice: core elements of an MTM service model (version 2.0). J Am Pharm Assoc. 2008;48(3):341-353.
6. Chisholm-Burns MA, Kim Lee J, Spivey CA, Slack M, Herrier RN, Hall-Lipsy E, et al. US pharmacists' effect as team members on patient care: systematic review and meta-analyses. Med Care. 2010;48(10):923-933.
7. Ramalho de Oliveira D, Brummel AR, Miller DB. Medication therapy management: 10 years of experience in a large integrated health care system. J Manag Care Pharm. 2010;16(3):185-195.
8. Lounsbery JL, Green CG, Bennett MS, Pedersen CA. Evaluation of pharmacists' barriers to the implementation of medication therapy management services. J Am Pharm Assoc. 2009;49(1):51-58.
9. Pellegrino AN, Martin MT, Tilton JJ, Touchette DR. Medication therapy management services: definitions and outcomes. Drugs. 2009;69(4):393-406.
10. Smith M, Bates DW, Bodenheimer T, Cleary PD. Why pharmacists belong in the medical home. Health Aff (Millwood). 2010;29(5):906-913.

CHAPTER 8

PATIENT EDUCATION AND COUNSELLING

Author

Dr. Farheen Malik, Assistant Professor, Department of Pharmacy Practice, Sir C.R. Reddy College of Pharmaceutical Sciences, Eluru, Andhra Pradesh, India

Abstract

Patient education and counseling skills fundamentally transform medication knowledge into improved health behaviors through effective communication strategies addressing diverse patient needs. Counseling techniques employ patient-centered approaches including show-and-tell demonstrations, teach-back verification, and prioritized information delivery focused on essential action-oriented content rather than exhaustive details. Health literacy assessment guides communication complexity through recognition of literacy barriers, numeracy challenges, and comprehension limitations requiring plain language, visual aids, and simplified instructions appropriate for diverse populations. Medication adherence enhancement addresses intentional and unintentional non-adherence through multifaceted interventions including regimen simplification, reminder systems, side effect management, and affordability solutions tailored to specific barriers. Educational materials development incorporates design principles including appropriate reading level, visual reinforcement, cultural relevance, and practical organization enhancing comprehension and retention. Motivational interviewing techniques facilitate behavior change through collaborative exploration of ambivalence, resistance reduction, and intrinsic motivation enhancement rather than confrontational approaches or simple information provision. These integrated skills enable pharmacists to effectively communicate medication information while addressing psychological, social, and practical barriers to optimal medication use.

Keywords: *Patient-Centered Communication, Adherence Support, Health Behavior Change, Therapeutic Alliance, Medication Literacy*

Learning Objectives

After completion of the chapter, the learners should be able to:

- Apply patient-centered counseling techniques including show-and-tell demonstration, teach-back method, and chunking information to enhance comprehension and retention.
- Assess patient health literacy levels and adapt communication approaches accordingly using plain language, visual aids, and appropriate complexity.
- Implement evidence-based strategies to improve medication adherence addressing intentional and unintentional non-adherence through targeted interventions.
- Develop patient education materials incorporating appropriate reading level, visual reinforcement, and cultural relevance for diverse patient populations.
- Demonstrate motivational interviewing techniques including open-ended questioning, affirmations, reflective listening, and summaries to facilitate behavior change.
- Evaluate the effectiveness of patient education interventions through appropriate assessment techniques and outcome measures.

COUNSELING TECHNIQUES

Personalization strategies adapt counseling content and delivery to individual needs, preferences, and circumstances rather than delivering standardized information regardless of patient characteristics. Autonomy support respects patient decision-making authority through presentation of options, transparent discussion of benefits and risks, and acceptance of informed choices even when they differ from provider recommendations. Relationship development establishes trust through authentic engagement, demonstrated competence, and continuity over time, creating foundation for effective education beyond transactional information delivery.

Structured Counseling Frameworks

Indian Health Service model implements a systematic approach including opening the session (establishing purpose and rapport), obtaining information (assessing current knowledge and concerns), providing information (addressing specific medication details), verifying understanding (confirming comprehension), and closing the session (summarizing key points and establishing follow-up). USP medication counseling framework addresses essential elements including medication name and indication, dose and administration, special instructions, side effects, storage requirements, and refill information through organized delivery ensuring comprehensive coverage. AHRQ Ask Me 3 approach focuses patient engagement around three fundamental questions: What is my main problem? What do I need to do? Why is it important for me to do this?

Table 8.1: Patient Counseling Techniques and Applications

Counseling Technique	Description	Application
Show and Tell Method	Physical demonstration with narration followed by patient practice	Device training, administration techniques, self-monitoring
Teach-Back Method	Having patients explain information in their own words	Critical safety information, complex regimens, high-risk medications
Indian Health Service Model	Systematic 3-Prime Questions approach (What did your doctor tell you? How/when will you use? What results do you expect?)	New prescriptions, medication changes, comprehensive education
Chunking and Checking	Presenting information in digestible segments with comprehension verification	Complex information, multiple medications, limited attention span
Visual Reinforcement	Using pictures, diagrams, or models alongside verbal information	Abstract concepts, mechanism explanations, spatial relationships
Motivational Interviewing	Collaborative conversation eliciting behavior change motivation	Adherence challenges, lifestyle modifications, preventive behaviors
Personalized Relevance	Connecting information to patient's specific situation and concerns	Preventive medications, lifestyle changes, symptom management
Shared Decision Making	Collaborative decision process incorporating patient values and preferences	Preference-sensitive decisions, multiple reasonable options, value-based choices

Communication Technique Enhancement

Active listening demonstrates engaged attention through verbal and non-verbal behaviors including eye contact, attentive posture, reflective responses, and minimal interruptions, establishing foundation for effective information exchange. Plain language communication employs everyday vocabulary, short sentences, direct phrasing, and concrete examples rather than medical terminology, complex sentence structures, or abstract concepts that impede understanding. Teachback verification asks patients to explain key information in their own words through questions like "To make sure I explained clearly, could you tell me how you'll take this medication?" identifying and addressing comprehension gaps immediately rather than assuming understanding.

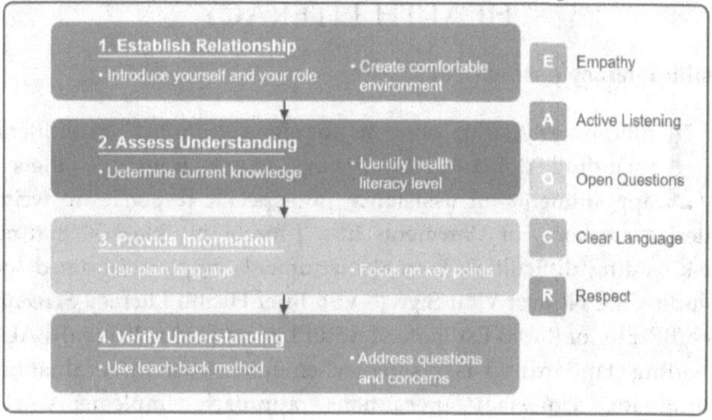

Figure 8.1: Effective Patient Counseling Process

Difficult Conversation Management

Medication safety concern discussions address potentially sensitive topics including high-risk medications, serious adverse effects, or error prevention strategies without creating unnecessary anxiety or undermining confidence in therapy through balanced, contextual presentation. Adherence barrier exploration investigates challenges through non-judgmental questioning about specific difficulties rather than general compliance inquiries, distinguishing between different non-adherence patterns requiring tailored interventions. Denial and resistance navigation responds to information rejection through reflection of concerns, continued engagement without confrontation, and finding common ground through shared goals even when complete agreement remains unachieved.

Special Population Considerations

Pediatric counseling adapts approaches for different developmental stages while appropriately engaging both children and caregivers, including age-appropriate explanations for children while ensuring comprehensive information for those responsible for administration. Geriatric communication accommodates potential sensory limitations (hearing, vision), cognitive changes, and longer processing time requirements through appropriate adjustments to pace, volume, visual aids, and repetition without infantilizing older adults. Language barrier management employs professional interpreters (preferably trained medical interpreters rather than family members) for limited English proficiency, utilizing best practices including first-person speech, manageable information segments, and direct patient engagement.

HEALTH LITERACY

Health Literacy Assessment

Informal evaluation observes for signs of limited health literacy including difficulty completing forms, bringing others to appointments for assistance, non-specific responses to written material questions, or statements like "I forgot my glasses" that may mask reading difficulties. Formal instruments employ validated tools including the Newest Vital Sign (NVS), Brief Health Literacy Screening Tool (BRIEF), or Rapid Estimate of Adult Literacy in Medicine (REALM) providing standardized assessment when more structured evaluation is appropriate. Universal precautions approach implements clear communication strategies for all patients regardless of presumed literacy level, recognizing that health literacy assessment tools identify only some individuals with challenges while literacy fluctuates under stress regardless of baseline capability.

Table 8.2: Health Literacy Assessment and Adaptation Strategies

Literacy Component	Assessment	Patient Indicators	Adaptation
Reading Literacy	Validated tools (REALM, NVS), educational level proxy, comprehension checks	Difficulty with forms, avoidance of reading tasks, "forgot glasses" excuse	Plain language (5th-6th grade level), limited text, bullet points, adequate font size
Numeracy Skills	Dosing calculations, risk interpretation, quantitative tasks	Confusion with numbers, inability to describe quantitative concepts	Visual aids (pill charts, pictographs), simplified dosing, concrete examples
Medical Vocabulary	Term recognition, concept explanation, teach-back assessment	Misuse of terms, vague descriptions, nodding without understanding	Everyday language, consistent terminology, plain language substitutions

Literacy Component	Assessment	Patient Indicators	Adaptation
Document Navigation	Form completion observation, information location tasks	Incomplete forms, random marking, disorganized approach	Simplified formats, step-by-step instructions, visual cues, form assistance
Technological Literacy	Device use observation, electronic resource navigation, comfort assessment	Avoidance of technology, inability to navigate interfaces, anxiety with devices	Simplified interfaces, hands-on training, alternative non-digital options
Oral Communication	Comprehension of verbal instructions, question formulation ability	Limited questioning, inappropriate responses, passivity	Slow pace, teach-back verification, limited content per session
Cultural Health Literacy	Understanding of health system, cultural concepts of illness, traditional practices	Misalignment with medical model, unexplained non-adherence, cultural references	Culturally adapted explanations, cultural broker involvement, integrated approaches
Navigational Literacy	Ability to access resources, follow referrals, navigate health system	Missed appointments, unused resources, system frustration	Step-by-step instructions, resource navigation assistance, system orientation

Communication Adaptation Strategies

Readability enhancement employs techniques including short sentences, active voice, common words, limited statistics, and concrete examples rather than abstract concepts, generally aiming for 5th-6th grade reading level for most patient materials. Numerical concept simplification presents statistical information through consistent denominators, absolute risk formats, natural frequencies, and visual representations rather than percentages, relative risks, or complex probability expressions. Medical terminology management explains necessary technical terms using plain language definitions, provides context for unavoidable medical vocabulary, and consistently uses the same term rather than introducing synonyms that create confusion.

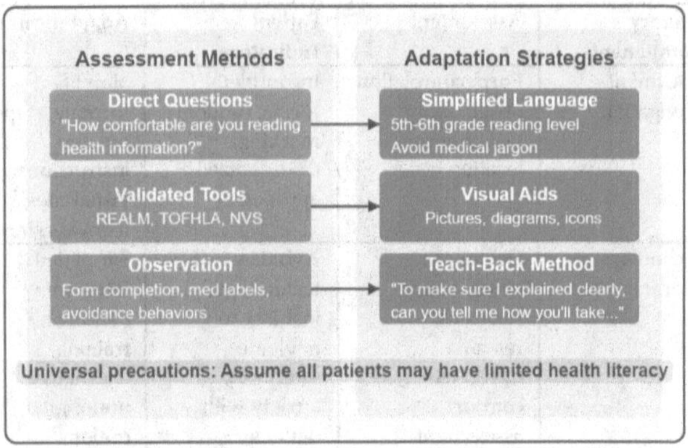

Figure 8.2: Health Literacy Assessment and Adaptation

Teach-Back Implementation

Question formulation phrases verification as assessment of teaching effectiveness rather than patient testing through statements like "I want to be sure I explained this clearly" rather than "Do you understand?" which often elicits automatic affirmative responses regardless of comprehension. Comprehension assessment focuses on application understanding rather than fact repetition through questions about how medications will be taken, what side effects warrant contact, or when follow-up should occur rather than simply repeating drug names or general purposes. Clarification techniques address identified misunderstandings through alternative explanations, demonstrations, or analogies rather than simply repeating the original information that proved ineffective.

Educational Material Enhancement

Visual aid integration incorporates pictures, diagrams, icons, or videos demonstrating key concepts including administration techniques, monitoring procedures, or expected appearance of medications enhancing understanding beyond text-based information alone. White space utilization employs adequate margins, paragraph breaks, and spacing between content sections reducing cognitive overload and enhancing readability compared to dense, text-heavy formats. Prioritization strategies emphasize most critical information through positioning (beginning of materials), visual cues (highlighting, boxes, larger font), and explicit importance statements ensuring essential content receives attention even when complete material review exceeds capacity.

Organizational Health Literacy Improvement

Systems approach implements structural improvements beyond individual provider efforts, including simplified forms, consistent signage, clear wayfinding, and organizational plain language policies supporting comprehensive health literacy-friendly environments. Technology utilization employs multimedia platforms including videos, interactive tutorials, and mobile applications providing alternative learning channels beyond traditional written materials, particularly valuable for those with limited reading skills. Staff training develops consistent health literacy competencies across team members including reception staff, pharmacy technicians, and all patient-facing personnel beyond clinical providers alone.

MEDICATION ADHERENCE

Adherence Assessment Methods

Self-report evaluation employs structured questions including validated instruments (Morisky Medication Adherence Scale, Brief Medication Questionnaire) or targeted inquiry about specific missed doses, administration challenges, or intentional adjustments revealing different non-adherence patterns. Refill pattern analysis examines prescription claims data calculating measures including proportion of days covered, medication possession ratio, or gaps in therapy revealing potential adherence issues before clinical deterioration. Direct measurement methods include therapeutic drug monitoring (blood levels), electronic monitoring devices (recording package openings), or direct observation of administration in specific situations requiring definitive adherence verification.

Adherence Barrier Identification

Practical obstacle assessment identifies logistics-based challenges including complex regimens, physical limitations, transportation difficulties, or financial constraints contributing to unintentional non-adherence despite willingness to take medications as prescribed. Knowledge deficit evaluation examines understanding gaps including confusion about directions, uncertainty about importance, or misunderstanding of expected benefits potentially addressed through educational interventions. Belief and perception exploration investigates concerns about necessity (questioning need for medication), concerns about harm (side effect worries, long-term consequence fears), or treatment-related identity issues (medication use conflicting with self-perception) requiring different approaches than practical barriers.

Table 8.3: Medication Adherence Barriers and Interventions

Adherence Barrier Category	Specific Barriers	Assessment	Targeted Interventions
Practical Barriers	Complex regimens, physical limitations, scheduling challenges, forgetfulness	Brown bag review, daily routine analysis, physical ability assessment	Simplification, pill organizers, timing with daily activities, reminder systems
Knowledge Barriers	Misunderstanding directions, purpose confusion, unclear expectations	Teach-back assessment, demonstration observation, knowledge questionnaires	Clear instructions, visual aids, indication labeling, regular reinforcement
Attitudinal Barriers	Medication concerns, perceived lack of necessity, fear of dependence	Beliefs about Medicines Questionnaire, motivation assessment, concern exploration	Address specific concerns, emphasize personal benefits, align with values
Financial Barriers	High cost, insurance issues, copayment burden, coverage gaps	Cost assessment, insurance review, affordability evaluation	Generic substitution, patient assistance programs, therapeutic alternatives
Social/Cultural Barriers	Stigma, cultural beliefs, family influence, language barriers	Cultural assessment, family dynamics evaluation, language needs	Cultural adaptation, family involvement, language services, cultural mediators
Health System Barriers	Poor provider communication, multiple prescribers, access limitations	Provider inventory, access assessment, communication evaluation	Care coordination, provider communication, telehealth options, mail delivery
Condition-Related Barriers	Symptom absence, cognitive impairment, depression, changing severity	Symptom assessment, cognitive screening	Symptom-benefit connection, cognitive aids, depression

Adherence Barrier Category	Specific Barriers	Assessment	Targeted Interventions
Therapy-Related Barriers	Side effects, delayed benefits, administration challenges	Side effect assessment, benefit perception, administration challenges	Side effect management, immediate benefit emphasis, administration assistance

Tailored Intervention Selection

Forgetfulness countermeasures implement reminder systems including technology-based alerts, visual cues (placement near routine activities), linking with daily habits, or specialized packaging with day/time indicators specifically addressing unintentional adherence challenges. Regimen simplification strategies reduce complexity through consolidated administration times, extended-release formulations when appropriate, combination products, or synchronized refill schedules reducing cognitive and practical burden. Motivational approaches address intentional non-adherence through exploration of personal goals, perceived benefits, and alignment of medication therapy with individual priorities rather than simply providing factual information.

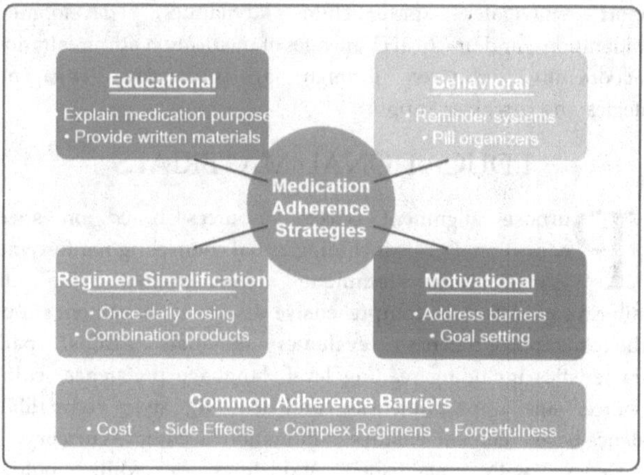

Figure 8.3: Strategies to Improve Medication Adherence

Technology-Based Support

Mobile application utilization leverages smartphone-based tools providing customizable reminders, medication logs, educational information, and sometimes connectivity with healthcare providers or family members supporting adherence. Smart packaging employs technology-embedded containers recording openings, providing reminders, or transmitting adherence data to monitoring systems, though balancing potential benefits against cost and complexity. Automated refill management implements systems for prescription synchronization, early refill alerts, or automatic renewal processing addressing logistical barriers to medication continuity.

Special Adherence Considerations

Chronic asymptomatic condition management addresses particular challenges with preventive medications for conditions like hypertension or hyperlipidemia where absence of perceptible benefit combined with potential side effects creates unfavorable risk-benefit perception requiring specific adherence support. Psychiatric medication approaches address unique challenges including condition-related adherence barriers (depression reducing motivation, paranoia creating medication suspicion), stigma concerns, and substantial side effect profiles requiring specialized adherence strategies. Pediatric adherence support navigates parent-child dynamics, developmental considerations, and practical challenges of medication administration to non-cooperative children through age-appropriate engagement strategies and caregiver support.

EDUCATIONAL MATERIALS

Purpose alignment selects resources based on specific educational goals including initial counseling reinforcement, administration technique demonstration, side effect monitoring guidance, or comprehensive disease management support. Audience appropriateness evaluates materials against patient characteristics including reading level, language preference, cultural relevance, age appropriateness, and learning style compatibility. Evidence-based content ensures information accuracy, currency, and consistency with established guidelines, avoiding outdated recommendations or unsubstantiated claims regardless of professional appearance or engaging presentation.

Written Material Development

Content organization implements information hierarchy with most critical points first, logical progression between related concepts, and clear section demarcation through headings, numbering, or visual separation enhancing navigation and comprehension. Design enhancement employs adequate white space, sufficient font size (minimum 12-point), high contrast colors, and limited use of all capitals or italics supporting readability particularly for those with visual limitations. Action-oriented approach emphasizes specific behaviors rather than general concepts through concrete instructions, explicit next steps, and clear expectations regarding medication use, monitoring, and follow-up.

Visual Aid Effectiveness

Pictogram utilization employs standardized visual representations of administration timing, techniques, or precautions enhancing understanding across literacy and language barriers when designed according to best practices. Demonstration tool selection provides models, placebo devices, or actual medication packaging allowing hands-on practice with administration techniques for inhalers, injections, or other complex delivery systems. Video resource development creates visual demonstrations of medication preparation, administration, storage, or monitoring procedures providing consistent, repeatable instruction available outside clinical settings.

Cultural Adaptation Considerations

Language translation implements professional conversion of materials beyond literal word replacement, considering cultural context, health belief systems, and communication norms appropriate to target populations. Cultural appropriateness ensures content respects diverse values, family structures, decision-making approaches, and health beliefs while avoiding assumptions based on majority cultural perspectives. Visual representation inclusion depicts diverse individuals reflecting various racial, ethnic, age, and gender characteristics creating identification and relevance across different patient populations.

Digital Resource Integration

Mobile health resource curation selects evidence-based, user-friendly applications supporting specific educational needs including medication identification, drug information access, administration reminders, or symptom tracking with appropriate privacy protections. Interactive tool implementation employs technologies allowing personalization, self-assessment, feedback on understanding, and tailored content delivery based on individual needs and preferences. Accessibility enhancement ensures digital resources comply with standards supporting users with disabilities including screen reader compatibility, alternative text for images, appropriate color contrast, and keyboard navigation options beyond mouse-dependent interfaces.

Table 8.4: Effective Educational Materials Development

Material Component	Design Principles	Evaluation Criteria	Examples
Readability	5th-6th grade level, short sentences, active voice, common words	SMOG or Flesch-Kincaid scoring, patient feedback, comprehension testing	"Take one pill in the morning" vs. "The medication should be administered once daily in the A.M."
Visual Design	Adequate white space, consistent layout, visual hierarchy, sufficient contrast	Usability testing, reader tracking, comprehension assessment	Organized sections, bulleted lists, appropriate font size (12pt minimum)
Information Organization	Need-to-know first, logical flow, chunked information, prioritized content	Information recall, task completion, navigation efficiency	Most important safety information first, sequenced by use timeline
Action Orientation	Clear instructions, specific steps, concrete behaviors	Behavior performance, action completion, self-efficacy measurement	"Check your feet daily" vs. "Diabetic foot care is important"
Visual Reinforcement	Purposeful images, realistic pictures, informative graphics	Image comprehension, information retention, concept understanding	Pill identification images, administration technique sequences, body location diagrams
Accessibility	Multiple formats, screen reader compatibility, adaptive options	Usability across disabilities, format preference assessment	Large print options, audio versions, digital adaptive formats
Consistency with Verbal Counseling	Reinforces key points, uses same terminology, supports counseling	Alignment assessment, terminology consistency, reinforcement effect	Matching verbal counseling key points, consistent terminology for doses and timing

MOTIVATIONAL INTERVIEWING

Core Principles Application

Partnership establishment creates collaborative relationship viewing the patient as the expert on their own life while the provider contributes specialized knowledge, avoiding authoritarian approaches undermining autonomous motivation. Acceptance demonstrates respect for patient autonomy, acknowledges the validity of their perspective, and recognizes their capacity for growth and self-direction regardless of current choices. Compassion maintains genuine interest in patient welfare and priorities, distinguishing motivational interviewing from manipulation by ensuring focus remains on outcomes benefiting the patient rather than achieving provider-determined compliance. Evocation draws forth patient's own motivations, values, and solutions rather than imposing external reasons or strategies, recognizing that internally generated motivation proves more sustainable than externally imposed directives.

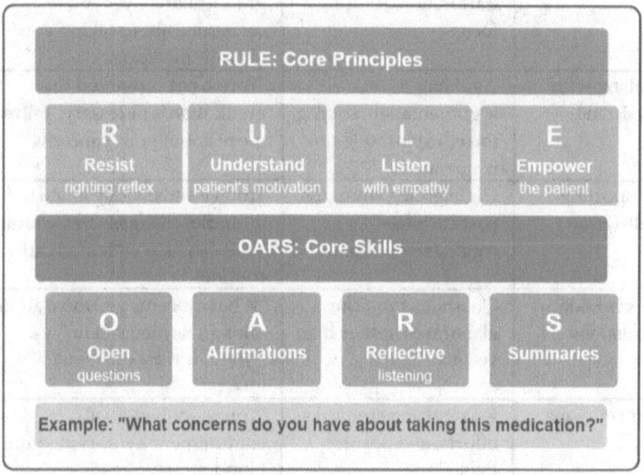

Figure 8.4: Motivational Interviewing

Foundational Skills Implementation

Open-ended questioning employs inquiries requiring more than yes/no or simple factual responses, inviting deeper exploration through questions beginning with how, what, or why rather than closed inquiries that limit response options. Affirmation recognizes and acknowledges strengths, efforts, values, and positive qualities building self-efficacy and reinforcing capabilities rather than focusing exclusively on problems or deficiencies. Reflective listening demonstrates understanding through statements rather than questions, ranging from simple repetition to complex reflection capturing underlying meanings and emotions beyond explicit content. Summarization periodically consolidates discussion, highlighting key points, patterns, and connections while providing opportunity for correction or elaboration ensuring shared understanding before proceeding.

Table 8.5: Motivational Interviewing Techniques in Medication Management

MI Component	Techniques	Application Examples
Expressing Empathy	Reflective listening, validation, nonjudgmental approach	"It sounds like taking multiple medications feels overwhelming to you."
Developing Discrepancy	Exploring goals vs. behaviors, values clarification, future focus	"You've mentioned wanting to be active with your grandchildren, yet you're concerned about taking your arthritis medication."
Rolling with Resistance	Avoiding argumentation, shifting focus, exploration not confrontation	"You're not convinced this medication is necessary. Tell me more about your concerns."
Supporting Self-Efficacy	Highlighting strengths, past successes, confidence building	"You've successfully managed your diet changes - those same skills can help with medication routines."
Open-Ended Questions	Questions requiring elaboration rather than yes/no	"What concerns you most about taking this medication?" vs. "Are you worried about side effects?"
Affirmations	Recognizing strengths, efforts, and positive behaviors	"You're showing real commitment by tracking your blood pressure readings."
Reflective Listening	Restating content, reflecting feelings, deepening meaning	"You're worried that starting insulin means your diabetes is getting worse."
Summarizing	Collecting key points, linking discussions, reinforcing change talk	"You've mentioned concerns about cost and side effects, but also recognize the importance of preventing another stroke."

Change Talk Identification and Reinforcement

Desire statements express wanting, wishing, or preferring change including phrases like "I want to," "I wish I could," or "I hope to" indicating internal motivation beyond mere recognition of external pressure. Ability language acknowledges capability for change through statements like "I could," "I can," or "I might be able to" reflecting self-efficacy rather than merely recognizing importance. Reason expressions articulate specific benefits or advantages anticipated from change including health improvements, enhanced functioning, or alignment with personal values. Need articulation communicates urgency or necessity through statements like "I have to," "I need to," or "I must" indicating internal imperative rather than external obligation.

Resistance Management

Rolling with resistance responds to opposition non-defensively, avoiding argumentation, acknowledging concerns, and exploring rather than confronting ambivalence or hesitation. Developing discrepancy gently highlights contradictions between current behavior and important personal values or goals without accusation, allowing patient to recognize inconsistencies independently. Permission requesting precedes information provision or advice offering through questions like "Would it be helpful if I shared some information about..." respecting autonomy and reducing defensive reactions to unsolicited recommendations. Autonomy support explicitly acknowledges patient decision-making authority through statements emphasizing their choice, right to reject recommendations, and ultimate control over their health decisions.

Motivational Interviewing in Brief Encounters

Agenda setting collaboratively determines conversation focus within time constraints, prioritizing issues most important to both patient and provider rather than attempting comprehensive coverage in limited encounters. Brief action planning facilitates concrete next steps through collaborative identification of specific, achievable actions patients feel confident implementing, enhancing probability of successful behavior change between visits. Strategic focusing concentrates on aspects of medication use where patient demonstrates readiness for change rather than addressing all potential issues simultaneously, maximizing impact of limited interaction time. Efficiency enhancement employs targeted implementation of motivational interviewing elements rather than full protocol application, strategically incorporating key components within time-limited clinical interactions.

Summary

- Effective counseling techniques include assessing baseline knowledge, using plain language, demonstrating proper medication use, and verifying understanding through teach-back.
- Health literacy considerations require tailoring information to the patient's comprehension level, avoiding medical jargon, and using visual aids when appropriate.
- Strategies to improve medication adherence include simplifying regimens, addressing barriers, using adherence aids, and providing clear instructions on medication purpose and benefits.
- Educational materials should be evidence-based, culturally appropriate, accessible at appropriate reading levels, and available in multiple formats to meet diverse patient needs.
- Motivational interviewing techniques help patients explore and resolve ambivalence about medication use through reflective listening, open questioning, and supporting self-efficacy.
- Tailoring counseling to patient-specific factors such as age, cognitive status, cultural background, and learning preferences improves information retention and adherence.
- Addressing psychosocial and economic barriers to medication adherence is as important as providing clinical information during patient education sessions.

Multiple Choice Questions

1. Which counseling technique is MOST effective for assessing patient understanding of medication instructions?
   A) Asking "Do you have any questions?"
   B) Providing detailed written materials
   C) Using the teach-back method
   D) Having patients sign a counseling form
2. A pharmacist is counseling a patient with low health literacy about a new medication. Which approach is MOST appropriate?
   A) Providing comprehensive technical information about the drug
   B) Using simple language and focusing on key points with visual aids

C) Speaking very slowly and loudly to ensure understanding
D) Providing only written information for the patient to review at home

3. Which of the following is the BEST indicator that a patient education handout is appropriate for most patients?
A) It contains all possible information about the medication
B) It is written at a 5th to 6th grade reading level with clear formatting
C) It includes extensive medical terminology with definitions
D) It is comprehensive enough to replace verbal counseling

4. When using motivational interviewing to address medication nonadherence, which approach is MOST effective?
A) Directly telling the patient why they need to take their medication
B) Focusing on the negative consequences of nonadherence
C) Exploring the patient's own motivations for medication adherence
D) Providing statistics about risks of untreated conditions

5. A patient reports, "I don't think I need to take my blood pressure medication when my pressure is normal." Which response best demonstrates effective counseling?
A) "You must take your medication as prescribed or you could have a stroke."
B) "I understand you feel that way, but could you tell me more about your concerns?"
C) "Your doctor wouldn't have prescribed it if you didn't need it."
D) "Let me explain how blood pressure medications work in the body."

6. Which of the following is the MOST reliable method for assessing medication adherence?
A) Asking the patient if they take their medication regularly
B) Reviewing prescription refill records
C) Having the patient complete an adherence questionnaire
D) No single method is completely reliable; multiple approaches should be used

7. When counseling a patient about a medication with significant adverse effects, the MOST appropriate approach is to:
   A) Minimize discussion of side effects to avoid alarming the patient
   B) Focus only on common side effects that occur in at least 10% of patients
   C) Emphasize serious side effects that require immediate attention and provide balanced information
   D) Tell the patient to read the package insert for complete information
8. Which of the following statements about cultural competency in patient education is MOST accurate?
   A) Cultural beliefs rarely impact medication-taking behaviors
   B) Pharmacists should adapt their approach based on cultural considerations specific to each patient
   C) Standard counseling approaches are equally effective across all cultural groups
   D) Cultural factors only affect traditional or herbal medicine use
9. The Indian Health Service medication counseling model includes which of the following key components?
   A) Focus primarily on side effects
   B) Three prime questions about indication, administration, and expectations
   C) Emphasis on cost-saving strategies
   D) Extended counseling sessions of at least 30 minutes
10. When providing education about a new insulin regimen, which of the following should receive the HIGHEST priority?
   A) The pharmacology of different insulin types
   B) Insurance coverage and prior authorization requirements
   C) Proper administration technique and hypoglycemia recognition/management
   D) The history of insulin development

Self-Assessment Questions

1. Describe the teach-back method, including how to implement it effectively and why it's superior to simply asking "Do you understand?"
2. Explain three strategies pharmacists can use to assess a patient's health literacy level without causing embarrassment or discomfort.
3. Describe the relationship between health literacy and medication adherence, and discuss approaches to address both simultaneously.
4. Explain the core principles of motivational interviewing and how they can be applied to improve medication adherence.
5. Discuss three barriers to effective patient education and strategies to overcome each barrier.
6. Explain how written educational materials should be designed to accommodate patients with different health literacy levels.
7. Compare and contrast patient education approaches for acute medications versus chronic medications, highlighting key differences in counseling priorities.
8. Describe three methods to assess medication adherence, including the advantages and limitations of each method.
9. Explain how cultural factors might influence medication-taking behaviors and how pharmacists should adapt their counseling approach accordingly.
10. Discuss strategies for effectively educating patients about high-risk medications, including what information should be prioritized.

Bibliography

1. Berger BA. Communication skills for pharmacists: building relationships, improving patient care. 3rd ed. Washington DC: American Pharmacists Association; 2009.
2. Wolf MS, Davis TC, Shrank W, Rapp DN, Bass PF, Connor UM, et al. To err is human: patient misinterpretations of prescription drug label instructions. Patient Educ Couns. 2007;67(3):293-300.
3. Schillinger D, Piette J, Grumbach K, Wang F, Wilson C, Daher C, et al. Closing the loop: physician communication with diabetic patients who have low health literacy. Arch Intern Med. 2003;163(1):83-90.
4. Sabaté E. Adherence to long-term therapies: evidence for action. Geneva: World Health Organization; 2003.
5. Doak CC, Doak LG, Root JH. Teaching patients with low literacy skills. 2nd ed. Philadelphia: J.B. Lippincott; 1996.
6. Miller WR, Rollnick S. Motivational interviewing: helping people change. 3rd ed. New York: Guilford Press; 2013.
7. Osterberg L, Blaschke T. Adherence to medication. N Engl J Med. 2005;353(5):487-497.
8. Weiss BD. Health literacy and patient safety: help patients understand. Manual for clinicians. 2nd ed. Chicago: American Medical Association Foundation; 2007.
9. Touchette DR, Shapiro NL. Medication compliance, adherence, and persistence: current status of behavioral and educational interventions to improve outcomes. J Manag Care Pharm. 2008;14(6 Suppl S-d):S2-S10.
10. Kripalani S, Yao X, Haynes RB. Interventions to enhance medication adherence in chronic medical conditions: a systematic review. Arch Intern Med. 2007;167(6):540-550

CHAPTER 9

DRUG THERAPY OPTIMIZATION

Author

Dr. Nayyar Parvez, Professor & HOD, Department of Pharmaceutics, School of Pharmacy, Sharda University, Greater Noida, Uttar Pradesh, India

Abstract

Drug therapy optimization represents the systematic process of maximizing therapeutic benefits while minimizing risks through personalized medication selection and management strategies. Dosing considerations incorporate pharmacokinetic principles, physiological variations, and disease-specific factors requiring individualized adjustment based on renal function, hepatic status, age, weight, and genetic factors affecting drug disposition. Drug interaction management addresses pharmacokinetic and pharmacodynamic mechanisms requiring systematic screening, clinical significance assessment, and mitigation strategies including dose adjustment, spacing administration, or alternative therapy selection. Adverse effect prevention and management employs risk factor identification, proactive monitoring, and intervention protocols balancing therapeutic benefits against potential harms through structured assessment tools and documentation systems. Special population adaptation addresses unique considerations for pediatric, geriatric, pregnant, and physiologically compromised patients requiring specific dosing algorithms, monitoring parameters, and safety precautions. Cost consideration strategies integrate economic factors with clinical decision-making through formulary management, therapeutic interchange, assistance program navigation, and value assessment methodologies. This comprehensive approach ensures patients receive medications optimally matched to their specific needs, characteristics, and circumstances.

Keywords: *Pharmacokinetic Optimization, Patient-Specific Dosing, Polypharmacy Management, Benefit-Risk Assessment, Therapeutic Individualization*

Learning Objectives

After completion of the chapter, the learners should be able to:

- Calculate and adjust medication dosages based on patient-specific factors including renal function, hepatic status, weight, age, and pharmacogenetic considerations.
- Identify clinically significant drug interactions and implement appropriate management strategies including dose adjustment, scheduling changes, or alternative therapy selection.
- Develop comprehensive plans for preventing, monitoring, and managing medication adverse effects through risk factor identification and systematic monitoring.
- Modify drug therapy approaches for special populations including pediatric, geriatric, pregnant, and physiologically compromised patients requiring specialized dosing and monitoring.
- Implement cost-effectiveness strategies including formulary management, therapeutic interchange, and assistance program utilization to optimize medication affordability.
- Integrate pharmacokinetic principles into patient-specific dosing regimens for narrow therapeutic index medications requiring individualized approaches.

DOSING CONSIDERATIONS

Weight-based dosing implements appropriate calculations based on actual, ideal, or adjusted body weight depending on medication characteristics, with lipophilic drugs (e.g., benzodiazepines, phenytoin) typically using actual weight while hydrophilic medications (e.g., aminoglycosides, many antimicrobials) may require adjusted calculations for obese patients. Age-related adjustments account for physiological changes across the lifespan, with pediatric dosing based on weight, body surface area, or age bands reflecting developmental pharmacokinetics, while geriatric dosing often requires reduction due to decreased renal function, altered body composition, and increased sensitivity to many medications. Organ function considerations adjust dosing based on elimination pathway impairment, with medications cleared renally requiring systematic modification based on creatinine clearance or eGFR, while hepatically metabolized drugs may require empiric dose reduction or monitoring based on liver function parameters.

Table 9.1: Patient-Specific Dosing Considerations

Dosing Factor	Assessment Parameters	Adjustment	Monitoring
Renal Function	Serum creatinine, eGFR (CKD-EPI, Cockcroft-Gault), urinary markers	Dose reduction, interval extension, alternative agent	Renal function trends, drug levels, efficacy/toxicity markers
Hepatic Function	Liver enzymes, Child-Pugh score, albumin, coagulation	Dose reduction, empiric adjustment, alternative agent	Liver function tests, drug levels, clinical toxicity signs
Age-Related Factors	Physiological age, organ function, frailty assessment	Start low-go slow approach, geriatric-specific guidelines	Enhanced adverse effect monitoring, functional assessments
Body Size/Composition	Actual vs. ideal body weight, BMI, body surface area, lean body mass	Weight-based calculations, capping doses, composition adjustments	Therapeutic response, concentration monitoring, effect assessment
Genetic Variations	Pharmacogenetic testing, ancestry considerations, response history	Genotype-guided dosing, alternative pathway drugs, dose adjustments	Enhanced monitoring for variant phenotypes, efficacy/toxicity assessment
Comorbid Conditions	Disease states affecting PK/PD, organ function impact, drug-disease interactions	Disease-specific adjustments, alternative agents, enhanced monitoring	Disease-specific parameters, drug response in comorbidity context
Pregnancy/Lactation	Trimester, physiological changes, placental transfer, breast milk excretion	Pregnancy-specific dosing, risk-benefit assessment, alternative agents	Maternal/fetal monitoring, postpartum adjustment, infant observation

Dosing Factor	Assessment Parameters	Adjustment	Monitoring
Pediatric Considerations	Age, weight, body surface area, developmental stage	Weight-based dosing, age-specific formulations, developmental adjustments	Growth parameters, developmental assessments, age-appropriate monitoring
Extracorporeal Therapy	Dialysis modality, CRRT settings, dialyzer characteristics, timing	Supplemental doses, timing relative to dialysis, alternative agents	Pre/post-dialysis levels, clinical response monitoring, residual function

Pharmacokinetic Principles

Loading dose calculation implements appropriate initial administrations establishing therapeutic concentrations rapidly for medications with long half-lives or delayed onset, with amount typically based on volume of distribution and target concentration independent of elimination function. Maintenance dose determination balances drug input with elimination based on clearance parameters, dosing interval, and desired steady-state concentrations, adjusting for individual patient factors affecting drug disposition. Dosing interval selection considers pharmacokinetic properties including half-life, therapeutic index, and concentration-effect relationships, with narrow therapeutic index drugs often requiring more frequent administration to minimize peak-trough fluctuations compared to medications with wider safety margins.

Specialized Dosing Approaches

Extended-interval dosing implements less frequent administration of larger doses based on concentration-dependent efficacy and post-antibiotic effect, particularly valuable for aminoglycosides (once-daily versus traditional three-times daily) reducing nephrotoxicity while maintaining effectiveness. Individualized pharmacokinetic dosing employs patient-specific parameters in formal pharmacokinetic models, using Bayesian approaches incorporating population parameters, individual drug levels, and patient characteristics to optimize therapy for narrow therapeutic index medications including vancomycin, aminoglycosides, and anticonvulsants. Continuous infusion strategies maintain consistent drug concentrations for medications where constant levels optimize effect (e.g., beta-lactam antibiotics, some anticoagulants), potentially improving efficacy while reducing toxicity compared to intermittent administration.

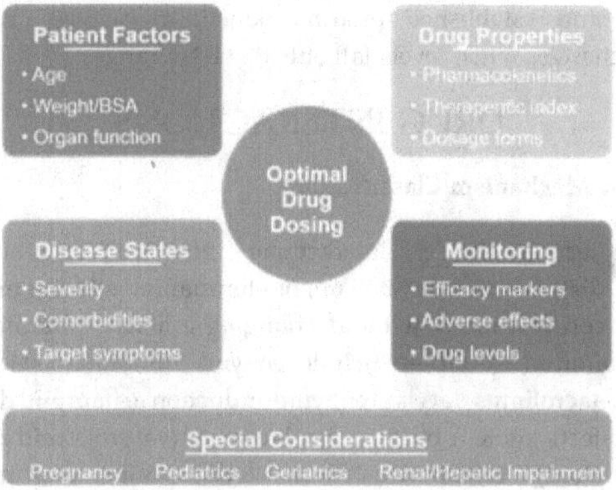

Figure 9.1: Dosing Considerations

Route of Administration Considerations

Bioavailability adjustment accounts for incomplete absorption of many oral medications compared to intravenous administration, with dose increases typically necessary when converting from parenteral to oral therapy for medications with poor bioavailability including many fluoroquinolones, antifungals, and immunosuppressants. First-pass metabolism considerations address extensive hepatic extraction reducing systemic availability of orally administered medications including morphine, propranolol, and many antipsychotics, potentially requiring higher oral doses or alternative routes when hepatic function changes. Alternative route selection evaluates options including subcutaneous, intramuscular, transdermal, sublingual, or rectal administration when conventional routes are unavailable or inappropriate, with each alternative requiring specific dose adjustments based on absorption characteristics and onset differences.

Therapeutic Drug Monitoring Implementation

Sampling strategy optimization collects specimens at appropriate times relative to dose administration based on specific questions being addressed, typically trough levels immediately before doses for most medications, but occasionally peak measurements or alternative timing for specific agents. Target range interpretation applies appropriate concentration goals based on indication, infection site, organism susceptibility, or disease severity rather than fixed ranges, particularly important for antimicrobials where targets may vary based on infection characteristics. Adjustment algorithm implementation modifies dosing regimens systematically based on measured concentrations, patient response, and established pharmacokinetic principles rather than arbitrary changes when levels fall outside target ranges.

DRUG INTERACTIONS

Interaction Mechanism Classification

Pharmacokinetic interactions affect drug absorption, distribution, metabolism, or elimination, altering medication concentrations without changing inherent pharmacological effects. Common examples include enzyme inhibition (ketoconazole increasing tacrolimus levels), enzyme induction (rifampin decreasing warfarin effect), protein binding displacement (valproic acid increasing free phenytoin), transporter effects (cyclosporine affecting statin disposition), and absorption alterations (calcium binding tetracyclines). Pharmacodynamic interactions involve drugs affecting the same physiological system with additive, synergistic, or antagonistic effects without altering concentrations. Examples include increased bleeding risk with combined anticoagulants and antiplatelets, enhanced QT prolongation with multiple QT-prolonging agents, and beta-blocker antagonism of beta-agonist bronchodilators.

Clinical Significance Assessment

Severity evaluation categorizes potential outcomes ranging from minor effects requiring monitoring to life-threatening consequences necessitating complete avoidance, with consideration of patient-specific risk factors potentially increasing vulnerability to particular interactions. Evidence quality assessment examines interaction documentation foundation including well-controlled studies, case reports, theoretical predictions, or in vitro data, recognizing that management decisions should reflect the strength of supporting evidence rather than treating all reported interactions equally. Temporal considerations evaluate interaction onset timing based on mechanism, with enzyme inhibition often occurring rapidly while induction develops over days to weeks, and offset timing following discontinuation varying similarly based on underlying mechanism.

Table 9.2: Drug Interaction Mechanisms and Management

Interaction Type	Mechanism	Clinical Significance	Management
Pharmacokinetic (Absorption)	Chelation, pH alteration, P-glycoprotein effects, gastric motility changes	Magnitude of absorption change, therapeutic index, clinical consequences	Separation timing, administration adjustments, monitoring, dose adjustments
Pharmacokinetic (Distribution)	Protein binding displacement, tissue distribution changes	Displaced drug characteristics, free fraction effects, clinical relevance	Dose adjustments, enhanced monitoring, alternative agents
Pharmacokinetic (Metabolism)	Enzyme induction/inhibition (CYP450, UGT), competing pathways	Inhibition/induction potency, affected drug's therapeutic index, timeline	Dose adjustments, alternative pathway drugs, therapeutic monitoring
Pharmacokinetic (Excretion)	Transporter inhibition, pH effects, excretion competition	Excretion dependency, alternative pathways, clinical consequences	Dose adjustments, monitoring, alternative agents, renal function monitoring
Pharmacodynamic (Additive)	Similar or complementary effects at same or related targets	Combined effect magnitude, benefit vs. risk, therapeutic intent	Dose adjustments of one/both agents, enhanced monitoring, therapeutic intent
Pharmacodynamic (Antagonistic)	Opposing effects at same or functional targets	Therapeutic failure risk, clinical impact, antagonism degree	Separation if possible, alternative agents, efficacy monitoring
Pharmacodynamic (Synergistic)	Potentiated effects beyond simple addition	Safety margin, benefit vs. risk, intended vs. unintended	Dose reduction of one/both agents

Management Strategy Selection

Therapeutic alternative substitution replaces one interacting medication with a non-interacting agent in the same therapeutic class when available, such as replacing simvastatin with pravastatin when combined with strong CYP3A4 inhibitors. Dose modification implements empiric adjustments based on expected interaction magnitude, such as preemptively reducing tacrolimus dose when initiating azole antifungals or increasing levothyroxine when starting enzyme inducers. Administration time separation addresses interactions involving physical or chemical incompatibility or altered gastrointestinal absorption, such as separating fluoroquinolones from multivalent cations by several hours to prevent chelation reducing antibiotic absorption.

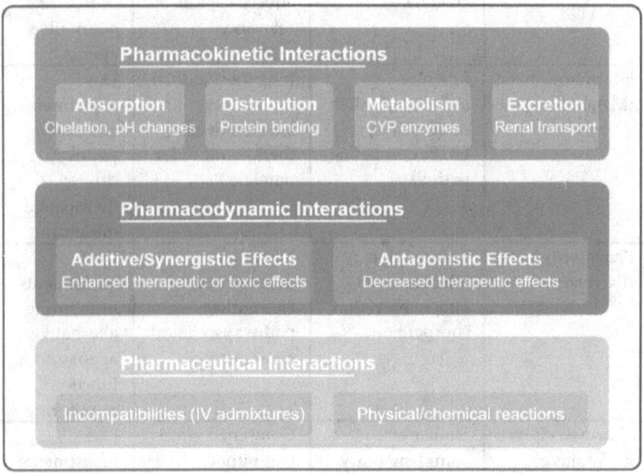

Figure 9.2: Mechanisms of Drug Interactions

Monitoring Plan Development

Parameter selection identifies appropriate indicators for detecting interaction consequences including laboratory values (INR, drug concentrations, electrolytes), physiological measurements (blood pressure, heart rate, blood glucose), or symptom assessment targeted to the specific interaction of concern. Frequency determination establishes appropriate monitoring intervals based on interaction onset expectations, effect severity, and adjustment capability, with higher-risk combinations requiring more intensive surveillance. Duration planning establishes monitoring continuation periods based on interaction persistence, including extended monitoring for enzyme induction effects that may continue weeks after inducer discontinuation compared to shorter monitoring for interactions with rapid offset.

Interaction Information Systems

Clinical decision support optimization configures electronic alerting systems balancing comprehensiveness against alert fatigue through appropriate severity thresholds, suppression of clinically insignificant interactions, and contextual relevance filtering based on patient-specific factors. Resource selection guidance directs practitioners to appropriate interaction information sources including comprehensive databases (Micromedex, Lexicomp), primary literature for emerging interactions, and specialized references for specific interaction types including herbal-drug or food-drug combinations not well-covered in standard references. Documentation standards establish consistent approaches for recording interaction assessments, management decisions, and monitoring plans ensuring information transfer across care settings and providers.

ADVERSE EFFECTS

Signal detection identifies potential adverse effects through systematic approaches including targeted questioning about expected reactions, open-ended inquiry about new symptoms since therapy initiation, physical examination for objective findings, and laboratory monitoring for subclinical effects. Causality assessment employs structured evaluation frameworks including temporal relationship, dechallenge/rechallenge response, dose-relationship, alternative explanations, and known reaction patterns to establish likelihood of medication causation versus coincidental occurrence. Severity classification categorizes reactions from mild (no intervention required, minimal discomfort) through moderate (requiring treatment, possibly extending hospitalization) to severe (life-threatening, causing persistent disability), guiding appropriate response proportional to impact.

Prevention Strategies

Risk factor identification recognizes patient characteristics increasing vulnerability to specific adverse effects including age, genetics, organ function, comorbidities, and previous reaction history, allowing preventive measures targeting high-risk individuals rather than universal precautions. Preemptive intervention implements prophylactic measures preventing expected adverse effects including antiemetics before chemotherapy, laxatives with opioid initiation, or potassium supplementation with potassium-depleting diuretics. Careful initiation employs conservative dosing approaches including lower starting doses, gradual titration, or divided dosing schedules reducing peak-related adverse effects during initial tolerance development.

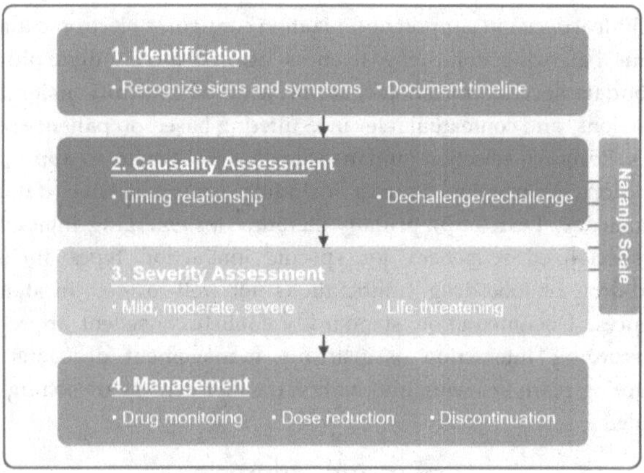

Figure 9.3: Assessment of Adverse Effects

Management Approaches

Supportive care provides symptomatic relief for reactions that can be appropriately managed without therapy modification, including antihistamines for mild drug rashes, hydration for minor gastrointestinal disturbances, or analgesics for headache while continuing necessary therapy. Dosage modification reduces drug exposure through dose reduction, extended intervals, or formulation changes maintaining therapeutic benefit while minimizing adverse effects when relationship is dose-dependent. Medication discontinuation implements immediate cessation for severe, potentially progressive, or idiosyncratic reactions where continued exposure risks significant harm outweighing potential benefits of therapy continuation.

Specific Adverse Effect Considerations

Dermatologic reaction management distinguishes between predictable, mild manifestations (fixed drug eruptions, exanthems) versus severe, potentially life-threatening reactions (Stevens-Johnson syndrome, toxic epidermal necrolysis, DRESS syndrome) requiring immediate recognition and intervention. Gastrointestinal effect mitigation addresses common tolerance issues through administration timing optimization (with/without food), formulation changes (extended-release, enteric-coated), or adjunctive therapy (acid suppressants, antiemetics) maintaining necessary treatment while minimizing discomfort.

Table 9.3: Adverse Effect Prevention and Management

Adverse Effect Category	Prevention Strategies	Monitoring Parameters	Management Approaches
Predictable/Dose-Related	Appropriate dosing, titration schedules, therapeutic drug monitoring	Drug levels, dose-related markers, clinical symptoms	Dose reduction, schedule adjustment, concentration-guided dosing
Hypersensitivity/Allergic	History taking, cross-reactivity awareness, genetic screening when applicable	Allergic symptoms, rash characteristics, organ involvement	Discontinuation, desensitization protocols, alternative agents
Idiosyncratic Reactions	Genetic screening, risk factor assessment, baseline testing	Specific organ function tests, symptom monitoring, biomarkers	Prompt discontinuation, supportive care, alternative classes
Cumulative Toxicity	Lifetime dose tracking, interval monitoring, risk factor assessment	Cumulative dose calculations, organ-specific monitoring	Planned drug holidays, dose limits, alternative strategies
Delayed Effects	Long-term monitoring plans, patient education, vigilance programs	Delayed manifestation signs, scheduled assessments	Early intervention, preventive strategies, alternative agents
Drug-Disease Interactions	Comprehensive disease assessment, risk-benefit analysis	Disease-specific parameters, exacerbation markers	Alternative agents, enhanced monitoring, preventive strategies
Withdrawal Effects	Tapering protocols, cross-dependence assessment, education	Withdrawal symptom scales, physiological parameters	Gradual tapering, supportive therapy, temporary substitution
Teratogenic Effects	Pregnancy testing, contraception programs, registry enrollment	Pregnancy status, contraceptive adherence, fetal monitoring	Planned pregnancy approaches, alternative agents, risk counseling

Neuropsychiatric symptom approaches address cognitive effects, mood changes, and behavioral manifestations through timing adjustments (bedtime dosing for sedating effects), dose modifications, or supportive interventions depending on severity and therapeutic necessity.

Reporting and Documentation

Adverse event reporting submits significant, unexpected, or severe reactions to appropriate systems including FDA MedWatch, facility incident reporting, and manufacturer programs, particularly important for serious reactions, newly marketed medications, or unusual manifestations advancing collective knowledge beyond individual patient management. Documentation standards establish comprehensive recording of reaction characteristics, assessment findings, management decisions, and communication with other providers ensuring appropriate information transfer across care transitions. Patient education provides clear guidance about experienced reactions including future avoidance instructions, medical alert needs, and cross-reactivity concerns for related medications preventing recurrence through informed decision-making.

SPECIAL POPULATIONS

Pediatric Considerations

Developmental pharmacokinetics addresses age-dependent changes in absorption, distribution, metabolism, and elimination requiring different approaches across developmental stages from premature neonates through adolescence rather than simply scaled-down adult regimens. Weight-based calculations implements appropriate dosing based on total body weight, body surface area, or age-specific recommendations depending on medication characteristics and developmental considerations. Formulation selection addresses administration challenges including inability to swallow tablets, taste preferences affecting acceptance, and availability of appropriate concentrations for accurate dose measurement in small children.

Geriatric Approaches

Polypharmacy management addresses the common challenge of multiple medication use in older adults through systematic deprescribing assessment, therapeutic duplication elimination, and regimen simplification reducing cognitive burden and adverse effect risks. Functional impact assessment evaluates medication effects on capabilities essential to independence including cognition, mobility, and balance, recognizing that preserving function may sometimes outweigh conventional therapeutic targets in older adults. Anticholinergic burden reduction identifies and minimizes medications with cumulative anticholinergic effects contributing to confusion, constipation, urinary retention, and dry mouth particularly problematic in elderly patients with reduced cholinergic reserve.

Table 9.4: Special Population

Population	**Physiological Considerations**	**Medication Adaptations**	**Monitoring Priorities**
Neonates /Infants	Immature hepatic/renal systems, blood-brain barrier development, body composition	Weight-based dosing, reduced metabolism consideration, appropriate formulations	Growth parameters, developmental milestones, age-specific toxicities
Children /Adolescents	Developing organ systems, growth considerations, weight changes	Weight/BSA-based dosing, age-appropriate formulations, developmental consideration	Growth velocity, pubertal development, age-specific effects
Pregnant Women	Expanded blood volume, altered metabolism, placental transfer	Pregnancy risk categories, trimester-specific adjustments, fetal benefit-risk	Maternal/fetal parameters, pregnancy-specific changes, fetal development
Lactating Women	Milk transfer, infant exposure, maternal needs	Lactation compatibility, timing strategies, infant monitoring	Infant effects, maternal therapeutic levels, breastfeeding success
Geriatric Patients	Reduced organ function, altered body composition, multiple comorbidities	Reduced starting doses, simplified regimens, geriatric-specific guidelines	Functional assessments, cognitive status, falls risk, comprehensive geriatric assessment
Renal Impairment	Reduced elimination, metabolite accumulation, altered protein binding	CrCl/GFR-based adjustments, alternative agents, dialysis considerations	Renal function trends, drug levels when applicable, uremic symptoms

Population	Physiological Considerations	Medication Adaptations	Monitoring Priorities
Hepatic Dysfunction	Altered metabolism, reduced protein synthesis, portal hypertension effects	Child-Pugh guided adjustments, alternative pathways, protein binding considerations	Liver function tests, encephalopathy signs, coagulation parameters
Critically Ill	Altered perfusion, organ dysfunction, extreme physiological states	Adjusted loading doses, more frequent monitoring, pathophysiological considerations	Organ function parameters, hemodynamic stability, drug levels
Obesity	Altered distribution, clearance changes, dosing weight selection	Ideal vs. actual weight considerations, distribution characteristics, altered clearance	Therapeutic response, concentration monitoring, obesity-specific complications

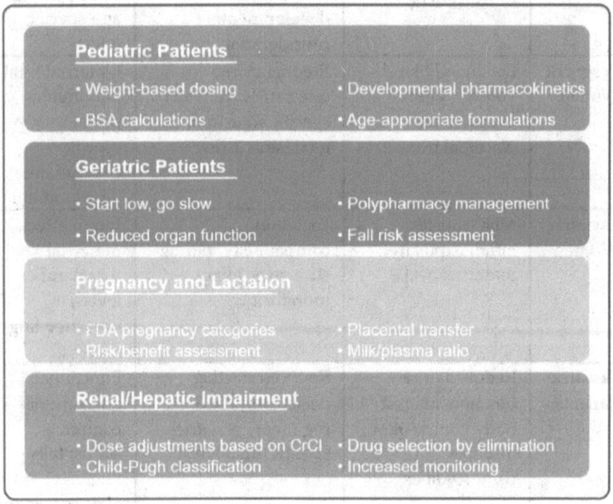

Figure 9.4: Drug Therapy Optimization

Pregnancy and Lactation

Risk categorization systems applies current FDA Pregnancy and Lactation Labeling Rule information replacing former letter categories with descriptive risk summaries based on available human experience, animal data, and pharmacological characteristics. Trimester-specific considerations addresses varying risks across pregnancy stages, recognizing different vulnerability periods for structural teratogenesis (primarily first trimester) versus functional development or growth effects (throughout pregnancy). Lactation compatibility assessment evaluates medication transfer into breast milk based on physicochemical properties (molecular weight, protein binding, lipophilicity), relative infant dose, and potential infant effects balancing maternal treatment needs against breastfeeding benefits.

Renal Impairment

Kidney function assessment employs appropriate estimation methods including Cockcroft-Gault for most medication dosing decisions, recognizing limitations of various formulas in specific populations including obesity, advanced age, and rapidly changing function. Dosing adjustment strategies implements appropriate modifications including dose reduction, interval extension, or combination approaches based on drug elimination characteristics, therapeutic index, and degree of renal impairment. Dialysis considerations addresses supplemental dosing requirements for medications significantly removed during hemodialysis, with replacement strategies based on specific clearance parameters, dialysis duration, and timing relative to scheduled doses.

Hepatic Dysfunction

Classification system application employs Child-Pugh or MELD scoring appropriately categorizing hepatic impairment severity guiding empiric dosage adjustments when specific guidelines unavailable. Pathway-specific considerations recognizes that hepatic impairment differentially affects various metabolic processes, with some pathways (e.g., CYP2D6) relatively preserved even in advanced disease while others (e.g., CYP1A2, CYP3A4) show more significant impairment requiring individualized assessment. Pharmacodynamic sensitivity addresses increased responsiveness to many central nervous system medications in hepatic dysfunction including sedatives, opioids, and psychotropics beyond pharmacokinetic changes alone, often requiring more conservative dosing approaches than suggested by standard hepatic adjustment guidelines.

COST CONSIDERATIONS

Therapeutic alternative evaluation compares clinical outcomes, adverse effect profiles, monitoring requirements, and acquisition costs across treatment options within therapeutic classes, identifying opportunities for equivalent outcomes at reduced expenditure. Generic substitution implements appropriate use of bioequivalent alternatives, recognizing situations where generic substitution is appropriate versus circumstances where brand formulations may be necessary due to narrow therapeutic index, unique delivery systems, or documented bioequivalence concerns. Step therapy implementation begins with most cost-effective options progressing to more expensive alternatives only after documented failure, intolerance, or contraindication to initial therapy when supported by clinical evidence and patient-specific factors.

Patient Financial Impact Assessment

Insurance coverage evaluation determines benefit design details including formulary status, prior authorization requirements, quantity limits, step therapy requirements, and specific exclusions affecting medication accessibility beyond simple covered/non-covered determinations. Out-of-pocket calculation estimates patient financial responsibility including copayments, coinsurance percentages, deductible considerations, and coverage gaps providing realistic expectations of treatment affordability. Affordability impact assessment examines medication costs within patient's overall financial circumstances, recognizing that identical copayments represent dramatically different burden depending on income, other healthcare expenses, and competing financial priorities.

Table 9.5: Cost Optimization Strategies

Cost Strategy	Implementation Approaches	Patient Impact Assessment	Quality Considerations
Therapeutic Substitution	Evidence-based alternatives, class equivalents, efficacy-comparable options	Out-of-pocket cost difference, formulary tier changes, long-term savings	Therapeutic equivalence evidence, outcome comparability, safety profile comparison
Generic Utilization	Brand to generic conversion, preferred generics, therapeutic equivalence	Cost reduction percentage, affordability improvement, sustainability	Bioequivalence standards, manufacturer considerations, patient perception
Dose Optimization	Tablet splitting, once-daily formulations, extended-release when appropriate	Overall regimen cost, adherence impact, convenience factors	Safety of manipulation, appropriate candidates, appropriate medications
Patient Assistance Programs	Manufacturer programs, foundation	Qualification likelihood, coverage gaps addressed,	Program stability, coverage comprehensiveness,

Cost Strategy	Implementation Approaches	Patient Impact Assessment	Quality Considerations
	assistance, copay cards	application burden	renewal requirements
Insurance Optimization	Formulary matching, prior authorization navigation, tier exceptions	Coverage improvement, reduced rejections, decreased delays	Administrative burden, approval likelihood, long-term sustainability
Appropriate Duration	Evidence-based duration, unnecessary therapy discontinuation, appropriate courses	Total therapy cost, unnecessary exposure reduction, resistance prevention	Outcome equivalence, relapse risk, individualized assessment
Procurement Strategies	Mail order utilization, pharmacy comparison, bulk purchasing	Total cost savings, convenience value, time savings	Quality assurance, appropriate storage, authentication verification
Preventive Focus	Preventing costly outcomes, adherence support, exacerbation prevention	Long-term economic benefit, indirect cost reduction, productivity impact	Outcome quality, preventive evidence, appropriate risk-benefit

Assistance Program Navigation

Manufacturer patient assistance programs connect eligible patients with pharmaceutical company-sponsored access to medications at reduced or no cost based on financial need, insurance status, and specific program criteria. Copayment assistance initiatives identify foundation-based and manufacturer-sponsored programs reducing out-of-pocket costs for insured patients facing high copayments or coinsurance percentages. Community resource connection links patients with local and national organizations providing medication assistance including charitable pharmacies, disease-specific foundations, and state pharmaceutical assistance programs supplementing conventional insurance coverage.

Cost-Minimization Strategies

Pill-splitting implementation identifies appropriate candidates for tablet division including scored medications with linear pharmacokinetics and adequate safety margins, while recognizing situations where splitting is inappropriate including extended-release formulations, enteric coatings, or narrow therapeutic index drugs. Quantity optimization adjusts prescription duration matching maintenance medication supply with follow-up intervals, insurance quantity allowances, and package sizes minimizing waste and dispensing fees while maintaining appropriate monitoring. Mail order utilization implements appropriate use of extended-supply options through mail service pharmacies when consistent with medication stability, monitoring requirements, and patient capabilities providing cost savings for suitable chronic medications.

System-Level Cost Management

Formulary management develops medication coverage frameworks balancing clinical effectiveness, safety, and cost considerations through evidence-based evaluation rather than acquisition cost alone, ideally involving clinical pharmacist expertise in decision-making processes. Utilization management implements appropriate constraints on high-cost therapies including prior authorization requirements, quantity limits, and specialist prescribing restrictions matching resource intensity with clinical necessity while maintaining access for appropriate patients. Medication assistance coordination establishes systematic approaches for identifying financial need, connecting patients with appropriate resources, and providing navigation support through complex assistance programs rather than addressing financial barriers reactively or inconsistently.

Summary

• Dosing considerations include patient-specific factors such as age, weight, organ function, genetics, comorbidities, and concomitant medications that may necessitate individualized dosing.

• Drug interaction management requires screening for potential interactions, assessing clinical significance, implementing preventive strategies, and monitoring for unexpected outcomes.

• Strategies for managing adverse effects include dose adjustments, alternative therapy selection, prophylactic treatment, and monitoring parameters for early detection.

• Special populations requiring customized pharmacotherapy approaches include pediatric and geriatric patients, pregnant women, and those with renal or hepatic impairment.

• Cost considerations in therapy selection involve balancing clinical efficacy, formulary status, patient affordability, and the value of interventions relative to overall healthcare costs.

• Deprescribing principles guide the process of tapering or discontinuing medications when potential harms outweigh benefits, particularly in elderly patients or those with polypharmacy.

• Therapeutic substitution and formulary management strategies optimize drug therapy while containing costs and ensuring appropriate medication access.

Multiple Choice Questions

1. Which of the following is the MOST appropriate approach to medication dosing in a patient with renal impairment?
   A) Reduce the dose of all medications by the same percentage
   B) Adjust doses based on the specific drug's dependence on renal elimination
   C) Switch all medications to alternatives that are not renally cleared
   D) Use loading doses for all medications to achieve therapeutic levels faster
2. A 78-year-old patient with declining renal function is prescribed enoxaparin for DVT prophylaxis. Which method provides the MOST accurate dosing guidance for this patient?
   A) Cockcroft-Gault equation using actual body weight
   B) Cockcroft-Gault equation using ideal body weight
   C) eGFR from the EPI-CKD equation
   D) Most recent serum creatinine value alone
3. Which of the following drug interactions would be considered the MOST clinically significant?
   A) Concurrent use of simvastatin and grapefruit juice
   B) Concurrent use of warfarin and a high-vitamin K diet
   C) Concurrent use of warfarin and a NSAID in a patient with normal renal function
   D) Concurrent use of lisinopril and hydrochlorothiazide
4. A patient experiences dry cough after starting lisinopril. Which of the following is the MOST appropriate intervention?
   A) Recommend discontinuation of lisinopril and substitution with an ARB
   B) Add an antitussive medication to manage the cough
   C) Reduce the dose of lisinopril by 50%
   D) Switch to a different ACE inhibitor
5. When optimizing drug therapy for a patient with hepatic cirrhosis (Child-Pugh Class C), which of the following is the MOST appropriate approach?
   A) Avoid all medications metabolized by the liver
   B) Start with reduced doses of hepatically cleared medications and titrate carefully
   C) Use standard doses but monitor more frequently
   D) Focus only on medications that cause direct hepatotoxicity
6. A pharmacist is reviewing therapy for a morbidly obese patient (BMI 45 kg/m^2). Which of the following statements

about dosing is MOST accurate?

A) All medications should be dosed based on ideal body weight

B) All medications should be dosed based on actual body weight

C) Dosing weight depends on the specific drug's physicochemical properties

D) Standard adult doses are appropriate regardless of weight

7. Which of the following represents the MOST appropriate application of pharmacogenetic testing in clinical practice?

A) Testing all patients before initiating any medication therapy

B) Testing patients who will receive medications with known actionable gene-drug interactions

C) Using testing only for medications with narrow therapeutic indices

D) Applying test results to all medications in the same therapeutic class

8. When considering cost in drug therapy optimization, which approach is MOST appropriate?

A) Always selecting the lowest cost option regardless of other factors

B) Considering cost only after efficacy and safety have been established

C) Focusing exclusively on drugs covered by the patient's insurance

D) Leaving cost considerations to the patient to decide

9. Which of the following statements about drug therapy in pregnancy is MOST accurate?

A) All medications should be avoided throughout pregnancy

B) The first trimester is generally the period of lowest teratogenic risk

C) Risk categories are absolute and apply uniformly to all pregnant women

D) Risk-benefit assessment should consider maternal and fetal well-being

10. A patient with multiple chronic conditions is taking 12 different medications. The MOST appropriate initial approach to optimize this patient's therapy would be to:

A) Discontinue all unnecessary medications based on lack of FDA-approved indications

B) Conduct a comprehensive medication review to identify inappropriate medications

C) Switch all medications to once-daily formulations

D) Combine medications into fixed-dose combinations whenever possible

Self-Assessment Questions

1. Explain three important physiological changes that occur with aging and how these changes impact medication dosing and selection in geriatric patients.
2. Describe the four main types of drug interactions (pharmacokinetic and pharmacodynamic), providing an example of each and appropriate management strategies.
3. Explain how renal function should be assessed for medication dosing, including the limitations of different estimation methods.
4. Discuss three approaches to managing adverse drug effects, including when each approach would be most appropriate.
5. Explain how pharmacists should approach medication dosing in pregnancy, including risk assessment and trimester-specific considerations.
6. Describe three important considerations when optimizing drug therapy for patients with hepatic impairment.
7. Explain how pharmacogenetic information can be used to optimize drug therapy, providing specific examples of drug-gene pairs.
8. Discuss strategies for balancing medication effectiveness, safety, and cost when optimizing drug therapy.
9. Explain the concept of deprescribing, including when it is appropriate and how to implement it safely.
10. Describe three special considerations for drug therapy optimization in pediatric patients compared to adults.

Bibliography

1. DiPiro JT, Talbert RL, Yee GC, Matzke GR, Wells BG, Posey LM. Pharmacotherapy: a pathophysiologic approach. 11th ed. New York: McGraw-Hill Education; 2020.
2. Hanlon JT, Schmader KE, Samsa GP, Weinberger M, Uttech KM, Lewis IK, et al. A method for assessing drug therapy appropriateness. J Clin Epidemiol. 1992;45(10):1045-1051.
3. Matzke GR, Aronoff GR, Atkinson AJ Jr, Bennett WM, Decker BS, Eckardt KU, et al. Drug dosing consideration in patients with acute and chronic kidney disease—a clinical update from Kidney Disease: Improving Global Outcomes (KDIGO). Kidney Int. 2011;80(11):1122-1137.
4. Verbeeck RK. Pharmacokinetics and dosage adjustment in patients with hepatic dysfunction. Eur J Clin Pharmacol. 2008;64(12):1147-1161.
5. Hansten PD, Horn JR. Drug interactions analysis and management. St. Louis: Wolters Kluwer Health; 2014.
6. Budnitz DS, Lovegrove MC, Shehab N, Richards CL. Emergency hospitalizations for adverse drug events in older Americans. N Engl J Med. 2011;365(21):2002-2012.
7. Koren G, Pastuszak A, Ito S. Drugs in pregnancy. N Engl J Med. 1998;338(16):1128-1137.
8. Kearns GL, Abdel-Rahman SM, Alander SW, Blowey DL, Leeder JS, Kauffman RE. Developmental pharmacology—drug disposition, action, and therapy in infants and children. N Engl J Med. 2003;349(12):1157-1167.
9. Relling MV, Evans WE. Pharmacogenomics in the clinic. Nature. 2015;526(7573):343-350.
10. Scott IA, Hilmer SN, Reeve E, Potter K, Le Couteur D, Rigby D, et al. Reducing inappropriate polypharmacy: the process of deprescribing. JAMA Intern Med. 2015;175(5):827-834.

CHAPTER 10

AMBULATORY CARE PRACTICE

Author

Miss. Hyndavi Trylockya Nagumantri, PharmD Scholar, Department of Pharmacy Practice, Koringa College of Pharmacy, Korangi, Kakinada, Andhra Pradesh, India

Abstract

Ambulatory care pharmacy practice focuses on longitudinal patient care in outpatient settings, emphasizing chronic disease management, preventive services, and care coordination across the healthcare continuum. Chronic disease management implements comprehensive approaches for conditions including diabetes, hypertension, dyslipidemia, and respiratory disorders through collaborative practice agreements, protocol-driven care, and self-management support enhancing clinical outcomes and quality of life. Preventive care services encompass immunization delivery, health screening coordination, medication-related prevention strategies, and lifestyle modification support addressing modifiable risk factors before disease development. Collaborative practice models establish formalized relationships between pharmacists and physicians through scope of practice definitions, communication protocols, and responsibility delineation enabling comprehensive, team-based patient care. Care transition management addresses vulnerable periods between care settings through medication reconciliation, regimen simplification, access assurance, and post-discharge follow-up preventing adverse events and readmissions. Quality measurement methodologies demonstrate impact through standardized metrics addressing process improvement, clinical outcomes, patient satisfaction, and healthcare utilization. This patient-centered approach positions pharmacists as essential primary care team members optimizing medication therapy in longitudinal, community-based settings.

Keywords: *Chronic Care Management, Preventive Pharmacotherapy, Collaborative Drug Therapy Management, Care Coordination, Quality Improvement*

Learning Objectives

After completion of the chapter, the learners should be able to:

- Implement comprehensive chronic disease management protocols for conditions including diabetes, hypertension, dyslipidemia, and asthma/COPD through evidence-based approaches.
- Provide preventive care services including immunizations, health screenings, and risk reduction strategies in outpatient settings.
- Develop collaborative practice protocols defining scope, communication methods, and clinical responsibilities between pharmacists and other healthcare providers.
- Design care transition interventions addressing medication reconciliation, regimen simplification, and post-discharge follow-up to prevent adverse events and readmissions.
- Apply quality measurement methodologies to evaluate and improve ambulatory care pharmacy services using standardized metrics and continuous improvement approaches.
- Implement patient self-management support strategies promoting active patient engagement in chronic disease management.

CHRONIC DISEASE MANAGEMENT

Diabetes management implements comprehensive approaches addressing glycemic control, cardiovascular risk reduction, and complication prevention through medication optimization, monitoring protocols, and self-management support. Services typically include insulin initiation and adjustment, continuous glucose monitoring interpretation, comprehensive medication review, and complication screening coordination with documented improvements in HbA1c (average 1-2% reduction), hospitalizations (30-50% decrease), and adherence to standards of care. Anticoagulation services provide systematic management of warfarin and direct oral anticoagulants through dose adjustment, monitoring coordination, perioperative management, and drug interaction evaluation. These services consistently demonstrate improved time in therapeutic range (15-20% increase), reduced bleeding and thrombotic complications (40-60% decrease), and enhanced patient satisfaction compared to usual care.

Protocol Implementation

Collaborative practice agreements establish formal relationships between pharmacists and physicians authorizing specific patient care functions including medication initiation, discontinuation, or adjustment within defined parameters, laboratory ordering, and referral coordination based on established protocols. Delegation authority varies significantly by state practice acts, institution policies, and individual physician comfort level, requiring careful documentation, communication systems, and quality assurance processes. Standing order development creates standardized approaches for specific clinical situations including vaccination administration, emergency response, and routine monitoring, ensuring consistent implementation while reducing unnecessary variation through evidence-based intervention pathways appropriate for ambulatory care implementation.

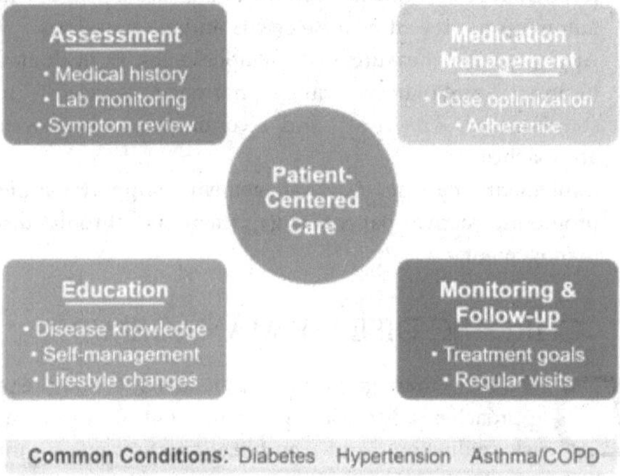

Figure 10.1: Chronic Disease Management

Population Health Management

Risk stratification categorizes patients based on disease severity, complication risk, medication complexity, or social determinants of health, allocating resources proportionally with highest-intensity services directed toward highest-risk individuals. Panel management implements systematic approaches to monitoring entire patient populations including identification of care gaps, preventive service needs, and quality measure opportunities beyond individual visit-based care. Outreach program development creates systematic approaches for engaging patients between scheduled visits through various modalities including telephone contact, secure messaging, home monitoring integration, and scheduled follow-up based on risk level and intervention needs.

Table 10.1: Chronic Disease Management Models in Ambulatory Care

Disease State	Management	Collaborative Protocols	Outcome Measures
Diabetes Mellitus	SMBG review, medication adjustment, complication screening, lifestyle modification	A1C management protocol, insulin adjustment algorithm, hypoglycemia protocol	A1C goals achieved, hypoglycemia rates, complication reduction, DSMES completion
Hypertension	BP monitoring review, medication titration, lifestyle counseling, sodium restriction	JNC/AHA-based protocols, medication titration algorithms, resistant HTN protocol	BP goal achievement, CV events reduction, medication adherence rates, lifestyle changes
Dyslipidemia	Lipid panel review, ASCVD risk calculation, statin intensity adjustment, non-statin therapy	ASCVD risk-based therapy protocol, statin intolerance algorithm, follow-up monitoring	LDL-C reduction, ASCVD event rates, statin adherence, goal attainment rates
Anticoagulation	INR monitoring, warfarin dose adjustment, DOAC monitoring, bleed risk assessment	Warfarin dosing nomogram, bridging protocol, DOAC selection algorithm	TTR for warfarin, bleeding events, thrombotic events, transition success rates
Asthma/COPD	Spirometry review, inhaler technique, symptom assessment, exacerbation management	Step-up/step-down therapy protocol, exacerbation action plan, device selection	Exacerbation rates, emergency visits, symptom control scores, device technique mastery

Disease State	Management	Collaborative Protocols	Outcome Measures
Heart Failure	Volume assessment, medication optimization, symptom monitoring, dietary adherence	GDMT titration protocol, diuretic adjustment algorithm, symptom response pathway	Hospitalization rates, NYHA class improvement, medication optimization rates, QOL scores
Mental Health	Symptom assessment, medication monitoring, therapy coordination, side effect management	PHQ-9 based intervention protocol, medication titration, referral criteria	Symptom scale improvement, remission rates, adherence rates, functional improvement
Pain Management	Pain assessment, functional impact, risk stratification, multi-modal approach	Stepped therapy algorithm, opioid monitoring protocol, non-pharmacologic integration	Pain scores, functional improvement, opioid dose reduction, quality of life measures

Self-Management Support

Action plan development creates personalized strategies for managing condition fluctuations, including specific parameters triggering medication adjustments or provider contact, appropriate for conditions with variable symptoms including asthma, heart failure, or diabetes. Home monitoring implementation establishes appropriate self-assessment programs including blood pressure measurement, blood glucose monitoring, peak flow assessment, or symptom tracking with clear recording systems, interpretation guidance, and response protocols. Behavioral goal setting employs collaborative approaches establishing specific, measurable, achievable, relevant, and time-bound objectives addressing health behaviors including medication adherence, dietary patterns, physical activity, or self-monitoring practices.

Care Model Integration

Patient-centered medical home incorporation positions pharmacists as core team members within primary care practices, providing comprehensive medication management integrated with physician, nursing, and behavioral health services rather than fragmented consultation. Shared medical appointment facilitation implements group-based care combining efficiency with peer support for conditions including diabetes, hypertension, or heart failure, with pharmacists typically addressing medication management, monitoring interpretation, and self-care education components. Care manager collaboration coordinates pharmacist medication expertise with nurse care managers, social workers, or community health workers addressing broader health needs including social determinants, care coordination, and navigation of complex healthcare systems.

PREVENTIVE CARE

Vaccination assessment evaluates immunization status against current recommendations based on age, medical conditions, occupational exposures, and previous vaccination history, identifying appropriate vaccines while avoiding unnecessary administration. Administration protocols implement proper storage, preparation, injection technique, documentation, and monitoring procedures ensuring safe and effective vaccination delivery with appropriate emergency response capability for rare adverse reactions. Barrier reduction strategies address common obstacles including misconceptions about vaccine safety, scheduling challenges, or financial concerns through evidence-based communication approaches, convenient access models including walk-in availability, and assistance program navigation.

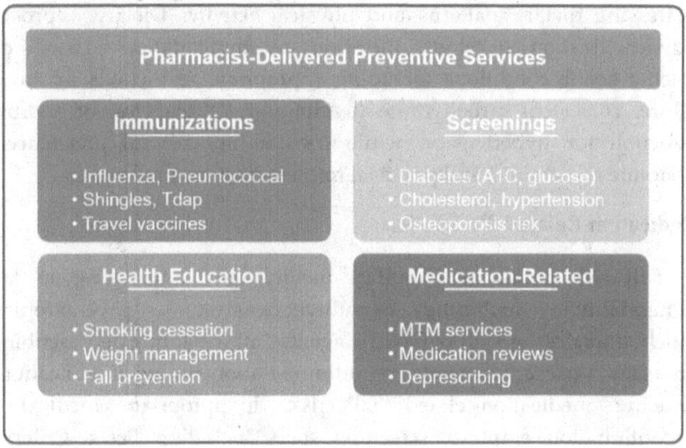

Figure 10.2: Preventive Care Services in Ambulatory Settings

Screening Program Implementation

Cardiovascular risk assessment employs validated tools including Atherosclerotic Cardiovascular Disease (ASCVD) Risk Calculator, Framingham Risk Score, or QRISK3 to identify appropriate candidates for preventive interventions including statin therapy, aspirin consideration, or intensive lifestyle modification. Cancer screening coordination ensures appropriate implementation of evidence-based recommendations including colorectal, breast, cervical, and lung cancer screening through systematic prompts, referral facilitation, and result tracking appropriate to age, risk factors, and previous screening history. Mental health screening implements validated instruments including PHQ-9 for depression, GAD-7 for anxiety, or AUDIT for alcohol use disorders with appropriate follow-up pathways for positive findings including referral coordination, treatment initiation, or monitoring protocols.

Lifestyle Modification Support

Tobacco cessation programs implement evidence-based interventions including pharmacotherapy selection (nicotine replacement, varenicline, bupropion), behavioral support strategies, relapse prevention planning, and systematic follow-up protocols significantly increasing quit rates compared to unassisted attempts. Weight management support provides personalized approaches to healthy weight achievement through medication review for agents contributing to weight gain, appropriate pharmacotherapy consideration when indicated, and lifestyle modification strategies addressing dietary patterns and physical activity. Dietary approach individualization develops nutrition recommendations based on specific health conditions including appropriate restrictions for heart failure, consistent carbohydrate distribution for diabetes, or sodium reduction for hypertension while considering cultural preferences, economic constraints, and practical implementation challenges.

Medication-Related Prevention

Fall risk reduction identifies medications contributing to fall vulnerability including antihypertensives, psychotropics, anticholinergics, and hypoglycemic agents, implementing deprescribing strategies, dose adjustments, or administration timing modifications reducing medication-related fall risk. Inappropriate medication discontinuation employs screening tools including Beers Criteria, STOPP/START, or Medication Appropriateness Index identifying potentially inappropriate medications for deprescribing, particularly in older adults where medication-related adverse events cause significant preventable morbidity. Antibiotic stewardship implements appropriate prescribing practices for common ambulatory infections including respiratory tract infections, urinary tract infections, and skin/soft tissue infections, reducing unnecessary antimicrobial use while ensuring appropriate therapy for bacterial conditions.

Table 10.2: Preventive Care Services in Ambulatory Pharmacy Practice

Preventive Service	Pharmacy Implementation	Documentation Requirements	Quality Metrics
Immunization Services	Vaccine administration, documentation, registry reporting, recall systems	Vaccine product details, administration site, patient counseling, registry reporting	Vaccination rates, series completion, missed opportunity reduction, HEDIS measures
Health Screenings	Point-of-care testing, risk assessments, screening coordination	Screening results, risk scores, referral information, follow-up plan	Screening rate improvement, positive screen follow-up rates, disease detection rates
Medication-Related Prevention	High-risk medication review, fall risk assessment, deprescribing	Medication risk scores, intervention documentation, preventive recommendations	Reduction in high-risk medications, fall rate reduction, adverse drug event prevention
Lifestyle Modification	Smoking cessation, weight management, physical activity counseling	Behavioral assessment, goal setting, intervention specifics, follow-up plan	Quit rates, weight outcomes, health behavior change metrics, engagement rates
Travel Health	Travel medication consultations, immunization planning, health advisories	Destination analysis, recommended interventions, patient education, prophylaxis details	Pre-travel completion rates, travel-related illness prevention, traveler satisfaction
Disease Prevention Counseling	Cardiovascular risk reduction, diabetes prevention, osteoporosis prevention	Risk calculations, preventive strategies, goal-setting documentation, education details	Risk score improvement, disease development rates, prevention program completion

Preventive Service	Pharmacy Implementation	Documentation Requirements	Quality Metrics
Cancer Prevention	Medication-related strategies, screening coordination, risk assessment	Cancer risk assessment, prevention strategies, screening recommendations	Screening compliance rates, preventive medication utilization, risk reduction metrics
Public Health Initiatives	Needle exchange, naloxone distribution, community education campaigns	Service utilization, distribution metrics, educational outcomes, community impact	Harm reduction metrics, opioid overdose rates, community health indicators

Prevention Coordination

Healthcare maintenance tracking establishes systems monitoring preventive service needs across patient populations, identifying due or overdue services including vaccinations, screening tests, and monitoring parameters with systematic reminder generation. Referral management coordinates services beyond pharmacy scope including diagnostic imaging, specialist evaluation, or procedural interventions through systematic tracking ensuring completed referrals with appropriate result integration into comprehensive care plans. Community resource connection links patients with non-medical preventive services including nutrition assistance programs, physical activity resources, smoking cessation groups, and other community-based prevention programs addressing social determinants of health beyond clinical interventions alone.

COLLABORATIVE PRACTICE

Workflow integration establishes pharmacist involvement at appropriate points within care processes including pre-visit planning, huddle participation, concurrent patient evaluation, or post-visit follow-up rather than disconnected consultation. Responsibility delineation clearly defines roles and accountability distribution between team members including physicians, nurses, pharmacists, and support staff, ensuring comprehensive care without unnecessary duplication or critical gap creation. Communication protocol development establishes consistent approaches for information sharing including documentation standards, verbal communication expectations, and urgent versus routine distinction ensuring appropriate information transfer across team members.

Physician Collaboration Enhancement

Value demonstration establishes pharmacist contributions through outcome tracking, workload reduction measurement, and quality improvement documentation building physician recognition of tangible benefits beyond theoretical value. Complementary expertise positioning emphasizes unique pharmacist contributions including detailed pharmacotherapy knowledge, medication system navigation, and comprehensive medication management complementing rather than competing with physician skills. Relationship development invests in interpersonal connection through physical presence, participation in shared activities including education sessions or quality improvement projects, and demonstrated reliability building trust essential for effective collaboration.

Scope of Practice Optimization

Practice act utilization maximizes activities permitted under state pharmacy practice regulations including various levels of prescriptive authority, laboratory test ordering, physical assessment performance, and diagnostic interpretation appropriate to pharmacist training and competence. Privileging process development establishes formal credentialing mechanisms documenting specific clinical activities authorized within institutions based on education, training, experience, and demonstrated competence rather than arbitrary or traditional role limitations. Continuous expansion strategy implements progressive responsibility advancement beginning with well-established collaborative activities and systematically expanding scope as comfort, trust, and demonstrated outcomes support increased independence.

Interprofessional Education Integration

Student training coordination develops structured experiences for pharmacy, medical, nursing, and other health profession students experiencing collaborative practice models during formative educational periods establishing expectations for future team-based practice. Continuing education collaboration implements joint learning activities for practicing professionals addressing shared clinical topics from interdisciplinary perspectives rather than siloed professional development. Cross-disciplinary knowledge sharing provides bidirectional education with pharmacists offering medication-focused updates to physician colleagues while gaining diagnostic reasoning and physical assessment insights from medical team members enhancing mutual respect and capability recognition.

Table 10.3: Collaborative Practice Models

Model Component	Implementation Elements	Legal/Regulatory Considerations	Success Factors
Scope Definition	Included disease states, specific authorities, excluded activities	State pharmacy practice act alignment, prescriptive authority limits, facility policies	Clear boundaries, appropriate clinical competencies, evidence-based protocols
Provider Collaboration	Communication mechanisms, escalation pathways, collaborative decision-making	Supervision requirements, prescriber availability, documentation standards	Established relationships, mutual respect, complementary roles, regular communication
Protocol Development	Evidence-based guidelines, decision algorithms, documentation standards	Required approvals, review frequency, authorized interventions	Stakeholder input, evidence basis, operational feasibility, regular updates
Quality Assurance	Chart review process, outcome tracking, protocol adherence monitoring	Required reporting, performance metrics, continuous improvement	Regular review schedule, defined metrics, improvement methodology, transparency
Training Requirements	Initial competency assessment, continuing education, skills validation	Credentialing requirements, privileging standards, certification maintenance	Standardized training, competency demonstration, ongoing education requirements
Patient Enrollment	Eligibility criteria, referral process, consent procedures	Informed consent requirements, patient selection criteria, opt-out provisions	Clear patient communication, benefits explanation, referral process
Team Integration	Role definition, workflow integration, team communication	Scope delineation, responsibility boundaries, conflict resolution processes	Team-based training, shared goals, defined processes

Collaborative Documentation Approaches

Shared record utilization implements comprehensive documentation within common electronic health records accessible to all team members rather than separate pharmacy-specific systems creating information silos. Standardized format development establishes consistent documentation approaches including problem-oriented frameworks, standardized terminology, and structured templates facilitating efficient information extraction by different disciplines. Recommendation communication employs clear, actionable documentation of assessment findings, specific suggestions, and follow-up plans without ambiguity regarding responsibility or implementation expectations.

CARE TRANSITIONS

Medication reconciliation performs systematic comparison between pre-admission regimens, inpatient medications, and discharge prescriptions, identifying and resolving discrepancies before causing post-discharge adverse events. Post-discharge follow-up implements structured contact within 2-7 days after hospitalization through telephone calls, video visits, or in-person appointments focusing on medication understanding, adherence challenges, symptom monitoring, and initial response assessment. High-risk patient identification prioritizes transition support for individuals with complex regimens, recent high-risk medication changes, limited support systems, or cognitive impairment potentially benefiting most from pharmacist intervention during vulnerable transition periods.

Medication Access Assurance

Prior authorization management navigates insurance requirements for restricted medications through systematic documentation submission, follow-up communication, and alternative therapy identification when approvals remain unattainable despite appropriate clinical justification. Formulary transition addresses insurance coverage changes requiring therapeutic substitution, prior authorization coordination, or non-formulary exception requests maintaining treatment continuity despite benefit design limitations. Affordability evaluation assesses patient financial capability for prescribed regimens, implementing cost-reduction strategies including generic substitution, therapeutic alternatives, manufacturer assistance programs, or pharmacy comparison when financial barriers threaten adherence or treatment implementation.

Information Transfer Enhancement

Discharge summary review analyzes hospital documentation extracting critical medication information including therapy changes, monitoring requirements, limited-duration treatments, and follow-up expectations integrating hospital care decisions with ongoing ambulatory management. Community pharmacy communication establishes consistent information sharing with dispensing pharmacies regarding intentional therapy changes, monitoring expectations, or special administration requirements ensuring alignment between prescribing intentions and dispensing implementation. Primary care coordination ensures appropriate information transfer to longitudinal care providers including medication changes, follow-up requirements, and ongoing monitoring needs, particularly important when ambulatory care pharmacists practice in specialty settings separate from primary care.

Table 10.4: Care Transitions in Ambulatory Pharmacy Practice

Transition Type	Pharmacy Interventions	Risk Assessment Tools	Outcome Measures
Hospital to Home	Medication reconciliation, discharge counseling, follow-up scheduling	LACE Index, 8P Scale, BOOST risk tool	30-day readmission rates, medication discrepancy resolution
Primary Care to Specialty	Therapy coordination, pre-visit planning, information transfer	Medication complexity assessment, therapy goal alignment	Care coordination quality, information accuracy, medication duplication reduction
Home to Long-Term Care	Regimen simplification, formulary alignment, care plan transfer	FRAIL scale, medication appropriateness indices	Medication continuity, adverse event prevention, therapeutic resolution
Adult to Geriatric Care	Deprescribing assessment, geriatric-appropriate regimens	Beers Criteria, STOPP/START, medication burden indices	Inappropriate medication reduction, geriatric syndrome prevention, care plan continuity

Transition Type	Pharmacy Interventions	Risk Assessment Tools	Outcome Measures
Pediatric to Adult Care	Responsibility transfer, adult-dose transitions, self-management support	Transition readiness assessment, self-management capability	Successful transition completion, care continuity, therapy adherence maintenance
Insurance Coverage Changes	Formulary transition planning, prior authorization transfer, affordability solutions	Coverage gap assessment, out-of-pocket impact analysis	Therapy continuity, cost management, access maintenance, adherence preservation
Care Setting Transitions	Information transfer, medication access planning, monitoring continuity	Care setting compatibility assessment, access barriers evaluation	Medication access continuity, monitoring plan execution, information accuracy
Provider Transitions	Comprehensive medication history transfer, care plan communication	Care complexity assessment, handoff quality tools	Information accuracy, care plan continuity, provider satisfaction with handoff

Regimen Simplification and Education

Medication schedule consolidation reorganizes complex regimens to minimize daily administration episodes, aligning medication timing with established daily routines and reducing regimen complexity particularly following hospitalizations often creating fragmented administration schedules. Enhanced counseling provides comprehensive education about therapy changes, addressing knowledge gaps created during stressful transitions when information retention is compromised by illness, stress, and information overload. Monitoring plan development establishes clear expectations for post-transition assessment including specific parameters requiring evaluation, responsibility assignment, and communication pathways for concerning findings requiring intervention.

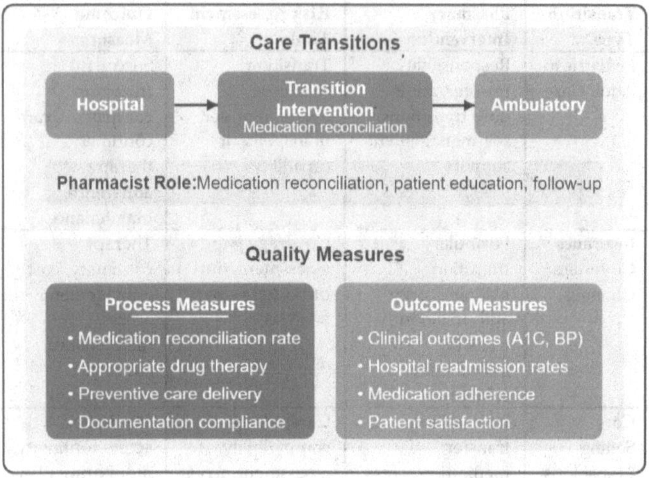

Figure 10.3: Care Transitions and Quality Measures

Care Transition Service Models

Transitions of care clinic establishes dedicated appointment availability specifically for recently discharged patients, providing focused medication review, regimen adjustment, monitoring implementation, and coordination with other post-discharge services including home health or rehabilitation services. Integrated discharge planning incorporates pharmacist involvement before hospital discharge through inpatient consultation, participation in discharge planning rounds, or direct communication with inpatient pharmacy teams ensuring continuity between inpatient and ambulatory medication management. Home visit programs provide transition support in patient residences, addressing environmental factors affecting medication management including storage conditions, organization systems, and practical administration challenges not apparent during facility-based encounters.

QUALITY MEASURES

HEDIS measure optimization addresses Healthcare Effectiveness Data and Information Set metrics including medication-related measures for diabetes, cardiovascular disease, asthma, and behavioral health conditions through systematic identification of non-adherent patients, therapy optimization, and documentation improvement. Star Rating improvement focuses on Medicare Part D measures including medication adherence for diabetes medications, renin-angiotensin system antagonists, and statins, along with high risk medication avoidance in elderly patients significantly affecting plan quality ratings and payment. Merit-Based Incentive Payment System (MIPS) advancement addresses quality metrics within the Centers for Medicare and Medicaid Services payment program, particularly medication-related measures within the quality, improvement activities, and promoting interoperability categories affecting physician reimbursement.

Table 10.5: Quality Measurement in Ambulatory Pharmacy Practice

Quality Category	Measurement	Data Collection Methods	Performance Improvement Approaches
Clinical Outcomes	Disease-specific goals (A1C, BP, LDL), event rates (hospitalizations, ED visits), complication reduction	EHR data extraction, patient registries, claims analysis	Population management, high-risk targeting, protocol optimization
Process Measures	Medication appropriateness, guideline adherence, monitoring completion rates	Chart review, quality dashboards, process tracking	Protocol standardization, workflow optimization, decision support
Access Measures	Time to appointment, service availability, geographic reach	Scheduling system data, patient surveys, geographic analysis	Extended hours, telehealth integration, outreach programs
Patient Experience	Satisfaction scores, perceived value, communication effectiveness	Standardized surveys (CG-CAHPS), focused questionnaires, interviews	Service design improvement, communication training, experience mapping

Quality Category	Measurement	Data Collection Methods	Performance Improvement Approaches
Efficiency Measures	Visit duration, provider productivity, resource utilization	Time tracking, productivity reports, resource allocation analysis	Workflow redesign, technology utilization, task distribution optimization
Safety Measures	Adverse drug events, medication errors, high-risk medication monitoring	Incident reports, trigger tool analysis, high-risk monitoring completion	Safety systems implementation, proactive risk assessment, near-miss analysis
Care Coordination	Information transfer completeness, referral completion, care plan alignment	Chart review, referral tracking, care plan assessment	Standardized handoffs, closed-loop communication, interface management
Health Equity	Care disparities, demographic-stratified outcomes, access equity	Demographic data analysis, outcome stratification, geographic mapping	Targeted outreach, cultural adaptation, barrier reduction strategies

Outcome Measurement Strategies

Clinical outcome tracking implements systematic monitoring of condition-specific parameters including blood pressure control rates, HbA1c goal achievement, lipid target attainment, or international normalized ratio therapeutic range maintenance documenting clinical impact of pharmacy services. Utilization impact assessment measures changes in healthcare resource use including emergency department visits, hospitalizations, or unplanned care attributable to pharmacy interventions, typically demonstrating 30-50% reductions in acute care utilization following comprehensive medication management implementation. Patient-reported outcome collection systematically gathers patient perspectives on symptom improvement, functional status enhancement, quality of life impact, and treatment satisfaction providing complementary evaluation beyond conventional clinical parameters.

Process Measure Development

Comprehensive medication review completion tracks the percentage of eligible patients receiving structured evaluation of complete medication regimens, typically targeting high-risk populations including those with multiple chronic conditions, polypharmacy, recent hospitalizations, or high-risk medication use. Care gap closure monitors identification and addressment of quality measure deficiencies, preventive care needs, and monitoring requirements with tracking of improvement rates following pharmacy intervention. Documentation quality assessment evaluates adherence to established standards including problem identification, assessment comprehensiveness, intervention specificity, and follow-up planning ensuring appropriate process implementation beyond outcome achievement alone.

Quality Improvement Methodology

Plan-Do-Study-Act cycles implement iterative improvement processes identifying intervention targets, developing specific changes, measuring impact, and refining approaches based on results before broader implementation. Root cause analysis examines underlying factors contributing to quality shortfalls, identifying systemic issues rather than individual performance gaps requiring process redesign rather than targeted interventions. Benchmark comparison evaluates performance against similar organizations, published standards, or historical baselines identifying relative strengths and improvement opportunities beyond isolated metric review.

Return on Investment Demonstration

Direct cost impact quantifies economic benefits including medication cost reductions through regimen optimization, unnecessary therapy discontinuation, or therapeutic substitution demonstrating tangible financial return beyond clinical outcomes. Indirect cost savings calculates broader economic effects including reduced emergency visits, hospitalizations, or unplanned care attributable to improved medication management beyond direct medication expenditures. Resource utilization efficiency measures service delivery costs against outcome achievement, optimizing staffing models, visit structures, and technology utilization maximizing results relative to resource investment supporting program sustainability beyond grant funding or initial implementation support.

Summary

- Chronic disease management in ambulatory care requires longitudinal patient relationships, systematic monitoring, and protocol-driven interventions for conditions like diabetes, hypertension, and dyslipidemia.
- Preventive care services provided by pharmacists include immunizations, health screenings, risk assessments, and education on lifestyle modifications to prevent disease progression.
- Collaborative practice agreements expand pharmacists' scope of practice, allowing for independent medication management, laboratory ordering, and treatment adjustments within defined protocols.
- Care transitions between inpatient and outpatient settings represent high-risk periods requiring medication reconciliation, patient education, and coordinated follow-up to prevent adverse events.
- Quality measures in ambulatory care pharmacy include HEDIS metrics, patient-reported outcomes, medication adherence rates, and clinical goal attainment for chronic disease states.
- Patient access considerations include extended hours, telehealth services, and multiple care delivery models to accommodate diverse patient needs and improve engagement.
- Population health management strategies employ risk stratification, targeted interventions, and data analytics to optimize outcomes across patient panels rather than focusing solely on individual encounters.

Multiple Choice Questions

1. Which of the following services is MOST appropriately provided by ambulatory care pharmacists under a collaborative practice agreement?
   A) Dispensing medications for acute conditions
   B) Independent prescribing of controlled substances
   C) Initiating and modifying medication therapy for chronic diseases
   D) Determining medical necessity for hospitalization
2. When managing a patient with type 2 diabetes in an ambulatory care setting, which of the following represents the MOST comprehensive approach?
   A) Focusing exclusively on glycemic control
   B) Addressing medication adherence only
   C) Comprehensive management including glycemic control, cardiovascular risk reduction, and complication prevention
   D) Referring all patients to endocrinology specialists
3. Which of the following is the MOST effective strategy for an ambulatory care pharmacist to improve care transitions?
   A) Providing discharge counseling only for new medications
   B) Performing medication reconciliation and follow-up within 7-14 days post-discharge
   C) Relying solely on the discharge summary for medication information
   D) Focusing primarily on insurance coverage issues
4. A key quality measure that ambulatory care pharmacists can directly impact is:
   A) Hospital-acquired infection rates
   B) Surgical complication rates
   C) Proportion of days covered (PDC) for chronic medications
   D) Emergency department wait times
5. Which of the following best describes the pharmacist's role in preventive care in ambulatory settings?
   A) Administering all types of vaccines regardless of state law
   B) Providing immunizations, screening services, and preventive medication recommendations
   C) Focusing exclusively on medication therapy
   D) Conducting annual physical examinations
6. In ambulatory care practice, which approach to chronic disease management is MOST effective?
   A) Episodic care based on acute exacerbations

B) Systematic, protocol-driven care with regular follow-up
C) Focusing primarily on medication dispensing
D) Independent management without physician collaboration

7. Which of the following is the MOST important factor in establishing a successful collaborative practice with physicians in ambulatory care?
A) Physical proximity to the physician's practice
B) Developing mutual trust and demonstrating value
C) Having independent prescriptive authority
D) Charging patients directly for pharmacy services

8. Which of the following is MOST important when implementing a pharmacist-managed anticoagulation service?
A) Having all patients switch to direct oral anticoagulants
B) Standardized protocols for dose adjustments and follow-up
C) Requiring all INR tests to be performed at the pharmacy
D) Managing anticoagulation without physician involvement

9. The MOST appropriate approach to measuring the impact of ambulatory care pharmacy services is:
A) Tracking the number of patients seen per day
B) Measuring clinical, economic, and humanistic outcomes
C) Focusing exclusively on cost savings
D) Comparing services to national averages without local context

10. When managing care transitions from hospital to ambulatory care, which of the following is the MOST critical intervention?
A) Ensuring the patient has a follow-up appointment with their primary care provider
B) Comprehensive medication reconciliation to identify and resolve discrepancies
C) Providing the patient with a complete list of their diagnoses
D) Transferring all medical records to the outpatient pharmacy

Self-Assessment Questions

1. Describe the key components of a collaborative practice agreement in ambulatory care and how it expands the pharmacist's scope of practice.
2. Explain three strategies that ambulatory care pharmacists can use to improve medication adherence in patients with chronic diseases.
3. Discuss how pharmacists can effectively contribute to preventive care services in the ambulatory setting, including specific examples of services they can provide.
4. Explain the role of ambulatory care pharmacists in managing care transitions from hospital to home, including key interventions to reduce readmissions.
5. Describe three quality measures commonly used in ambulatory care practice and how pharmacists can impact these measures.
6. Explain the concept of population health management in ambulatory care and how pharmacists can contribute to improving outcomes for specific patient populations.
7. Discuss the implementation and management of a pharmacist-run anticoagulation service, including key monitoring parameters and quality indicators.
8. Explain how ambulatory care pharmacists can effectively collaborate with primary care providers in managing patients with multiple chronic diseases.
9. Describe the role of technology and telehealth in expanding ambulatory care pharmacy services, including benefits and limitations.
10. Discuss three challenges in implementing ambulatory care pharmacy services and potential strategies to overcome these challenges.

Bibliography

1. Carmichael JM, O'Connell MB, Devine B, Kelly HW, Ereshefsky L, Linn WD, et al. Collaborative drug therapy management by pharmacists. Pharmacotherapy. 1997;17(5):1050-1061.
2. Smith M, Bates DW, Bodenheimer T, Cleary PD. Why pharmacists belong in the medical home. Health Aff (Millwood). 2010;29(5):906-913.
3. Fera T, Bluml BM, Ellis WM, Schaller CW, Garrett DG. The diabetes ten city challenge: interim clinical and humanistic outcomes of a multisite community pharmacy diabetes care program. J Am Pharm Assoc. 2008;48(2):181-190.
4. Chisholm-Burns MA, Kim Lee J, Spivey CA, Slack M, Herrier RN, Hall-Lipsy E, et al. US pharmacists' effect as team members on patient care: systematic review and meta-analyses. Med Care. 2010;48(10):923-933.
5. Giberson S, Yoder S, Lee MP. Improving patient and health system outcomes through advanced pharmacy practice. A report to the U.S. Surgeon General. Office of the Chief Pharmacist. U.S. Public Health Service; 2011.
6. Santschi V, Chiolero A, Colosimo AL, Platt RW, Taffé P, Burnier M, et al. Improving blood pressure control through pharmacist interventions: a meta-analysis of randomized controlled trials.J Am Heart Assoc. 2014;3(2):e000718.
7. Phatak HM, Thomas J 3rd. Relationships between beliefs about medications and nonadherence to prescribed chronic medications. Ann Pharmacother. 2006;40(10):1737-1742.
8. Milone AS, Philbrick AM, Harris IM, Fallert CJ. Medication reconciliation by clinical pharmacists in an outpatient family medicine clinic. J Am Pharm Assoc. 2014;54(2):181-187.
9. Pincus KJ, Romitti MK, Feret B, Gold M, Cooper JB, Griffin DW, et al. Development and implementation of a collaborative medication therapy management service for patients with HIV. J Am Pharm Assoc. 2019;59(4S):S54-S60.
10. Hazen ACM, de Bont AA, Boelman L, Zwart DLM, de Gier JJ, de Wit NJ, et al. The degree of integration of non-dispensing pharmacists in primary care practice and the impact on health outcomes: a systematic review. Res Social Adm Pharm. 2018;14(3):228-240.

CHAPTER 11

ACUTE CARE PRACTICE

Author

Dr. Nitin Ambati, PG Medico, Illinois, Saint James School of Medicine, Chicago, United States

Abstract

Acute care pharmacy practice addresses complex medication needs in hospitalized patients through specialized knowledge, rapid intervention, and interdisciplinary collaboration across diverse clinical environments. Critical care pharmacotherapy optimizes life-sustaining medications including vasopressors, antimicrobials, sedatives, and nutrition support through precise pharmacokinetic dosing, advanced monitoring, and pathophysiologic-based decision-making in critically ill patients. Emergency medicine services provide time-sensitive medication management for trauma, cardiovascular emergencies, toxicological exposures, and acute exacerbations requiring rapid assessment, prioritization, and intervention coordination. Internal medicine practice addresses complex multimorbidity through comprehensive medication management, transitions of care coordination, and antimicrobial stewardship integrating evidence-based approaches with patient-specific factors. Surgical care management encompasses perioperative medication optimization, antimicrobial prophylaxis, thromboembolism prevention, and enhanced recovery protocols promoting favorable surgical outcomes while preventing complications. Pain management strategies implement multimodal analgesia, opioid stewardship, and patient-specific approaches addressing acute, chronic, and procedural pain through appropriate medication selection, administration techniques, and monitoring protocols. This specialized practice area requires advanced clinical knowledge, rapid decision-making, and effective interdisciplinary communication to optimize medication therapy in acutely ill patients.

Keywords: *Hospital Pharmacy Practice, Critical Illness Pharmacotherapy, Perioperative Medication Management, Antimicrobial Stewardship, Emergency Pharmaceutical Care*

Learning Objectives

After completion of the chapter, the learners should be able to:

- Apply specialized pharmacotherapy knowledge to optimize medication therapy in critically ill patients including vasopressor selection, antimicrobial management, and nutrition support.
- Implement emergency medication protocols for time-sensitive conditions including cardiac arrest, stroke, sepsis, and toxicological emergencies.
- Develop comprehensive medication management approaches for complex internal medicine patients with multiple comorbidities and polypharmacy issues.
- Optimize perioperative medication management including antimicrobial prophylaxis, thromboembolism prevention, and transition planning for surgical patients.
- Implement multimodal pain management strategies balancing effective analgesia with appropriate opioid stewardship and adverse effect prevention.
- Participate effectively in interprofessional rounding and decision-making processes within acute care settings.

CRITICAL CARE

Vasopressor selection addresses different shock states through targeted pharmacological effects: norepinephrine as first-line for most shock types due to balanced alpha/beta effects, vasopressin for catecholamine-resistant vasodilatory shock, epinephrine for cardiogenic shock with low cardiac output, and phenylephrine for specific situations requiring pure alpha-adrenergic effects. Inotropic therapy implementation supports cardiac output in cardiogenic shock or cardiac dysfunction through agents including dobutamine (primarily beta-1 effects improving contractility), milrinone (phosphodiesterase inhibition with combined inotropic and vasodilatory properties), or epinephrine (combined inotropic and vasopressor effects for profound shock). Continuous infusion management establishes standardized concentrations, compatibility evaluation, and titration protocols with clearly defined hemodynamic targets including mean arterial pressure goals, cardiac index targets, or peripheral perfusion parameters.

Mechanical Ventilation Support

Sedation strategy development emphasizes targeted light sedation with daily interruption protocols to minimize ventilator duration and delirium risk, selecting appropriate agents including propofol (rapid onset/offset but hypotension risk), benzodiazepines (effective but delirium association), or dexmedetomidine (preserved respiratory drive but bradycardia concerns). Analgesia optimization implements appropriate pain control essential for ventilator tolerance and patient comfort while minimizing respiratory depression through opioid selection, adjunctive agents, and regular reassessment using appropriate scales for non-verbal patients. Neuromuscular blockade management addresses appropriate indications including refractory hypoxemia, ventilator dyssynchrony, and elevated intracranial pressure, with monitoring for complications including prolonged weakness and adequate concurrent sedation.

Infection Management

Empiric therapy selection addresses likely pathogens based on infection site, hospital ecology, and patient risk factors for resistant organisms, while balancing broad coverage against antimicrobial stewardship principles particularly important in critically ill patients where inadequate initial therapy significantly increases mortality. Pharmacokinetic/pharmacodynamic optimization employs extended infusions for time-dependent antibiotics (beta-lactams), appropriate loading doses for hydrophilic agents in fluid-shifted patients, and therapeutic drug monitoring for narrow therapeutic index antimicrobials (vancomycin, aminoglycosides) accounting for critical illness alterations in drug disposition. De-escalation protocols guide systematic narrowing of antimicrobial coverage based on culture results, clinical response, and biomarker trends, ensuring appropriate stewardship without compromising patient outcomes.

Table 11.1: Critical Care Pharmacy Interventions

Clinical Focus	Assessment Parameters	Pharmacist Interventions	Outcome Measures
Hemodynamic Support	MAP, CO/CI, vasopressor doses, hemodynamic monitoring, tissue perfusion	Vasopressor selection/titration, inotrope optimization, fluid resuscitation support	Time to MAP goals, vasopressor weaning success, organ perfusion markers
Respiratory Support	Ventilation parameters, oxygenation, sedation requirements, lung mechanics	Sedation/paralytic protocols, lung-protection, ventilator-associated pneumonia prevention	Ventilator days, successful extubation rates, sedation goal achievement, VAP rates

Antimicrobial Therapy	Culture results, susceptibilities, PK/PD parameters, infection markers	Empiric therapy selection, de-escalation, dose optimization, therapeutic drug monitoring	Clinical cure rates, pathogen eradication, resistance development, C. difficile rates
Renal Replacement	RRT modality, drug clearance, dosing adjustments, fluid status	Medication dosing during CRRT/HD, replacement fluid composition, drug removal assessment	Medication-related adverse events, therapeutic goal achievement, fluid balance targets
Nutrition Support	Metabolic requirements, feeding tolerance, micronutrient status	TPN formulation, enteral feeding optimization, drug-nutrient interactions	Nitrogen balance, prevention of refeeding syndrome, nutritional goal achievement
Neurologic Emergencies	ICP, cerebral perfusion, seizure activity, neurologic assessment	Brain injury protocols, anti-seizure therapy, neuroprotective strategies	ICP control, seizure prevention, neurologic outcome measures, Glasgow outcome score
Toxicology Management	Toxidrome recognition, decontamination needs, antidote requirements	Antidote selection/dosing, enhanced elimination strategies, supportive care	Time to clinical improvement, complication rates, successful decontamination
Trauma/Burn Care	Injury severity, resuscitation status, coagulation, metabolic demands	Massive transfusion support, coagulation management, hypermetabolic management	Resuscitation goal achievement, complication rates, wound healing metrics

Neurologic Emergencies

Acute ischemic stroke management implements time-sensitive protocols for thrombolytic therapy including alteplase dosing (0.9 mg/kg, maximum 90mg), inclusion/exclusion criteria assessment, blood pressure management (≤185/110 mmHg before treatment, ≤180/105 mmHg during/after), and post-thrombolytic monitoring for hemorrhagic transformation. Status epilepticus treatment follows stepwise progression from benzodiazepines (lorazepam, midazolam) to loading doses of antiepileptic drugs (fosphenytoin, valproate, levetiracetam) and potentially to anesthetic infusions (midazolam, propofol, ketamine, pentobarbital) for refractory cases. Intracranial pressure management employs osmotic agents (mannitol, hypertonic saline) with precise osmolality targets and timing, while minimizing medications exacerbating intracranial hypertension through appropriate selection and dosing.

Renal Replacement Therapy

Drug removal assessment evaluates medication characteristics affecting dialyzability, including molecular weight (<500 Da more readily removed), protein binding (<80% binding increases removal), volume of distribution (<0.7 L/kg more significantly affected), and existing clinical dialysis data guiding therapy adjustments. Dosing strategy implementation addresses different replacement modalities including supplemental doses after intermittent hemodialysis, continuous renal replacement therapy adjustments based on effluent rates, and hybrid approaches for prolonged intermittent therapies requiring different considerations than conventional methods. Administration timing coordination positions critical medications relative to dialysis sessions, administering highly dialyzable drugs after treatment while scheduling pre-dialysis medications requiring controlled removal.

Nutrition Support

Parenteral nutrition formulation designs patient-specific macronutrient and micronutrient compositions based on metabolic requirements, organ function, and disease state, with particular attention to modified requirements in critical illness including appropriate protein provision (1.2-2.0 g/kg/day), moderate caloric delivery avoiding overfeeding, and electrolyte adjustments accounting for organ dysfunction. Enteral therapy selection addresses specialized formulation needs for specific conditions including renal failure (reduced electrolytes, modified protein), hepatic encephalopathy (branched-chain amino acid enrichment), respiratory insufficiency (modified carbohydrate:fat ratio), and hyperglycemia (diabetes-specific formulations) beyond standard enteral nutrition. Medication-nutrition interaction management prevents physical incompatibilities, absorption alterations, and metabolic effects when medications and nutrition therapies are co-administered.

Toxicological Emergencies

Decontamination approach selection evaluates appropriate interventions including activated charcoal for recent ingestions of absorbable toxins, whole bowel irrigation for extended-release preparations or body packers, or various enhanced elimination techniques based on specific toxin characteristics, timing, and patient condition. Antidote selection and dosing addresses specific toxins with available reversal agents, including N-acetylcysteine for acetaminophen, naloxone for opioids, flumazenil for benzodiazepines (with appropriate seizure precautions), digoxin-specific antibody fragments for cardiac glycosides, and various chelating agents for heavy metals. Enhanced elimination implementation considers hemodialysis for toxins meeting criteria of low molecular weight, low protein binding, small volume of distribution, and limited endogenous clearance, including substances like methanol, ethylene glycol, salicylates, and lithium.

Multidisciplinary Team Integration

Daily interdisciplinary rounds incorporate pharmacist medication review, therapeutic recommendations, and intervention planning as standard components rather than consultative add-ons, with pharmacist participation demonstrating significant reductions in preventable adverse drug events and improved adherence to quality measures. Protocol development leadership engages pharmacist expertise in creating standardized approaches to common critical care scenarios including sedation management, glycemic control, and thromboprophylaxis, establishing evidence-based interventions while reducing unnecessary practice variation. Emergency response team participation includes pharmacist presence during cardiac arrests, trauma activations, and other time-sensitive emergencies requiring immediate medication management and preparation.

EMERGENCY MEDICINE

Resuscitation Pharmacotherapy

Code response responsibilities include medication preparation, dose calculation verification, administration timing recommendations, and documentation during cardiac arrest resuscitation, with ACLS algorithm adherence enhanced by pharmacist participation ensuring appropriate drug selection, dosing, and sequence during high-stress situations. Rapid sequence intubation support involves preparing appropriate induction and paralytic agents based on patient-specific factors including hemodynamic stability, neurologic status, and difficult airway characteristics, selecting between etomidate, ketamine, propofol, or midazolam paired with appropriate neuromuscular blockers. Post-cardiac arrest care implements targeted temperature management protocols, vasopressor optimization, and neuroprotective strategies including appropriate sedation and seizure prophylaxis following return of spontaneous circulation.

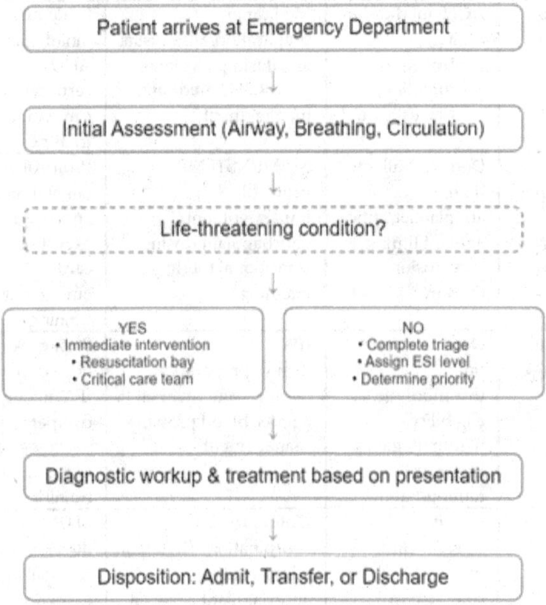

Figure 11.1: Emergency Medicine Triage Algorithm

Time-Sensitive Condition Management

Acute coronary syndrome protocols include appropriate antiplatelet loading (aspirin plus P2Y12 inhibitor), anticoagulation initiation (unfractionated heparin, enoxaparin, or bivalirudin), and preparation for emergent procedures with attention to timing and dosing precision, particularly for STEMI requiring immediate reperfusion. Stroke management involves tissue plasminogen activator (tPA) preparation, inclusion/exclusion criteria review, blood pressure management, and hemorrhagic transformation monitoring, with door-to-needle time targets under 60 minutes requiring efficient pharmacist integration into stroke teams. Status epilepticus intervention follows stepwise algorithms requiring rapid sequential medication administration when initial therapies fail, with pharmacist preparation of multiple agents potentially needed within short timeframes while ensuring appropriate dosing and administration.

Table 11.2: Emergency Medicine Pharmacy Services

Clinical Scenario	Time-Critical Elements	Pharmacist Roles	Preparedness Requirements
Cardiac Arrest	ACLS medication timing, defibrillation coordination, post-arrest care	Medication preparation/administration, dosing calculations, post-ROSC medication management	Code cart maintenance, ACLS certification, simulation training
Acute Coronary Syndrome	Door-to-balloon time, antiplatelet/anticoagulant timing, reperfusion therapy	STEMI/NSTEMI protocol implementation, anticoagulant dosing, transitional therapy planning	Protocol development, anticoagulant expertise, cardiac emergency training
Stroke Management	Door-to-needle time, thrombolytic eligibility, hemorrhagic vs. ischemic differentiation	tPA dosing/preparation, hemorrhage reversal agents, blood pressure management	Stroke protocol development, tPA mixing competency, neurological assessment training
Trauma Resuscitation	Massive transfusion protocol, coagulation support, damage control	Blood product coordination, TXA administration, anticoagulant reversal	MTP development, reversal agent expertise, trauma certification
Sepsis/Septic Shock	Time to antibiotics, early source control, appropriate fluid resuscitation	Empiric antibiotic selection, prompt preparation, vasopressor initiation	Sepsis bundle development, antimicrobial stewardship, sepsis certification
Toxicological Emergencies	Antidote availability, decontamination timing, enhanced elimination	Antidote stocking/preparation, decontamination recommendations, elimination strategy implementation	Toxicology resources, poison center relationships, antidote inventories

Clinical Scenario	Time-Critical Elements	Pharmacist Roles	Preparedness Requirements
Status Epileptic us	Time to benzodiazepine, sequential therapy timing, refractory status management	Anti-seizure medication preparation, refractory protocol implementation, continuous EEG monitoring support	Status epilepticus protocol development, neurological emergency training
Acute Respirat ory Failure	Rapid sequence intubation, mechanical ventilation initiation, noninvasive ventilation	RSI medication preparation, post-intubation sedation/analgesia, paralytic management	Airway cart maintenance, RSI protocol development, ventilator management training

Toxicology Management

Toxidrome recognition assists in identifying specific poisoning patterns when history is limited or unreliable, including anticholinergic (hyperthermia, dry mucous membranes, urinary retention, tachycardia), cholinergic (bronchorrhea, bradycardia, diarrhea, miosis), opioid (respiratory depression, miosis, decreased consciousness), and sympathomimetic (hypertension, tachycardia, hyperthermia, agitation) presentations guiding initial management approaches. Antidote preparation and dosing addresses high-risk, low-frequency interventions including N-acetylcysteine for acetaminophen toxicity (150 mg/kg loading dose followed by 50 mg/kg over 4 hours, then 100 mg/kg over 16 hours), sodium bicarbonate for sodium channel blocker poisoning, hydroxocobalamin for cyanide exposure, and fomepizole for toxic alcohols. Decontamination method selection weighs benefits against risks for interventions including activated charcoal, whole bowel irrigation, and enhanced elimination techniques.

Trauma Pharmacotherapy

Massive transfusion protocol implementation includes coordination of blood products, coagulation factor concentrates, antifibrinolytics (tranexamic acid 1g over 10 minutes, then 1g over 8 hours within 3 hours of injury), and reversal agents for anticoagulated patients, optimizing hemostasis during significant hemorrhage. Rapid sequence intubation for traumatic brain injury employs neuroprotective strategies minimizing secondary injury including appropriate pretreatment (fentanyl), careful induction agent selection (etomidate or ketamine with appropriate precautions), and controlled post-intubation parameters preventing harmful physiological fluctuations. Pain management balances adequate analgesia against respiratory depression risks and diagnostic concerns in acutely injured patients, selecting appropriate agents including fentanyl, ketamine, or regional anesthesia techniques depending on injury pattern and patient status.

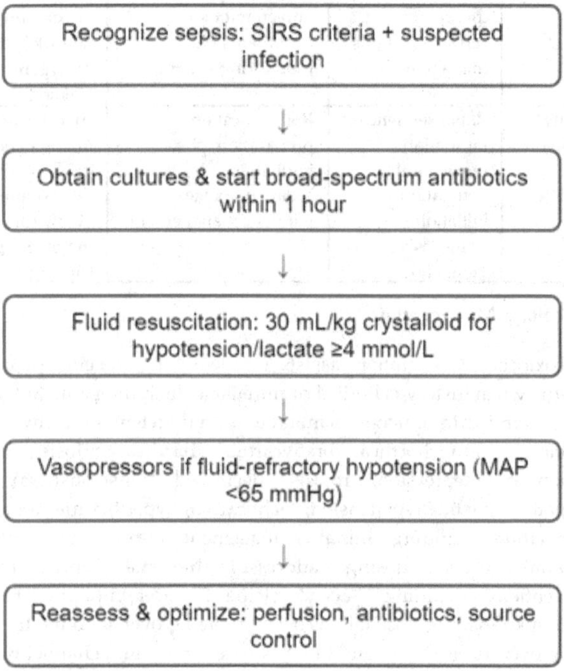

Figure 11.2: Sepsis Management Protocol in Critical Care

Pediatric Emergencies

Dosing calculations utilize appropriate weight-based formulas with verification processes preventing mathematical errors during high-stress situations, employing resources including length-based tapes (Broselow), pre-calculated references, or electronic tools reducing cognitive burden during pediatric resuscitations. Medication preparation addresses the need for dilution of adult formulations to appropriate concentrations for pediatric administration, particularly for critical medications including epinephrine, antiarrhythmics, and anticonvulsants requiring precise concentrations for safe delivery. Pediatric-specific emergency protocols address conditions including status asthmaticus, diabetic ketoacidosis, and febrile seizures with age-appropriate medication selection and dosing strategies.

Antimicrobial Stewardship

Empiric therapy protocols provide guidance for common infectious presentations including pneumonia, urinary tract infections, skin/soft tissue infections, and intra-abdominal infections based on local resistance patterns and patient risk factors for resistant organisms, balancing appropriate empiric coverage against unnecessary broad-spectrum therapy. Culture-guided intervention enables appropriate modification of initial therapy based on preliminary and final microbiology results, ensuring timely de-escalation to targeted therapy or appropriate broadening if initial coverage proves inadequate. Penicillin allergy assessment distinguishes true IgE-mediated reactions from non-allergic intolerances to expand therapeutic options, particularly important for serious infections where beta-lactams represent optimal therapy.

Transition of Care Coordination

Admission medication reconciliation aligns emergency interventions with home medications while resolving discrepancies for patients requiring hospitalization, identifying critical chronic medications requiring continuation despite acute illness while preventing unintentional duplications or omissions during transition. Discharge prescription review addresses appropriateness, affordability, and accessibility before patients leave the emergency department, ensuring necessary treatments including antibiotics, analgesics, or short-term symptom management medications can be obtained and correctly used following discharge. Outpatient follow-up planning ensures appropriate monitoring for high-risk medications initiated in the emergency setting, including arrangements for laboratory testing, specialist evaluation, or primary care follow-up within appropriate timeframes.

Clinical Care Area Coverage

Critical care pods receive support for high-acuity patients requiring intensive intervention and monitoring, including advanced cardiac life support, ventilator management, vasopressor therapy, and complex medication regimens requiring specialized pharmaceutical expertise. Observation units receive medication management for patients requiring extended evaluation or short-term therapy before disposition decisions, including chest pain rule-outs, transient ischemic attack monitoring, or parenteral therapy completion for conditions not requiring full inpatient admission. Fast-track areas receive support for lower acuity conditions still requiring appropriate medication selection and patient education, including uncomplicated infections, minor trauma, or exacerbations of chronic conditions amenable to short-term intervention.

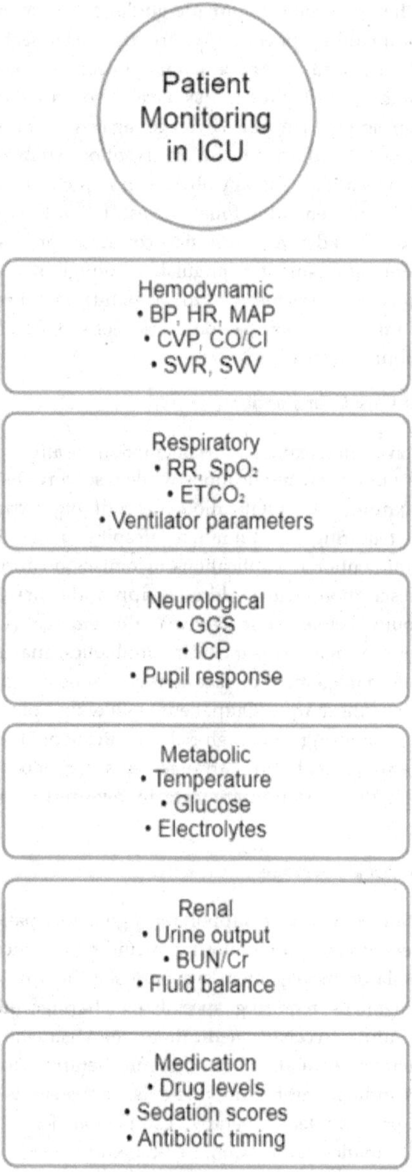

Figure 11.3: Critical Care Monitoring Parameters

INTERNAL MEDICINE

Admission medication reconciliation resolves discrepancies between pre-admission regimens and initial inpatient orders, identifying unintentional omissions, duplications, and dosing errors occurring during the transition to hospital care through systematic comparison of medication sources including patient/family reports, outpatient records, pharmacy dispensing data, and previous hospitalizations. Daily medication profile review systematically evaluates appropriateness, effectiveness, safety, and necessity for all active medications, generating specific optimization recommendations addressing issues beyond the primary admission diagnosis. Therapeutic duplication identification prevents unintentional overlap of similar agents resulting from multiple prescriber involvement, particularly common with analgesics, gastrointestinal medications, and cardiovascular drugs where different formulations or terminology may obscure redundancy.

Table 11.3: Internal Medicine Pharmacotherapy Management

Clinical Focus	Assessment Approaches	Therapeutic Interventions	Monitoring Parameters
Multimorbidity Management	Comprehensive geriatric assessment, condition prioritization, goal alignment	Therapy rationalization, regimen simplification, integrated care plans	Goal attainment, adverse event rates, patient-reported outcomes
Antimicrobial Stewardship	Infection probability assessment, culture evaluation, PK/PD analysis	De-escalation, IV-to-PO conversion, duration optimization, therapeutic drug monitoring	Appropriate utilization rates, resistance patterns, C. difficile rates
Thromboprophylaxis	VTE risk assessment, bleeding risk stratification, contraindication screening	Prophylactic anticoagulant selection, mechanical prophylaxis integration, risk-appropriate dosing	VTE events, bleeding complications, prophylaxis appropriateness rates

Clinical Focus	Assessment Approaches	Therapeutic Interventions	Monitoring Parameters
Stress Ulcer Prophylaxis	GI bleed risk factors, indication assessment, appropriate discontinuation	Risk-appropriate agent selection, duration limitation, step-down therapy	Stress ulcer bleeding rates, inappropriate continuation rates, C. difficile rates
Glycemic Management	Glycemic pattern analysis, insulin resistance assessment, hypoglycemia risk	Basal-bolus insulin protocols, correction factor adjustment, transition planning	Time in target range, hypoglycemia rates, hyperglycemia resolution
Delirium Management	CAM-ICU assessment, precipitating factor evaluation, non-pharmacologic strategies	Medication reconciliation, deliriogenic drug elimination, appropriate pharmacotherapy	Delirium duration, severity reduction, antipsychotic utilization rates
Medication Reconciliation	Admission/discharge discrepancy identification, therapeutic duplication assessment	Best possible medication history, reconciliation documentation, transition planning	Discrepancy resolution rates, medication error reduction, readmission rates
Renal/Hepatic Dosing	Organ function assessment, drug clearance evaluation, accumulation risk	Dose adjustments, interval modifications, alternative agent selection	Therapeutic goal achievement, toxicity prevention, organ function trends

Antimicrobial Stewardship

Empiric therapy selection matches antimicrobial coverage to likely pathogens based on infection site, hospital resistance patterns, and patient risk factors for resistant organisms, balancing appropriate initial therapy against unnecessary broad-spectrum coverage. Definitive therapy optimization adjusts initial regimens based on culture results, employing the narrowest effective therapy for identified pathogens while ensuring appropriate coverage for documented infections. Duration management prevents unnecessarily prolonged antimicrobial courses through evidence-based recommendations and automatic stop-date provisions, encouraging reassessment at key timepoints rather than default prolonged durations. Intravenous-to-oral conversion identifies candidates for early transition to oral therapy when appropriate clinical criteria are met, including clinical improvement, functioning gastrointestinal tract, and suitable oral alternatives.

Anticoagulation Management

Therapeutic anticoagulation protocols guide selection between various agents (unfractionated heparin, low molecular weight heparins, direct oral anticoagulants, warfarin) based on indication, patient characteristics, and transition planning, with particular attention to renal function, drug interactions, and bleeding risk assessment. Dosing individualization accounts for renal function, hepatic status, age, weight, and drug interactions affecting anticoagulant response, particularly important for direct oral anticoagulants where standard dosing may be inappropriate for patients with characteristics not well-represented in clinical trials. Monitoring protocol implementation ensures appropriate laboratory assessment including anti-Xa levels, activated partial thromboplastin time, or INR monitoring based on specific anticoagulant selection, with frequency determined by stability, recent changes, and risk factors.

Pain and Sedation Management

Multimodal analgesia implementation employs combinations of non-opioid analgesics (acetaminophen, NSAIDs), adjuvant agents (gabapentinoids, antidepressants), and targeted opioid therapy to maximize pain control while minimizing opioid-related risks, tailoring approaches to specific pain etiologies rather than defaulting to opioid monotherapy. Opioid stewardship applies appropriate selection, initial dosing, and titration strategies while implementing risk mitigation measures for patients requiring opioid therapy, including bowel regimen initiation, respiratory depression monitoring, and naloxone availability for high-risk patients. Sedation minimization strategies prevent delirium and prolonged hospitalization through appropriate agent selection, targeted use, and daily interruption protocols, particularly important for elderly patients with high delirium vulnerability.

Transitions of Care Coordination

Discharge medication reconciliation systematically compares

admission medications with current inpatient therapy and planned discharge regimens to identify and resolve discrepancies, ensuring intentional changes are continued while unintentional differences are corrected before transition. Medication access evaluation addresses insurance coverage, affordability, and availability for new prescriptions before hospital discharge, preventing treatment delays or interruptions due to formulary restrictions, prior authorization requirements, or cost barriers identified proactively rather than after discharge. Patient education provides clear instructions regarding medication changes, administration techniques, and monitoring expectations using teach-back methodology to verify understanding, supplemented with written materials appropriate to health literacy level.

Complex Pharmacotherapy Management

Renal dosing adjustment implements appropriate medication selection and dosage modification for patients with acute kidney injury or chronic kidney disease based on current renal function and drug-specific elimination characteristics, using the most appropriate kidney function estimation method for the specific clinical scenario. Hepatic impairment management addresses altered medication metabolism and increased sensitivity in patients with liver dysfunction through appropriate agent selection and dosage adjustment based on severity classification (Child-Pugh or MELD) and specific metabolic pathway involvement rather than generalized approaches. Drug interaction management identifies clinically significant interactions requiring intervention while distinguishing these from theoretical concerns with limited practical significance, implementing appropriate strategies including dose adjustment, alternative agent selection, or monitoring intensification.

Interdisciplinary Team Integration

Daily rounds participation enables real-time medication evaluation, therapeutic recommendation development, and intervention implementation within the context of comprehensive care planning, with pharmacist involvement demonstrated to reduce medication errors by 66-80% compared to physician-only teams. Team-based decision making incorporates pharmaceutical perspective alongside medical, nursing, and other disciplines to develop coordinated care approaches addressing complex therapeutic problems through multifaceted intervention strategies. Electronic health record documentation ensures that pharmacist assessments, recommendations, and interventions are visible to all team members as part of the integrated patient record, facilitating communication across disciplines and care settings.

Quality Improvement Leadership

Adverse drug event monitoring identifies patterns requiring intervention beyond individual cases, implementing systematic prevention strategies for frequently occurring events including anticoagulant complications, hypoglycemia, electrolyte disturbances, and opioid-related adverse effects. Medication error reporting analysis reveals system vulnerabilities requiring process redesign rather than individual practice changes, addressing underlying causes of errors through standardization, simplification, forcing functions, and error-resistant systems. High-risk medication protocol development creates standardized approaches to narrow therapeutic index drugs requiring consistent management approaches, including insulin, anticoagulants, opioids, and electrolyte replacement therapies.

SURGICAL CARE

Antithrombotic management protocols guide timing of anticoagulant and antiplatelet agent discontinuation based on bleeding risk, thrombotic risk, and specific agent pharmacokinetics, including warfarin (typically stopped 5 days before surgery with INR <1.5), direct oral anticoagulants (generally 2-3 days before surgery depending on renal function and bleeding risk), and antiplatelet agents (5-7 days for clopidogrel and prasugrel, 3-5 days for ticagrelor). Chronic disease medication management addresses continuation decisions for antihypertensives (typically continued except angiotensin-converting enzyme inhibitors and angiotensin receptor blockers often held 24 hours before surgery), diabetes medications (insulin adjusted rather than omitted, oral agents typically held day of surgery), and psychiatric agents (generally continued through perioperative period to prevent withdrawal or decompensation).

Surgical Antimicrobial Prophylaxis

Agent selection matches antimicrobial coverage to likely contaminating organisms based on surgical site, institutional resistance patterns, and patient factors including cefazolin for most clean and clean-contaminated procedures, with alternatives for beta-lactam allergies or MRSA risk. Administration timing ensures maximal tissue concentration at incision time, typically 30-60 minutes before incision for most antibiotics, with exceptions for vancomycin and fluoroquinolones (120 minutes before) due to different infusion requirements. Intraoperative redosing protocols maintain adequate antimicrobial levels during prolonged procedures based on antibiotic half-life and procedure duration, typically redosing cefazolin after 4 hours, clindamycin after 6 hours, and vancomycin after 8-12 hours when procedures extend beyond these intervals.

Perioperative Pain Management

Multimodal analgesic protocols implement combinations of acetaminophen, NSAIDs, gabapentinoids, regional anesthesia, and targeted opioid therapy to provide effective pain control while minimizing opioid requirements, with scheduled non-opioid analgesics forming the foundation supplemented by opioids for breakthrough pain. Opioid-sparing strategies employ appropriate non-opioid alternatives as foundation therapy, reserving opioids for breakthrough pain and tapering as recovery progresses to minimize postoperative opioid consumption, particularly important for opioid-naïve patients at risk for persistent postoperative use. Patient-controlled analgesia management ensures appropriate agent selection, initial programming, monitoring parameters, and transition planning, with typical settings including morphine (1mg every 6 minutes, 10mg hourly maximum) or hydromorphone (0.2mg every 6 minutes, 2mg hourly maximum) adjusted based on age, renal function, and opioid tolerance.

Table 11.4: Perioperative Pharmacy Services

Perioperative Phase	Medication Considerations	Pharmacy Interventions	Quality Indicators
Preoperative Assessment	Medication reconciliation, hold/continue decisions, preoperative medication optimization	Anticoagulation bridging, chronic disease optimization, pre-anesthesia medication management	Surgical delay reduction, medication-related cancellations, preoperative goal achievement
Antimicrobial Prophylaxis	Appropriate selection, timing, weight-based dosing, redosing criteria	Protocol development, timing optimization, allergy assessment, MRSA risk evaluation	Surgical site infection rates, timing compliance, appropriate selection rates
Anesthesia Support	Controlled substance management, rapid sequence medications, emergency drugs	Medication preparation, shortage management, alternative protocol development	Medication availability, preparation accuracy, emergency response capabilities

Perioperative Phase	Medication Considerations	Pharmacy Interventions	Quality Indicators
Enhanced Recovery Protocols	Multimodal analgesia, PONV prophylaxis, early nutrition, minimized opioids	Protocol development, order set creation, multimodal strategy implementation	Protocol compliance, length of stay, opioid utilization, patient satisfaction
Venous Thromboembolism Prevention	Risk stratification, appropriate agent selection, mechanical prophylaxis	Protocol development, risk assessment integration, contraindication evaluation	VTE rates, appropriate prophylaxis rates, bleeding complications
Glycemic Management	Perioperative insulin protocols, hypoglycemia prevention, transition planning	Protocol development, glucose management algorithms, transition planning	Glycemic target achievement, hypoglycemia rates, hyperglycemia complications
Medication Continuity	Inpatient-to-home transition, discharge planning, medication access	Discharge medication reconciliation, outpatient conversion planning, medication access coordination	Medication continuity rates, post-discharge adherence, readmission rates
Postoperative Pain Management	Multimodal approaches, opioid stewardship, transition planning	Pain protocol development, opioid-sparing strategies, tapering plans	Pain scores, opioid consumption, functional recovery, chronic opioid conversion

Enhanced Recovery After Surgery (ERAS) Protocols

Preoperative carbohydrate loading provides metabolic preparation, reducing insulin resistance and catabolism following surgery through clear carbohydrate beverages (typically 50g carbohydrate) 2-3 hours before anesthesia, replacing traditional prolonged fasting with evidence-based alternatives. Prophylactic antiemetic protocols employ combinations of agents with different mechanisms to prevent postoperative nausea and vomiting based on patient-specific risk factors, typically including 5-HT3 antagonists, corticosteroids, and dopamine antagonists for high-risk patients. Early oral nutrition support facilitates gastrointestinal recovery through appropriate medication selection and timing to address ileus prevention and management, including alvimopan for bowel resection procedures, appropriate opioid minimization, and chewing gum as non-pharmacologic intervention.

Specialty Surgical Populations

Transplant surgery management addresses immunosuppression initiation, maintenance, and monitoring while coordinating complex medication regimens during the transition to post-transplant care, including induction therapy (anti-thymocyte globulin, basiliximab), maintenance immunosuppression (tacrolimus, mycophenolate, corticosteroids), and infection prophylaxis (antivirals, antifungals, antibacterials). Cardiac surgery requires specialized anticoagulation management for cardiopulmonary bypass, inotropic support protocols, and strategies addressing post-pump inflammation and coagulopathy, including heparin dosing/reversal with protamine, vasopressor/inotrope selection, and blood product/factor concentrate utilization. Neurosurgical care involves medication selection and administration that minimizes intracranial pressure effects while providing appropriate seizure prophylaxis when indicated, particularly for traumatic brain injury or procedures with high seizure risk.

Anesthesia-Related Medication Management

Malignant hyperthermia protocol development ensures immediate availability of dantrolene and supporting medications with clear administration guidelines for this rare but life-threatening condition, including dantrolene (2.5 mg/kg initial dose, repeated until symptoms resolve, typically requiring 10 mg/kg total), sodium bicarbonate for metabolic acidosis, and cooling measures. Local anesthetic systemic toxicity management includes lipid emulsion therapy preparation and administration protocols for this serious anesthetic complication, with 20% lipid emulsion bolus (1.5 mL/kg) followed by infusion (0.25 mL/kg/min) while supporting cardiovascular and central nervous system effects. Neuromuscular blockade monitoring guides appropriate dosing and reversal agent selection based on depth and duration of paralysis, with quantitative monitoring preferred over subjective assessment for determining appropriate timing of reversal agent administration.

Post-surgical Complications

Postoperative delirium prevention and management employs non-pharmacological approaches as first-line therapy while developing appropriate medication strategies when necessary, emphasizing agents with favorable side effect profiles (low-dose haloperidol, quetiapine) and avoiding medications that exacerbate confusion (benzodiazepines, anticholinergics) except in alcohol withdrawal. Stress ulcer prophylaxis implements appropriate agent selection and duration based on risk factor assessment rather than routine universal administration, reserving therapy for patients with specific risk factors including mechanical ventilation >48 hours, coagulopathy, or significant burn injury. Ileus prevention and management combines prokinetic medications with appropriate use of opioid-sparing analgesia and early enteral nutrition when feasible, implementing multimodal approaches rather than single-agent interventions.

Perioperative Medication Safety

High-alert medication protocols establish specialized procedures for handling particularly dangerous medications in the perioperative setting, including concentrated electrolytes, opioids, anticoagulants, and insulin with specific safeguards addressing the unique risks of surgical environments. Perioperative handoff communication tools ensure complete medication information transfer between preoperative, intraoperative, and postoperative care teams, addressing critical elements including allergies, medications given during each phase, and specific concerns requiring continued monitoring. Look-alike/sound-alike medication error prevention implements specialized labeling, storage separation, and verification procedures for easily confused medications in surgical settings, particularly important for emergency situations where time pressure increases error vulnerability.

PAIN MANAGEMENT

Multidimensional assessment incorporates pain intensity, quality, temporal patterns, functional impact, and psychosocial factors to develop complete pain profiles beyond simple numeric ratings, using validated tools appropriate to specific populations including verbal patients (Brief Pain Inventory, McGill Pain Questionnaire) and non-verbal patients (Critical Care Pain Observation Tool, Behavioral Pain Scale). Assessment tool selection matches specific instruments to patient populations and pain types, including specialized tools for non-verbal patients, pediatric populations, and cognitively impaired individuals such as PAINAD (Pain Assessment in Advanced Dementia) or FLACC (Face, Legs, Activity, Cry, Consolability) scale. Functional assessment emphasizes activity limitations, quality of life impact, and specific functional goals rather than focusing exclusively on pain intensity scores, establishing measurable objectives beyond pain reduction.

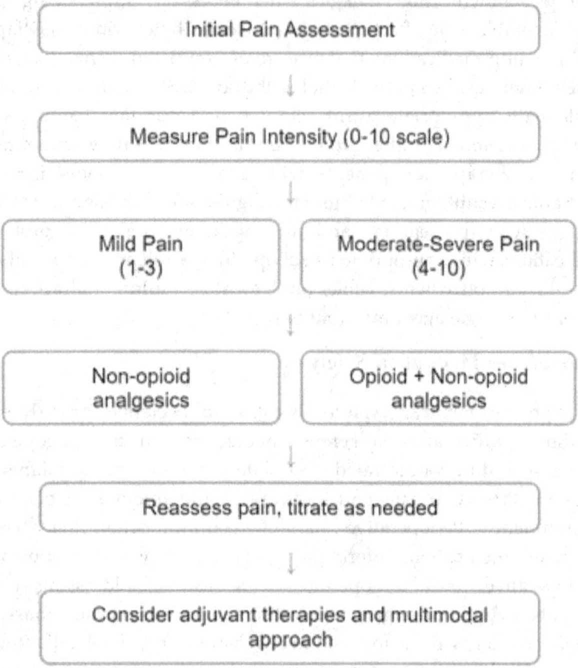

Figure 11.4: Acute Pain Assessment and Management Algorithm

Multimodal Analgesia

Non-opioid foundation therapy establishes acetaminophen and NSAIDs as baseline analgesics for nociceptive pain, providing opioid-sparing effects through different mechanisms including peripheral inflammation reduction, central prostaglandin inhibition, and modified central processing. Adjuvant analgesic optimization employs agents including antidepressants (duloxetine, amitriptyline), anticonvulsants (gabapentin, pregabalin), muscle relaxants, and topical therapies based on specific pain mechanisms and patient characteristics, particularly valuable for neuropathic and mixed pain syndromes. Interventional technique support coordinates pharmacotherapy with procedural approaches including nerve blocks, trigger point injections, and neurostimulation, ensuring appropriate medication adjustments following successful interventions while developing contingency plans for incomplete response.

Opioid Stewardship

Risk assessment implements standardized tools including the Opioid Risk Tool, DIRE score, or SOAPP-R to identify patients requiring enhanced monitoring or structured approaches, stratifying patients into low, moderate, and high-risk categories guiding appropriate safeguards proportional to identified concerns. Opioid selection matches specific agents to pain characteristics and patient factors, considering pharmacokinetics (immediate versus extended-release), metabolism pathways (avoiding codeine and tramadol in poor CYP2D6 metabolizers), formulation options, and specific risk factors including sleep-disordered breathing or concurrent benzodiazepine use. Naloxone co-prescribing provides overdose reversal capability for patients receiving high-dose therapy (>50 morphine milligram equivalents daily), concurrent benzodiazepines, or those with other risk factors including sleep apnea, pulmonary disease, or renal dysfunction.

Table 11.5: Pain Management Approaches in Acute Care

Pain Type	Assessment Tools	Pharmacological Strategies	Monitoring Parameters
Acute Postoperative	Numeric rating scale, functional assessment, opioid risk tools	Multimodal therapy (NSAIDs, acetaminophen, gabapentinoids, regional techniques), scheduled non-opioids, PRN opioids	Pain scores at rest/movement, functional recovery, opioid consumption, side effects
Chronic Pain Exacerbation	Brief Pain Inventory, pain diagrams, functional impact scales	Continuation of home regimens, adjuvant additions, breakthrough management, non-pharmacologic approaches	Baseline vs. acute pain, functional improvement, safe transitions, misuse behaviors
Neuropathic Pain	DN4, LANSS, neuropathic descriptors	Gabapentinoids, SNRIs, tricyclics, topical agents, targeted opioids	Pain quality changes, functional improvement, side effect management, sleep improvement

Pain Type	Assessment Tools	Pharmacological Strategies	Monitoring Parameters
Cancer-Related Pain	Brief Pain Inventory, breakthrough assessment, Edmonton system	WHO analgesic ladder, breakthrough dosing, adjuvant therapy, methadone considerations	Pain relief adequacy, breakthrough frequency, side effect management, quality of life
Procedural Pain	Procedural anxiety assessment, anticipated pain severity	Pre-procedural analgesia, conscious sedation, topical anesthetics, non-pharmacologic techniques	Procedural comfort, recovery time, patient satisfaction, complication rates
Trauma/Burn Pain	Critical care pain observation tool, functional pain assessment	Background analgesia, procedural coverage, anxiety management, wound care considerations	Background pain control, procedural tolerance, functional recovery, psychological impact
Opioid-Tolerant Patients	Opioid tolerance assessment, equianalgesic conversion, risk evaluation	Maintenance therapy, adjuvant emphasis, rotation strategies, withdrawal prevention	Pain control adequacy, withdrawal prevention, functional improvement, safe transitions
Non-pharmacologic Integration	Pain coping assessment, previous response history, preference evaluation	Integration with pharmacotherapy, cognitive techniques, physical modalities, psychological approaches	Technique effectiveness, patient engagement, opioid-sparing effect, sustainability

Non-pharmacological Intervention Integration

Physical modality coordination aligns pharmacotherapy with physical therapy, occupational therapy, and rehabilitation approaches to maximize functional improvement through complementary interventions addressing both symptoms and underlying physical contributors to pain. Psychological intervention integration ensures that pharmacotherapy complements cognitive-behavioral therapy, mindfulness practices, and other psychological approaches addressing pain catastrophizing, fear-avoidance behaviors, and maladaptive coping strategies frequently exacerbating chronic pain conditions. Complementary therapy coordination addresses interactions and complementary effects between conventional medications and approaches such as acupuncture, massage, and chiropractic care, ensuring safe integration while recognizing potential for both beneficial and adverse interactions.

Special Population Considerations

Geriatric pain management implements age-appropriate medication selection, conservative dosing, and enhanced monitoring addressing altered pharmacokinetics, pharmacodynamic sensitivity, and polypharmacy concerns, typically starting with one-third to one-half standard adult doses while titrating slowly based on response and tolerability. Substance use disorder approaches balance adequate pain control against recovery maintenance, employing structured agreements, frequent monitoring, and consultation with addiction specialists, recognizing that untreated pain may trigger relapse while inappropriate opioid management may exacerbate substance use disorders. Pregnancy and lactation management selects appropriate agents and timing to minimize fetal or infant exposure while providing necessary maternal pain control, typically prioritizing acetaminophen, category B analgesics, and lowest effective opioid doses when necessary while avoiding NSAIDs in later pregnancy.

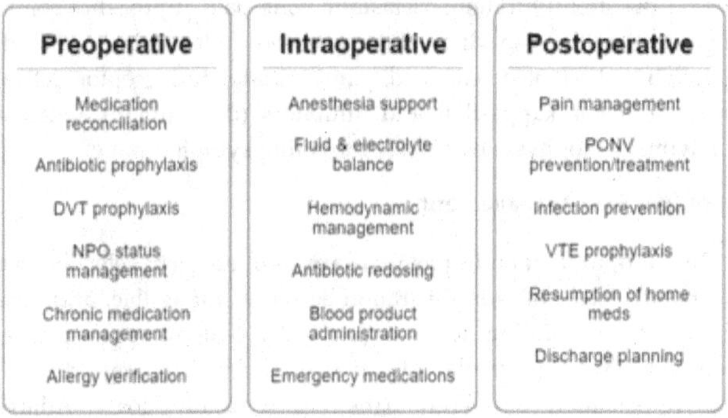

Figure 11.5 Role of Pharmacist in Perioperative Care

Chronic Non-cancer Pain Management

Neuropathic pain approaches emphasize anticonvulsants, selected antidepressants, and topical agents with established efficacy for conditions including diabetic neuropathy, post-herpetic neuralgia, and radiculopathy, typically employing duloxetine (60-120mg daily), gabapentin (1800-3600mg daily in divided doses), pregabalin (150-600mg daily in divided doses), or lidocaine patches (up to 3 patches for 12 hours daily) as first-line options. Inflammatory pain management employs disease-modifying agents for underlying inflammatory conditions while providing symptomatic relief through appropriate anti-inflammatory and analgesic therapy, addressing both acute symptoms and disease progression through complementary approaches. Functional improvement focus establishes specific activity goals and quality of life improvements as primary outcomes rather than pain elimination, recognizing that function often improves more significantly than pain intensity with effective management.

Cancer-Related Pain Management

Breakthrough pain management implements rapid-onset, short-duration interventions addressing transient pain exacerbations while maintaining stable background analgesia, typically employing immediate-release opioid formulations at 10-15% of total daily opioid dose with timing, frequency limitations, and reassessment protocols preventing overuse. Opioid rotation employs systematic conversion between different agents to address tolerance, adverse effects, or changing clinical situations while maintaining analgesic efficacy, using established equianalgesic tables with conservative initial dosing (typically 25-50% dose reduction from calculated equianalgesic dose) followed by careful titration. Metastatic bone pain approaches combine analgesics with specific bone-targeted therapies including bisphosphonates (zoledronic acid, pamidronate) and receptor activator of nuclear factor kappa-B ligand inhibitors (denosumab) addressing underlying pathophysiology while providing symptom relief.

End-of-life Pain Management

Opioid optimization implements appropriate agent selection, route conversion when oral administration becomes impossible, and dosage adjustments responding to changing pain patterns during disease progression, with particular attention to balancing comfort against excessive sedation based on patient and family goals. Adjuvant medication rationalization continues beneficial pain adjuncts while discontinuing unnecessary therapies that no longer contribute to comfort, simplifying regimens to essential interventions while ensuring comprehensive symptom management. Palliative sedation protocols establish clear guidelines for managing refractory symptoms when conventional approaches fail, including appropriate agent selection (typically midazolam, propofol, or phenobarbital), dosing strategies, and ethical implementation frameworks ensuring proportional intervention for genuinely refractory symptoms rather than inappropriate substitution for adequate pain management.

Summary

• Critical care pharmacy services focus on complex pharmacotherapy, including vasoactive medications, mechanical ventilation support, antimicrobial stewardship, and nutrition management.

• Emergency medicine pharmacy practice involves rapid assessment, preparation for high-risk medications, toxicology expertise, and participation in trauma and resuscitation teams.

• Internal medicine pharmacists address multiple disease states, medication reconciliation, transitions of care, and complex drug regimens in general hospital units.

• Surgical care pharmacy services include perioperative medication management, antimicrobial prophylaxis, venous thromboembolism prevention, and post-surgical pain management.

• Pain management approaches balance effective analgesia with risk mitigation strategies, employing multimodal therapy, opioid-sparing techniques, and appropriate monitoring.

• Antimicrobial stewardship is a core responsibility in acute care settings, focusing on appropriate selection, dosing, duration, and de-escalation of anti-infective therapy.

• Rapid response and code team participation allows pharmacists to provide critical medication expertise during emergent situations, including drug selection, dosing, preparation, and administration.

Multiple Choice Questions

1. Which of the following is the MOST important contribution of a pharmacist during multidisciplinary rounds in an ICU?
   A) Documenting the team's decisions
   B) Scheduling future consultations
   C) Providing real-time medication evaluation and recommendations
   D) Managing the unit's medication inventory
2. A pharmacist in the emergency department would MOST appropriately be involved in:
   A) Triage of incoming patients
   B) Time-sensitive medication preparation and dosing for critical patients
   C) Performing physical examinations
   D) Determining patient disposition
3. When optimizing sedation therapy for a mechanically ventilated patient, which of the following approaches is MOST appropriate?
   A) Maintaining deep sedation at all times to prevent ventilator asynchrony
   B) Using daily sedation interruption protocols and targeted sedation goals
   C) Relying exclusively on intermittent bolus dosing
   D) Avoiding analgesics to prevent respiratory depression
4. Which of the following best represents the pharmacist's role in antimicrobial stewardship in acute care?
   A) Restricting all broad-spectrum antibiotic use
   B) Ensuring appropriate empiric therapy, de-escalation, and duration optimization
   C) Approving all antibiotic orders before dispensing
   D) Performing all culture and sensitivity testing
5. The MOST appropriate role for a pharmacist in acute pain management is:
   A) Independently prescribing all analgesics
   B) Developing multimodal pain protocols and ensuring appropriate implementation
   C) Administering IV pain medications
   D) Focusing exclusively on opioid minimization regardless of pain severity

6. When providing pharmaceutical care to surgical patients, which of the following is MOST important?
   A) Perioperative antibiotic prophylaxis optimization
   B) Medication reconciliation throughout the surgical continuum of care
   C) Ensuring all medications are available in liquid form
   D) Converting all medications to IV formulations
7. In internal medicine units, pharmacists most effectively improve patient outcomes by:
   A) Managing all aspects of patient care independently
   B) Focusing exclusively on discharge medication counseling
   C) Providing comprehensive medication management throughout hospitalization
   D) Limiting interventions to high-cost medications
8. When managing vasoactive medications in shock states, which of the following pharmacokinetic considerations is MOST important?
   A) Hepatic first-pass metabolism
   B) Protein binding in normal physiologic states
   C) Altered volume of distribution and clearance in critical illness
   D) Drug absorption from intramuscular sites
9. The MOST appropriate pharmacist intervention for a critically ill patient with acute kidney injury would be:
   A) Discontinuing all medications with renal elimination
   B) Adjusting medication dosages based on degree of renal dysfunction and drug properties
   C) Converting all medications to oral formulations
   D) Recommending dialysis for medication clearance
10. In emergency medicine, the pharmacist's role in toxicologic emergencies most appropriately includes:
    A) Obtaining the patient's psychiatric history
    B) Performing gastrointestinal decontamination procedures
    C) Recommending appropriate antidotes and elimination strategies
    D) Determining patient disposition to psychiatric facilities

Self-Assessment Questions

1. Describe three key responsibilities of clinical pharmacists in critical care settings and how they contribute to patient outcomes.
2. Explain the pharmacist's role in antimicrobial stewardship in acute care, including specific interventions to optimize antimicrobial therapy.
3. Discuss the pharmacist's contribution to pain management in acute care, including assessment tools and multimodal approaches.
4. Explain how pharmacists can effectively participate in rapid response teams and code blue situations in the hospital setting.
5. Describe three strategies that acute care pharmacists use to identify and prevent medication errors during care transitions within the hospital.
6. Discuss the pharmacist's role in managing drug therapy in patients requiring renal replacement therapy in the ICU setting.
7. Explain how pharmacists contribute to medication management during perioperative care, including preoperative assessment and postoperative transitions.
8. Describe the role of the emergency department pharmacist, including time-critical interventions and medication safety initiatives.
9. Explain three approaches to dosing adjustments for critically ill patients with altered pharmacokinetics, including specific examples.
10. Discuss the clinical pharmacist's role in nutritional support services in acute care, including parenteral nutrition optimization.

Bibliography

1. MacLaren R, Bond CA, Martin SJ, Fike D. Clinical and economic outcomes of involving pharmacists in the direct care of critically ill patients with infections. Crit Care Med. 2008;36(12):3184-3189.
2. Leape LL, Cullen DJ, Clapp MD, Burdick E, Demonaco HJ, Erickson JI, et al. Pharmacist participation on physician rounds and adverse drug events in the intensive care unit. JAMA. 1999;282(3):267-270.
3. Eppert HD, Reznek AJ. ASHP guidelines on emergency medicine pharmacy services. Am J Health Syst Pharm. 2011;68(23):e81-e95.
4. Lada P, Delgado G Jr. Documentation of pharmacists' interventions in an emergency department and associated cost avoidance. Am J Health Syst Pharm. 2007;64(1):63-68.
5. Bond CA, Raehl CL. Clinical pharmacy services, pharmacy staffing, and hospital mortality rates. Pharmacotherapy. 2007;27(4):481-493.
6. Murphy EM, Oxencis CJ, Klauck JA, Meyer DA, Zimmerman JM. Medication reconciliation at an academic medical center: implementation of a comprehensive program from admission to discharge. Am J Health Syst Pharm. 2009;66(23):2126-2131.
7. American Society of Health-System Pharmacists. ASHP guidelines on surgery and anesthesiology pharmaceutical services. Am J Health Syst Pharm. 1999;56(9):887-895.
8. Chou R, Gordon DB, de Leon-Casasola OA, Rosenberg JM, Bickler S, Brennan T, et al. Management of postoperative pain: a clinical practice guideline from the American Pain Society, the American Society of Regional Anesthesia and Pain Medicine, and the American Society of Anesthesiologists' Committee on Regional Anesthesia, Executive Committee, and Administrative Council. J Pain. 2016;17(2):131-157.
9. Preslaski CR, Lat I, MacLaren R, Poston J. Pharmacist contributions as members of the multidisciplinary ICU team. Chest. 2013;144(5):1687-1695.
10. Schneider PJ, Pedersen CA, Montanya KR, Curran CR, Harpe SE, Bohenek W, et al. Improving the safety of medication administration using an interactive CD-ROM program. Am J Health Syst Pharm. 2006;63(1):59-64.

CHAPTER 12

SPECIAL POPULATION CARE

Author

Miss. Veera Naga Lalitha Nakkina, PharmD Scholar, Department of Pharmacy Practice, Koringa College of Pharmacy, Korangi, Kakinada, Andhra Pradesh, India

Abstract

Special population care addresses unique medication challenges in physiologically distinct patient groups requiring specialized knowledge, modified approaches, and heightened vigilance throughout the medication use process. Pediatric pharmacotherapy navigates developmental pharmacokinetics, weight-based dosing strategies, appropriate formulation selection, and age-specific monitoring parameters from neonates through adolescents with particular attention to medication safety and growth considerations. Geriatric medication management addresses pharmacokinetic alterations, pharmacodynamic sensitivity changes, polypharmacy challenges, and geriatric syndrome considerations through deprescribing methodologies, inappropriate medication avoidance, and simplified regimen development. Pregnancy and lactation pharmacotherapy balances maternal benefit against fetal or infant risk through teratogenicity assessment, placental transfer evaluation, lactation compatibility determination, and alternative therapeutic approaches when standard medications pose unacceptable risks. Renal impairment adaptations implement appropriate dosage adjustment methodologies, nephrotoxicity avoidance, dialysis considerations, and electrolyte management strategies based on kidney function assessment and medication clearance mechanisms. Hepatic dysfunction approaches address altered metabolism, protein binding changes, and encephalopathy risk through appropriate medication selection, dosage modification, and monitoring parameter adjustment based on liver disease severity classification. These specialized approaches ensure safe, effective medication use in populations with unique physiological considerations requiring modified pharmacotherapeutic strategies.

Keywords: *Developmental Pharmacokinetics, Altered Drug Disposition, Physiologic Adaptation, Vulnerable Populations, Organ Dysfunction*

Learning Objectives

After completion of the chapter, the learners should be able to:

- Apply pediatric-specific pharmacotherapy principles including weight-based dosing, appropriate formulation selection, and developmental considerations across pediatric age groups.
- Implement geriatric medication management strategies including deprescribing, falls risk reduction, and potentially inappropriate medication avoidance.
- Evaluate medication safety during pregnancy and lactation by assessing teratogenic potential, placental transfer, and breast milk excretion to optimize maternal-fetal outcomes.
- Adjust medication regimens appropriately for patients with renal impairment using established dosing algorithms, monitoring parameters, and nephrotoxicity prevention strategies.
- Modify drug therapy for patients with hepatic dysfunction based on liver disease severity, medication hepatic clearance mechanisms, and encephalopathy risk.
- Develop personalized therapeutic approaches addressing physiological alterations, pharmacokinetic changes, and specific monitoring requirements across special populations.

PEDIATRICS

Absorption variations include age-dependent gastric pH (relatively neutral in neonates, gradually acidifying to adult values by age 2), altered gastric emptying times, variable intestinal transit, and differences in transporter expression affecting drug uptake particularly for medications requiring active transport processes. Distribution changes include higher total body water percentage (80-85% in neonates versus 55-60% in adults), lower body fat proportion, reduced plasma protein concentrations affecting drug binding, and variable blood-brain barrier permeability allowing greater central nervous system penetration of many medications in neonates and young infants. Metabolism differences reflect immature hepatic enzyme systems in neonates with gradually developing activity, reaching adult capacity at variable ages depending on specific pathways (CYP3A4 approaches adult activity by 1 year, while CYP1A2 and CYP2D6 develop more slowly).

Dosing Strategies

Weight-based dosing calculates medication quantities based on total body weight (mg/kg), typically used for most pediatric medications but requiring consideration of maximum doses for larger children approaching or exceeding adult size to prevent excessive dosing. Body surface area approaches (mg/m^2) better approximate metabolic activity for selected medications, particularly chemotherapeutic agents and medications with significant pharmacokinetic differences between children and adults, generally calculated using the Mosteller formula (BSA = √[(height × weight)/3600]). Age-based dosing employs specific recommendations for different age categories, particularly for neonates and young infants where developmental pharmacology considerations significantly impact dosing requirements, sometimes using "step" approaches with distinct dosing for neonates, infants, children, and adolescents.

Table 12.1: Pediatric Pharmacotherapy Considerations

Age Group	Physiological Considerations	Dosing Approaches	Administration Challenges
Neonates (0-28 days)	Immature renal/hepatic systems, altered body composition, BBB permeability	Weight-based dosing, reduced clearance consideration, extended intervals	Limited IV access, small fluid volumes, accurate measurement challenges
Infants (1-12 months)	Developing enzyme systems, rapid growth, variable absorption	mg/kg dosing, developmental adjustments, organ maturation consideration	Taste considerations, liquid formulation needs, feeding coordination
Toddlers (1-3 years)	Increased clearance rates, activity levels, first-pass metabolism	BSA calculations, weight verification, frequent reassessment	Cooperation challenges, taste sensitivity, dosage form limitations
Children (4-11 years)	Approaching adult metabolism, growth variability, formulation needs	Weight or BSA-based, max dose considerations, growth monitoring	Swallowing ability development, school administration needs, taste importance
Adolescents (12-18 years)	Hormonal influences, adult-approaching clearance, compliance issues	Adult dose transitions, weight checks, adherence strategies	Autonomy development, privacy concerns, peer influence considerations

Medication Formulation Selection

Liquid formulation assessment evaluates concentration appropriateness, measuring device accuracy, taste characteristics, and excipient safety for young children unable to swallow solid dosage forms, with particular attention to potentially harmful preservatives including alcohol, propylene glycol, or benzyl alcohol in neonates and young infants. Extemporaneous compounding provides appropriate formulations when commercial liquid options are unavailable, including stability assessment, beyond-use dating, and palatability considerations with specific attention to appropriate vehicles, compatible flavoring agents, and physical stability throughout the intended use period. Alternative delivery systems include orally disintegrating tablets, chewable formulations, transdermal preparations, and intranasal options that may overcome administration challenges in specific pediatric populations.

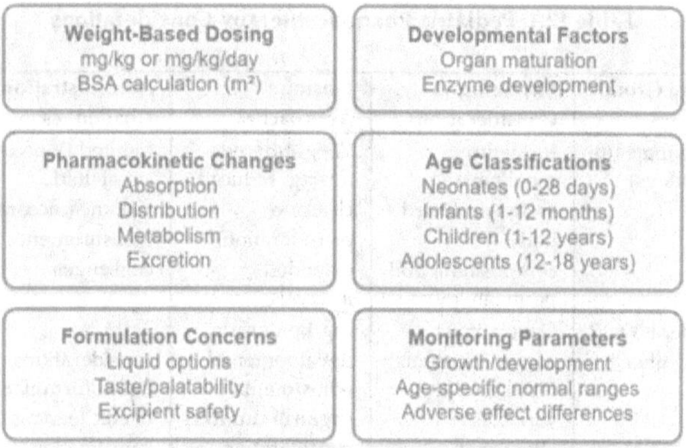

Figure 12.1: Pediatric Medication Dosing Considerations

Neonatal Intensive Care

Gestational age-based dosing adjusts medication selection and quantities based on developmental status, with significant differences between extremely premature (<28 weeks), moderately premature (28-34 weeks), late preterm (34-37 weeks), and term neonates (>37 weeks) reflecting varying degrees of organ system maturity affecting drug disposition. Parenteral nutrition design addresses the specialized nutritional needs of neonates with precise electrolyte, protein, and micronutrient requirements that differ substantially from older children, requiring careful calcium:phosphorus ratios, appropriate protein provision (2-4 g/kg/day depending on gestational age), and specific trace element considerations. Medication dilution protocols ensure appropriate concentration and volume for accurate administration of small doses while maintaining compatibility with limited fluid allowances.

Pediatric Infectious Disease Management

Empiric therapy selection matches antimicrobial coverage to age-specific pathogens and resistance patterns for common pediatric infections including otitis media, pharyngitis, pneumonia, and urinary tract infections, recognizing different pathogen distributions across age groups from neonates through adolescents. Antimicrobial dosing optimization ensures adequate drug exposure for common pediatric pathogens while accounting for developmental pharmacokinetic differences, often requiring weight-based dosing with careful maximum dose considerations and age-appropriate adjustments. Formulation palatability significantly impacts adherence for oral antimicrobials, requiring consideration of taste, texture, and administration volume alongside clinical efficacy, particularly important for longer treatment courses or younger children with limited cooperation capability.

Medication Safety Systems

Dose range checking implements automated or manual verification processes comparing calculated doses against age-appropriate reference ranges before dispensing or administration, flagging potential errors for additional verification before reaching patients. Weight-based double-checks verify both the weight measurement accuracy and the mathematical calculation of weight-based doses, employing independent calculations by different healthcare providers to identify potential errors before administration. Standardized concentrations establish consistent medication preparations across care areas, reducing the complexity that contributes to preparation errors, particularly important for high-risk medications including opioids, sedatives, anticonvulsants, and inotropes.

Chronic Disease Management

Growth and development monitoring tracks height, weight, and developmental milestones during chronic therapy, particularly for medications with potential growth effects including stimulants (possible growth velocity reduction) and corticosteroids (growth suppression with long-term systemic use), ensuring early detection and intervention for concerning trends. School-based medication administration coordinates treatment schedules with educational environments, addressing timing, administration supervision, and emergency medication access during school hours, particularly important for conditions requiring midday dosing including attention deficit hyperactivity disorder, diabetes, seizure disorders, and asthma. Transition planning prepares adolescents for eventual transfer to adult care services through gradually increasing medication self-management responsibility, knowledge development, and engagement in treatment decisions.

Pharmacogenomic Considerations

Developmental gene expression patterns show age-dependent activity for many pharmacogenetically relevant genes, with some polymorphisms having more significant effects during specific developmental periods, creating complex interactions between ontogeny and genetics requiring nuanced interpretation beyond adult pharmacogenomic models. Testing considerations include appropriate timing, interpretation differences across developmental stages, and ethical considerations regarding testing for adult-onset conditions, balancing immediate therapeutic decision needs against broader implications of genetic information. Medication selection incorporates available genetic information alongside developmental pharmacology principles, recognizing that genetic factors may alter expected developmental patterns of drug disposition and response.

GERIATRICS

Absorption changes include increased gastric pH, reduced gastrointestinal blood flow, decreased absorptive surface area, and delayed gastric emptying, collectively affecting drug dissolution and uptake particularly for medications requiring acidic environments for dissolution or exhibiting narrow absorption windows in specific intestinal segments. Distribution alterations include increased body fat percentage (affecting lipophilic drug distribution), decreased total body water (affecting hydrophilic drug concentration), reduced serum albumin affecting protein binding, and changes in tissue perfusion altering drug delivery to effect sites, collectively requiring consideration for initial dosing and volume of distribution estimates. Metabolism changes include reduced hepatic mass (approximately 1% reduction annually after age 40), decreased hepatic blood flow (reducing first-pass metabolism and clearance of flow-limited drugs), and altered activity of specific cytochrome P450 enzymes with variable age-related changes.

Table 12.2: Geriatric Medication Management

Geriatric Challenge	Assessment Tools	Intervention Strategies	Monitoring Approaches
Polypharmacy	Medication appropriateness index, STOPP/START criteria, medication count	Deprescribing protocols, therapeutic duplication elimination, prioritization frameworks	Medication count tracking, functional improvement, symptom resolution monitoring
Potentially Inappropriate Medications	Beers Criteria, STOPP/START, country-specific criteria	Alternative agent selection, dose reduction, risk mitigation strategies	Adverse effect resolution, functional improvement, symptom monitoring
Altered Pharmacokinetics	Cockcroft-Gault with ideal body weight, hepatic function tests, drug levels	Reduced initial doses, extended titration schedules, therapeutic drug monitoring	Concentration monitoring, response assessment, adverse effect vigilance
Altered Pharmacodynamics	Functional assessments, symptom reports, sensitivity indicators	Dose reduction, alternative selections, enhanced monitoring	Response magnitude, side effect emergence, cognitive impact assessment
Adherence Challenges	Pill counts, refill analysis, cognitive assessment, caregiver reports	Regimen simplification, adherence aids, caregiver integration	Adherence rate improvement, therapeutic outcome achievement, caregiver feedback
Falls Risk	Medication fall risk assessment, Timed Up and Go, fall history	High-risk medication reduction, dosage adjustment, non-pharmacologic alternatives	Fall incidence reduction, mobility improvement, fear of falling assessment

Geriatric Challenge	Assessment Tools	Intervention Strategies	Monitoring Approaches
Cognitive Impact	MMSE, Montreal Cognitive Assessment, caregiver reports	Anticholinergic burden reduction, cognitive-friendly alternatives, medication timing	Cognitive function trends, behavior changes, functional independence
Functional Independence	Activities of daily living, instrumental ADLs, functional assessment	Medication burden reduction, function-supporting selections, independence-oriented goals	Functional maintenance/improvement, quality of life measures, independence metrics

Pharmacodynamic Sensitivity Alterations

Increased sensitivity affects multiple drug classes including anticoagulants, cardiovascular agents, psychotropics, and analgesics through receptor density changes, altered signal transduction, and decreased homeostatic reserve creating exaggerated responses despite appropriate dosage adjustments based on pharmacokinetic changes alone. Specific sensitivity changes include enhanced response to central nervous system depressants (benzodiazepines, opioids), increased sensitivity to anticholinergic effects (cognitive impairment, constipation, urinary retention), greater orthostatic hypotension with cardiovascular agents, and enhanced analgesic response to opioids. Homeostatic mechanism impairment reduces compensatory responses to medication effects, including baroreceptor reflex blunting affecting blood pressure regulation, thermoregulatory response reduction, and glucose counter-regulatory mechanism impairment.

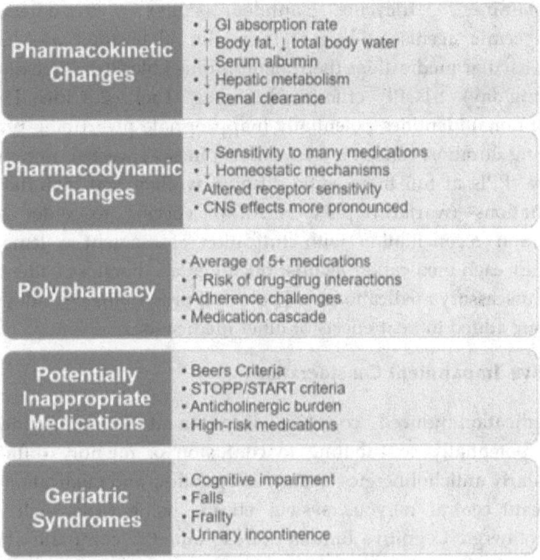

Figure 12.2: Geriatric Pharmacotherapy Considerations

Polypharmacy Management

Medication appropriateness assessment employs structured tools including the Beers Criteria, STOPP/START criteria, and Medication Appropriateness Index to identify potentially inappropriate medications based on age-related risks, drug-disease interactions, and therapeutic duplication, guiding systematic regimen evaluation beyond individual drug assessment. Deprescribing implements systematic approaches to medication discontinuation, including gradual tapering when appropriate, prioritization based on risk-benefit assessment, and monitoring for discontinuation syndromes or disease recurrence, targeting medications with unfavorable risk-benefit profiles, questionable ongoing indication, or minimal benefit relative to treatment burden. Regimen simplification reduces administration complexity through reduced frequency, combination products, and synchronization of administration timing to enhance adherence while reducing cognitive burden.

Potentially Inappropriate Medications (PIMs)

The Beers Criteria identifies medications associated with increased adverse effects in older adults, categorized by strength of evidence and severity of potential harm, including anticholinergics (first-generation antihistamines, tricyclic antidepressants), benzodiazepines, hypoglycemic agents (sliding scale insulin, glyburide), and selected cardiovascular medications (peripheral alpha-1 blockers, digoxin doses >0.125mg/day). STOPP criteria (Screening Tool of Older Person's Prescriptions) identifies potentially inappropriate prescribing practices including duration concerns (benzodiazepines >4 weeks), unnecessary therapy (PPIs at full therapeutic dose >8 weeks), and high-risk drug combinations (warfarin plus NSAIDs) specific to older adults. Medication reconciliation with indication assessment systematically evaluates each medication against documented diagnoses, identifying both unnecessary medications and potential prescribing cascades where drugs are added to treat effects of other medications.

Cognitive Impairment Considerations

Medication-induced cognitive impairment screening identifies agents potentially contributing to confusion or memory difficulties, particularly anticholinergics, sedative-hypnotics, and medications with significant central nervous system effects, using tools such as the Anticholinergic Cognitive Burden Scale to quantify cumulative burden across multiple medications. Adherence support strategies address the challenges of complex medication regimens in patients with memory impairment, including simplified regimens, medication organization systems, caregiver education, and technological reminder approaches ranging from simple pill boxes to electronic dispensing systems with programmable alerts. Pharmacotherapy for dementia implements appropriate agent selection, monitoring for behavioral and cognitive effects, and planned discontinuation when benefits no longer outweigh risks.

Geriatric Syndromes

Fall risk assessment screens medication regimens for agents associated with increased fall risk, including psychotropics (benzodiazepines, antipsychotics, antidepressants), antihypertensives (especially during initiation or dose changes), anticholinergics, and medications affecting alertness or balance, with particular attention to high-risk combinations potentiating fall potential. Urinary incontinence management addresses medications potentially contributing to or exacerbating incontinence, including diuretics (polyuria), anticholinergics (overflow incontinence), and CNS depressants (functional incontinence), while optimizing specific incontinence therapies when appropriate, balancing efficacy against anticholinergic burden and central nervous system effects. Frailty considerations include more conservative approaches to medication selection and dosing for vulnerable older adults with reduced physiological reserve, focusing on essential therapies while minimizing interventions with marginal benefit.

End-of-life and Palliative Considerations

Medication appropriateness reassessment evaluates preventive therapies and chronic disease medications based on time-to-benefit relative to life expectancy, discontinuing interventions unlikely to provide meaningful benefit within the patient's remaining lifespan, including statins for primary prevention, bisphosphonates, and tight glycemic control in advanced illness. Symptom management optimization ensures appropriate palliative medications addressing pain, dyspnea, nausea, anxiety, and other distressing symptoms while minimizing adverse effects, employing careful agent selection and conservative initial dosing with appropriate titration based on response and tolerability. Medication administration route adaptation implements appropriate alternatives when oral administration becomes difficult, including transdermal, sublingual, and parenteral options for essential therapies.

Transitions of Care

Care transition medication reconciliation addresses the high risk of discrepancies during transfers between healthcare settings, with particular attention to high-risk medications, recently changed therapies, and non-prescription products often omitted during transitions, preventing unintentional discontinuation of chronic medications or duplication when home medications are restarted alongside newly prescribed similar agents. Post-discharge follow-up provides continued support during the vulnerable period following hospitalization, addressing new medication questions, adherence challenges, and early adverse effects before serious consequences develop, particularly important for complex regimen changes or cognitively impaired patients with limited comprehension during hospitalization. Communication across settings ensures that medication changes, monitoring requirements, and follow-up plans transfer with the patient between care environments, preventing information gaps that commonly occur during transitions.

PREGNANCY AND LACTATION

The FDA Pregnancy and Lactation Labeling Rule (PLLR) replaced the former letter category system with descriptive risk summaries including available human and animal data, clinical considerations, and specific information regarding risks in different trimesters, requiring more nuanced interpretation beyond the simplified categorization of the previous system. International classification systems including the Australian categorization (A, B1, B2, B3, C, D, X) and European medicine evaluation frameworks provide alternative structured approaches to pregnancy risk evaluation, though all systems require integration with current evidence, individual clinical circumstances, and risk-benefit analysis specific to each maternal-fetal situation. Teratogenic mechanism understanding applies knowledge of critical developmental windows, with organogenesis (approximately weeks 3-8) representing particularly vulnerable periods for structural teratogenesis, while later exposure may affect functional development or growth.

Table 12.3: Pregnancy and Lactation Pharmacotherapy

Pregnancy Phase	Physiological Changes	Medication Considerations	Assessment Approaches
First Trimester (0-13 weeks)	Organogenesis, early placentation, hyperemesis	Teratogenicity risk highest, nausea management, folate needs	Risk category review, necessary vs. elective therapy, alternative considerations
Second Trimester (14-26 weeks)	Increased plasma volume, GFR increase, hepatic changes	Dose adjustments for volume changes, gestational condition emergence	Therapeutic monitoring, dose efficacy assessment, emerging condition management
Third Trimester (27-40 weeks)	Maximal blood volume, altered protein binding, impending delivery	Delivery considerations, dose increases, neonatal effect planning	Term proximity considerations, labor impact assessment, postpartum planning
Lactation Period	Milk production, maternal recovery, infant exposure	Milk transfer estimation, infant risk assessment, maternal need balancing	M:P ratio evaluation, infant age/health consideration

Maternal Pharmacokinetic Alterations

Absorption changes include delayed gastric emptying, reduced gastric acid secretion, and increased gastric mucus production affecting drug dissolution and uptake, potentially reducing rate but not extent of absorption for many medications. Distribution alterations include expanded plasma volume (30-50% increase), reduced plasma protein concentrations affecting drug binding, development of the maternal-placental-fetal unit creating an additional compartment, and increased total body water affecting concentration of hydrophilic medications requiring dosage adjustment for some therapeutic agents. Metabolism changes include altered hepatic enzyme activity with some pathways enhanced (CYP3A4, CYP2D6, UGT) and others reduced, producing variable effects on medication clearance throughout pregnancy, with most significant changes occurring in the third trimester requiring potential dose adjustments for medications with narrow therapeutic indices.

Category	Description
A	Adequate, well-controlled studies in pregnant women have not shown increased risk of fetal abnormalities.
B	Animal studies show no risk, but no adequate human studies; OR animal studies showed adverse effect not confirmed in human studies.
C	Animal studies show adverse effects, human studies inadequate; OR no animal or human studies. Potential benefits may justify potential risks.
D	Evidence of human fetal risk, but potential benefits may outweigh risks in serious situations where safer drugs ineffective.
X	Studies in animals or humans demonstrate fetal abnormalities or evidence of fetal risk. Risks clearly outweigh potential benefits.
Lactation	Key factors: Infant age, medication properties (protein binding, lipophilicity, half-life), milk:plasma ratio, maternal dose, and relative infant dose.

Figure 12.3: FDA Pregnancy Risk Categories & Lactation Considerations

Placental Transfer Mechanisms

Molecular characteristics affecting transfer include medication size (molecules <500 Daltons cross more readily), lipid solubility (lipophilic compounds transfer more extensively), protein binding (highly bound medications have reduced transfer), and ionization state (un-ionized forms cross more readily). Placental transport proteins including P-glycoprotein actively transport some medications back to maternal circulation, providing partial protection against fetal exposure, though this mechanism saturates at higher maternal concentrations and varies in efficiency throughout pregnancy. Developmental timing significantly influences risk, with different vulnerable periods for various organ systems and developmental processes, creating windows of specific concern depending on medication mechanism and fetal developmental stage during exposure.

Chronic Disease Management During Pregnancy

Hypertension management employs preferred agents including labetalol, nifedipine, and methyldopa with established safety profiles, while avoiding ACE inhibitors and ARBs due to established fetal risks including renal dysgenesis, oligohydramnios, and growth restriction, particularly in the second and third trimesters. Diabetes control implements insulin as primary therapy with select oral agents including metformin and glyburide as alternatives in specific situations, emphasizing tighter glycemic targets than non-pregnant patients (fasting <95 mg/dL, 1-hour postprandial <140 mg/dL, 2-hour postprandial <120 mg/dL) while avoiding hypoglycemia. Psychiatric disorder treatment maintains therapy for significant maternal conditions while selecting preferred agents with better-established safety profiles, including sertraline among SSRIs and lamotrigine among anticonvulsants used for mood stabilization, recognizing that untreated maternal mental illness poses significant risks to both mother and developing fetus.

Pregnancy-Specific Conditions

Nausea and vomiting of pregnancy (including hyperemesis gravidarum) management employs a stepwise approach beginning with pyridoxine (vitamin B6, 10-25mg three to four times daily) and doxylamine (12.5mg three to four times daily), progressing through phenothiazines, serotonin antagonists, and in severe cases, corticosteroids or total parenteral nutrition. Preeclampsia prevention and management includes low-dose aspirin prophylaxis (81mg daily) for high-risk women, magnesium sulfate for seizure prevention in established disease (4-6g loading dose followed by 1-2g/hour continuous infusion), and antihypertensive therapy for severe hypertension (systolic ≥160 mmHg or diastolic ≥110 mmHg). Preterm labor interventions include tocolytic agents for short-term delay allowing corticosteroid administration and maternal transfer when appropriate, with careful agent selection based on maternal comorbidities and gestational age.

Lactation Pharmacokinetics

Milk transfer mechanisms include passive diffusion of un-ionized, lipophilic medications and active transport through epithelial cells for some compounds and nutrients, with concentration in milk determined by maternal plasma level, medication characteristics, and breast tissue properties. The milk-to-plasma ratio expresses the relationship between drug concentration in milk relative to maternal plasma, though this static ratio inadequately represents the dynamic process of transfer over time and may vary with changes in maternal plasma levels throughout the dosing interval. Infant dose estimation calculates potential exposure through milk consumption volume (approximately 150 mL/kg/day) multiplied by medication concentration, with relative infant dose below 10% of maternal weight-adjusted dose generally considered acceptable for most medications.

Alternative Therapeutic Approaches

Medication selection prioritizes agents with established safety data, more favorable placental transfer characteristics, or reduced milk excretion depending on the reproductive stage, selecting medications with longer post-marketing experience and more extensive pregnancy registry data when multiple therapeutic options exist. Timing optimization spaces medication administration relative to breastfeeding sessions to minimize infant exposure, particularly for medications with short half-lives allowing strategic timing at typical feeding intervals, administering doses immediately after feeding or before the longest sleep interval to minimize peak concentration exposure. Non-pharmacological alternatives receive particular emphasis during pregnancy and lactation, including physical therapy, dietary modifications, and psychological interventions when appropriate for the condition.

Teratogen Information Services

MotherToBaby (formerly Organization of Teratology Information Specialists) offers free telephone consultation services with specialists in pregnancy and lactation pharmacology and teratology, providing evidence-based risk assessments for medication exposures during pregnancy and breastfeeding. Teratogen information databases including REPROTOX, Shepard's Catalog of Teratogenic Agents, and TERIS provide evidence summaries with risk evaluations based on available human and animal data, offering more comprehensive assessments than general drug information resources. Pregnancy registries collect prospective observational data on medication exposures during pregnancy, providing critical information on newer agents with limited published literature, with healthcare providers encouraged to enroll pregnant patients taking medications with established registries to expand the evidence base.

RENAL IMPAIRMENT

Kidney Function Assessment

Estimation method selection evaluates the relative utility of different kidney function calculations in specific clinical scenarios, including Cockcroft-Gault for traditional medication dosing, MDRD or CKD-EPI equations for staging chronic kidney disease, and measured creatinine clearance for high-risk situations requiring maximal precision. Body size adjustment addresses challenges in non-standard body habitus, with actual body weight typically used for underweight patients, while adjusted or ideal body weight may be more appropriate for obese individuals depending on the specific medication, recognizing that muscle mass significantly affects creatinine-based estimates. Dynamic assessment recognizes the fluctuating nature of kidney function in acute kidney injury, requiring frequent reassessment and dosage readjustment as renal function changes, potentially employing shorter dosing intervals with reassessment rather than extended modifications appropriate for stable chronic kidney disease.

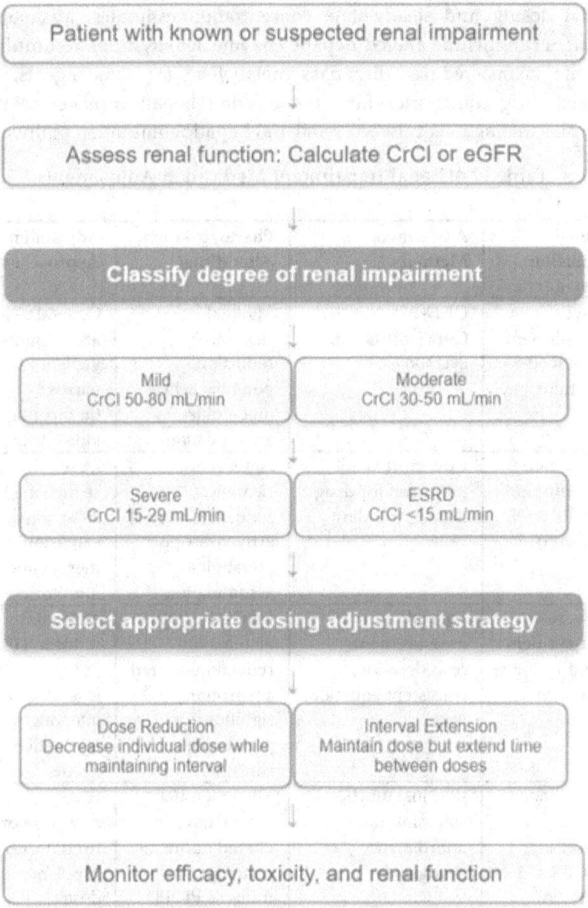

Figure 12.4: Medication Adjustment in Renal Impairment

Pharmacokinetic Alterations in Kidney Disease

Absorption changes may include altered gastric pH from uremia, phosphate binder interactions affecting drug availability, and edema affecting subcutaneous or intramuscular absorption, creating variable and sometimes unpredictable effects on medication uptake. Distribution alterations include reduced protein binding due to hypoalbuminemia and accumulated uremic toxins displacing medications from binding sites, altered tissue penetration from edema, and variable volume of distribution changes depending on fluid status, collectively affecting initial dosing and steady-state concentration estimates. Metabolism changes can include altered hepatic enzyme activity from accumulated uremic toxins, reduced first-pass metabolism for some agents, and altered drug transporter function affecting hepatic uptake, creating complex interactions between renal and hepatic elimination pathways.

Table 12.4: Renal Impairment Medication Adjustments

Renal Function Category	Assessment Methods	Pharmacokinetic Alterations	Adjustment Approaches
Mild Impairment (eGFR 60-89 ml/min)	CKD-EPI, Cockcroft-Gault, cystatin C	Minimal clearance reduction, potential active metabolite accumulation	Generally no adjustments, vigilance for narrow therapeutic index drugs
Moderate Impairment (eGFR 30-59 ml/min)	Cockcroft-Gault preferred for drug dosing, trending values	Significant clearance reduction, altered active transport, metabolite accumulation	Dose reduction (25-50%), interval extension, therapeutic monitoring
Severe Impairment (eGFR 15-29 ml/min)	Formal measurement consideration, consistent equation use	Marked elimination reduction, altered absorption, significant metabolite concerns	Major dose reduction (50-75%), extended intervals, alternative agents
End-Stage Renal Disease (eGFR <15 ml/min)	Residual function assessment, interdialytic changes	Minimal renal elimination, altered nonrenal clearance, multiple PK/PD changes	Severe reduction or fixed dosing, supplemental doses, alternative pathways
Renal Replacement Therapy	Modality characteristics, frequency/duration, filter properties	Extracorporeal clearance, session-related fluctuations, modality-specific removal	Supplemental post-dialysis doses, continuous therapy adjustments, timing strategies

Dosage Adjustment Methodologies

Dose reduction maintains the standard dosing interval while decreasing the amount administered, appropriate for medications where maintaining consistent blood levels is therapeutically important including many antimicrobials, anticonvulsants, and cardiovascular agents. Interval extension maintains the standard dose while increasing the time between administrations, suitable for medications with wider therapeutic indices where peak concentrations drive efficacy but trough accumulation creates toxicity concerns. Combined approaches adjust both dose and interval for medications requiring significant modification in severe renal impairment, balancing efficacy requirements against accumulation risks through individualized regimen design rather than applying standard formulas. Loading dose considerations address the need for normal initial doses regardless of renal function when rapid therapeutic concentrations are required, with subsequent maintenance doses adjusted for impaired elimination.

Medication Selection Modifications

Nephrotoxicity risk assessment evaluates mechanisms including direct tubular toxicity (aminoglycosides, cisplatin), crystal-induced injury (acyclovir, indinavir), hemodynamic alterations (NSAIDs, ACE inhibitors), and immune-mediated damage (drug-induced interstitial nephritis) to identify high-risk medications requiring avoidance or intensive monitoring. Alternative therapy selection identifies medications with predominantly non-renal clearance pathways when therapeutic alternatives exist within classes, such as selecting rosuvastatin over atorvastatin, ceftriaxone over cefazolin, or tramadol over morphine for patients with significant renal impairment. Renal-hepatic interplay consideration addresses situations where kidney disease affects hepatic metabolism through enzyme inhibition from accumulated uremic toxins, potentially altering clearance of medications traditionally considered "hepatically cleared" including propranolol, diazepam, or carvedilol.

Electrolyte and Acid-Base Management

Hyperkalemia management employs both acute interventions for dangerous elevations (calcium gluconate for membrane stabilization, insulin with glucose for intracellular potassium shifting, sodium bicarbonate for metabolic acidosis contribution) and chronic prevention strategies including medication adjustment, dietary modification, and binding agents when appropriate. Metabolic acidosis correction balances the risks of uncorrected acidemia against potential complications from alkali therapy, with particular attention to sodium content of correction agents in fluid-sensitive patients, employing sodium bicarbonate supplementation with dosing based on bicarbonate deficit calculation and ongoing acid production estimates. Bone and mineral disorder management addresses calcium, phosphorus, vitamin

D, and parathyroid hormone disturbances through integrated pharmacological approaches aligned with disease stage and biochemical parameters, including phosphate binders, vitamin D analogs, and calcimimetics.

Hemodialysis Considerations

Dialyzability assessment evaluates medication characteristics affecting removal during hemodialysis, including molecular weight (<500 Da more readily removed), protein binding (<80% binding increases removal), volume of distribution (<0.7 L/kg more significantly affected), and existing clinical dialysis data guiding therapy adjustments. Supplemental dosing implements appropriate post-dialysis administration for significantly removed medications, replacing the eliminated portion to maintain therapeutic concentrations, commonly required for antimicrobials including vancomycin, cefazolin, and meropenem after standard hemodialysis sessions. Administration timing relative to dialysis sessions optimizes therapy by scheduling highly dialyzable medications after treatment while positioning medications used to treat dialysis complications (antihypertensives, antiemetics) before sessions.

Continuous Renal Replacement Therapy (CRRT)

Clearance estimation considers the specific CRRT modality (CVVH, CVVHD, CVVHDF), effluent flow rate, blood flow rate, and filter characteristics to approximate the effective clearance for medication adjustment purposes, typically resulting in clearance between 25-50 mL/min depending on specific parameters. Dosing strategy implementation typically employs approaches intermediate between normal kidney function and conventional hemodialysis adjustments, recognizing the continuous but less efficient nature of these therapies compared to intermittent hemodialysis, often requiring higher doses or shorter intervals than would be used for similar GFR values in chronic kidney disease. CRRT-specific considerations include adsorption to filter materials, saturation of removal mechanisms over time, and potential for significant removal of highly water-soluble, minimally protein-bound medications regardless of molecular size.

Comorbidity Management

Cardiovascular disease approaches balance cardiac medication benefits against altered pharmacokinetics and increased adverse effect vulnerability, with particular attention to antihypertensives (reduced dosing, careful monitoring for hypotension), anticoagulants (reduced dosing for renally eliminated agents including enoxaparin, direct oral anticoagulants), and lipid-lowering therapies (dose limitations for statins, fibrates). Diabetes management adapts glycemic targets and agent selection based on kidney disease stage, with progressively fewer medication options and increased hypoglycemia risk as renal function declines, typically transitioning from metformin and sulfonylureas in early stages to insulin and dipeptidyl peptidase-4 inhibitors in advanced disease. Infectious disease treatment implements appropriate antimicrobial selection and dosing while considering both reduced elimination and increased susceptibility to adverse effects in the uremic patient.

HEPATIC DYSFUNCTION

Classification systems including Child-Pugh (categorizing dysfunction as Class A, B, or C based on bilirubin, albumin, INR, ascites, and encephalopathy) and MELD (Model for End-stage Liver Disease, using bilirubin, creatinine, INR, and etiology) provide structured approaches to severity assessment guiding empiric dosage adjustments when specific guidelines are unavailable. Laboratory parameter interpretation recognizes the significance of specific markers including transaminases (indicating hepatocellular injury), alkaline phosphatase and GGT (reflecting cholestatic patterns), bilirubin (measuring excretory function), albumin and coagulation factors (assessing synthetic function), and ammonia (related to metabolic capacity). Etiology consideration acknowledges different functional implications of various liver diseases, with conditions including alcoholic hepatitis, viral hepatitis, cirrhosis, and medication-induced injury affecting different hepatic functions to variable degrees.

Pharmacokinetic Alterations in Liver Disease

Absorption changes include altered gastrointestinal transit time, reduced first-pass extraction for highly metabolized drugs potentially increasing bioavailability up to 5-fold for some medications (propranolol, morphine, midazolam), and decreased bile production affecting fat-soluble vitamin and medication absorption. Distribution alterations include reduced albumin synthesis affecting protein binding (particularly significant for highly bound drugs including phenytoin, warfarin, valproic acid), expanded extracellular fluid volume from ascites and edema, and potentially altered blood-brain barrier permeability increasing CNS effects of some medications. Metabolism reductions affect phase I reactions (particularly oxidation, reduction, and hydrolysis) to a greater extent than phase II processes (conjugation), with specific cytochrome P450 enzyme activities declining at variable rates and to different degrees depending on liver disease etiology and severity.

Table 12.5: Hepatic Dysfunction Medication Management

Hepatic Status	Assessment Methods	Pharmacokinetic/Pharmacodynamic Effects
Mild Hepatic Impairment (Child-Pugh A)	Child-Pugh score 5-6, albumin, bilirubin, PT/INR	Mild metabolic reduction, potential protein binding changes
Moderate Hepatic Impairment (Child-Pugh B)	Child-Pugh score 7-9, MELD score consideration	Significant metabolic reduction, altered first-pass, protein binding reduction
Severe Hepatic Impairment (Child-Pugh C)	Child-Pugh score 10-15, MELD score, synthetic function tests	Severe metabolic impairment, significant bioavailability changes, multiple PK alterations
Acute Liver Injury	Liver enzyme trends, hepatocellular vs. cholestatic pattern, R factor	Rapidly changing metabolism, unpredictable alterations, temporary effects
Cirrhosis with Portal Hypertension	HVPG measurement, varices presence, ascites assessment	Altered drug distribution, portosystemic shunting, decreased first-pass effect

Dosage Adjustment Methodologies

Initial dose reduction addresses both altered pharmacokinetics and increased pharmacodynamic sensitivity common in liver disease, with typical recommendations of 25-50% reduction for Child-Pugh Class B and 50-75% reduction for Class C when specific guidelines are unavailable, particularly important for medications with significant hepatic metabolism or narrow therapeutic indices. Maintenance dose titration employs conservative approaches with close monitoring of both therapeutic and adverse effects, recognizing the significant inter-individual variability in hepatic dysfunction's impact on drug disposition, using more frequent reassessment and smaller adjustment increments than typically employed in patients with normal hepatic function. Interval adjustment considers prolonged half-lives of hepatically cleared medications, though used less commonly than dose reduction due to the complex and variable effects of liver disease on elimination.

Medication Selection Modifications

Hepatotoxicity risk assessment evaluates mechanisms including direct hepatocellular injury (acetaminophen, isoniazid), cholestatic patterns (amoxicillin-clavulanate, erythromycin), mitochondrial dysfunction (valproic acid, nucleoside reverse transcriptase inhibitors), and immune-mediated damage (phenytoin, sulfonamides) to identify high-risk medications requiring avoidance or intensive monitoring. Alternative therapy selection identifies medications with predominantly non-hepatic clearance pathways when therapeutic alternatives exist within classes, though recognizing that renal function may also be compromised in advanced liver disease (hepatorenal syndrome) limiting options with predominantly renal elimination. Formulation considerations include transdermal, sublingual, or parenteral routes that bypass first-pass metabolism when appropriate for specific agents with high hepatic extraction ratios, potentially requiring lower doses than typically employed for oral administration of the same agent.

Specific Medication Classes

Sedative and analgesic management employs conservative dosing of benzodiazepines, opioids, and other CNS depressants with high hepatic metabolism, while avoiding agents with toxic metabolites including meperidine (normeperidine accumulation) and morphine (potential morphine-6-glucuronide accumulation with concurrent renal impairment). Antimicrobial therapy addresses both altered pharmacokinetics of hepatically metabolized agents and potential for increased toxicity with agents having known hepatotoxic potential, requiring careful selection and monitoring particularly for antifungals (azoles), macrolides, rifamycins, and anti-tuberculosis medications. Cardiovascular medication adjustment considers reduced metabolism of beta-blockers (particularly propranolol, metoprolol, carvedilol), calcium channel blockers, and antiarrhythmics alongside hemodynamic alterations from portal hypertension affecting cardiovascular medication response.

Complication Management

Hepatic encephalopathy management employs ammonia-reducing strategies including lactulose (titrated to 2-3 soft bowel movements daily) and rifaximin (550mg twice daily), with careful avoidance of CNS depressants and attention to precipitating factors including medications, constipation, and electrolyte disturbances exacerbating neurological dysfunction. Ascites and edema treatment balances diuretic therapy effectiveness against risks of electrolyte disturbances, renal insufficiency, and encephalopathy exacerbation, typically employing spironolactone (starting 100mg daily, maximum 400mg daily) with or without furosemide (starting 40mg daily) at ratios maintaining sodium:potassium homeostasis. Coagulopathy considerations address both bleeding risk from reduced clotting factor synthesis and potential for thrombosis despite elevated INR due to concurrent reduction in anticoagulant proteins, requiring nuanced approaches to anticoagulation and procedural bleeding risk management.

Portal Hypertension Sequelae

Non-selective beta-blocker therapy employs propranolol or nadolol with careful dosage adjustment and monitoring for hemodynamic consequences, targeting heart rate reduction of 25% from baseline or maximum tolerated dose, demonstrating approximately 10-20% reduction in variceal bleeding risk through portal pressure reduction. Variceal bleeding management includes acute interventions with vasopressin analogs (terlipressin) and somatostatin derivatives (octreotide) alongside appropriate blood product support and infection prophylaxis with third-generation cephalosporins or fluoroquinolones reducing rebleeding and mortality. Secondary prophylaxis combines pharmacological approaches with endoscopic management to prevent recurrent bleeding following initial episodes, employing non-selective beta-blockers in combination with endoscopic band ligation for optimal risk reduction.

Liver Transplant Considerations

Pre-transplant optimization focuses on preventing further hepatic decompensation while managing complications and maintaining candidacy for transplantation through appropriate medication selection and monitoring, avoiding hepatotoxic agents while optimizing management of encephalopathy, ascites, and nutritional status. Immunosuppression management following transplantation implements complex regimens of calcineurin inhibitors (tacrolimus, cyclosporine), antimetabolites (mycophenolate), and corticosteroids with attention to numerous drug interactions, narrow therapeutic indices, and monitoring requirements including therapeutic drug monitoring and surveillance for specific toxicities. Rejection and infection prevention balances adequate immunosuppression against opportunistic infection risk through appropriate prophylactic regimens and monitoring strategies.

Summary

- Pediatric pharmacy care requires specialized knowledge of age-appropriate dosing, medication formulations, pharmacokinetic differences, growth and developmental considerations, and weight-based calculations.

- Geriatric pharmacy practice focuses on addressing polypharmacy, reducing inappropriate medications, managing drug-disease interactions, and adapting therapy to age-related physiological changes.

- Medication management during pregnancy and lactation requires balancing maternal benefit against fetal or infant risk using pregnancy category systems and lactation safety data.

- Patients with renal impairment need medication regimen adjustments based on kidney function, including dose reductions, interval extensions, and avoidance of nephrotoxic agents.

- Hepatic dysfunction necessitates special consideration for drugs with extensive hepatic metabolism, monitoring for drug-induced liver injury, and dose adjustments based on Child-Pugh classification.

- Genetic factors affecting drug response require pharmacogenomic considerations for medications with known genetic influences on metabolism, efficacy, or adverse effects.

- Culturally responsive care for diverse populations addresses language barriers, health beliefs, traditional practices, and social determinants that influence medication use patterns and outcomes.

Multiple Choice Questions

1. Which of the following is the MOST appropriate approach to weight-based dosing in pediatric patients?
   A) Always using ideal body weight for all medications
   B) Using total body weight for all medications
   C) Selecting the appropriate weight measure based on the drug's properties
   D) Using body surface area exclusively for all medications
2. When reviewing medication therapy for an 85-year-old patient, which of the following represents the BEST approach?
   A) Discontinuing all potentially inappropriate medications based on age alone
   B) Applying Beers Criteria while considering the individual risk-benefit assessment
   C) Maintaining all medications if the patient has been stable
   D) Switching all medications to geriatric-specific formulations
3. A pregnant patient in her first trimester needs treatment for bacterial pneumonia. The MOST appropriate approach would be to:
   A) Withhold all antibiotics due to universal teratogenic risk
   B) Select an antibiotic with established safety data in pregnancy
   C) Use the same antibiotic as would be used for non-pregnant patients
   D) Delay treatment until the second trimester when risks are lower
4. For a patient with estimated GFR of 25 mL/min, which of the following is the MOST appropriate approach to medication management?
   A) Discontinuing all renally cleared medications
   B) Reducing doses of renally cleared drugs and monitoring closely
   C) Using standard doses but increasing monitoring frequency
   D) Switching all medications to hepatically cleared alternatives
5. A patient with Child-Pugh Class C cirrhosis is prescribed a medication that is highly protein-bound and hepatically metabolized. The MOST appropriate intervention would be:
   A) Recommending standard doses with standard monitoring
   B) Suggesting a significant dose reduction with careful titration

C) Recommending against using the medication entirely

D) Increasing the dose to account for reduced bioavailability

6. Which of the following represents the MOST significant concern when managing medications for a 3-month-old infant?

   A) Risk of tablet aspiration

   B) Immature hepatic and renal function affecting drug clearance

   C) Ability to swallow capsules

   D) Medication adherence issues

7. When assessing medication appropriateness for an elderly patient, which of the following criteria would be MOST useful?

   A) Pediatric dosing guidelines

   B) Pregnancy risk categories

   C) STOPP/START criteria

   D) Standard adult dosing references

8. For a breastfeeding mother who requires medication therapy, the MOST appropriate approach is to:

   A) Discontinue breastfeeding for all medication use

   B) Evaluate the medication's milk-to-plasma ratio and infant exposure risk

   C) Time all medications immediately after breastfeeding

   D) Use only medications that are also approved for pediatric use

9. A patient with hepatorenal syndrome requires multiple medications. The MOST appropriate approach to medication management would be:

   A) Avoiding all medications until organ function improves

   B) Using standard doses but monitoring more frequently

   C) Careful selection and dosing adjustment based on both hepatic and renal parameters

   D) Focusing exclusively on renal function for dosing adjustments

10. For a pediatric patient requiring an antibiotic that lacks pediatric dosing information, the MOST appropriate approach would be:

   A) Using adult doses adjusted proportionally by weight

   B) Consulting pediatric references, specialists, and considering age-based physiologic factors

   C) Avoiding use of the medication regardless of need

D) Using 50% of the adult dose regardless of the child's age or weight

Self-Assessment Questions

1. Explain three key physiological differences between pediatric and adult patients that impact medication therapy, and how these differences affect dosing approaches.
2. Describe the major age-related physiological changes in geriatric patients and how these changes affect pharmacokinetics and pharmacodynamics.
3. Explain the considerations for medication use during pregnancy, including the limitations of pregnancy risk categories and current approaches to risk assessment.
4. Discuss three strategies for medication therapy management in patients with end-stage renal disease on dialysis, including specific considerations for drug dosing.
5. Explain how pharmacists should approach medication therapy in patients with hepatic cirrhosis, including assessment methods and dosing considerations.
6. Describe three medication safety concerns specific to pediatric patients and appropriate strategies to prevent medication errors in this population.
7. Discuss the application of the Beers Criteria and STOPP/START criteria in optimizing medication therapy for geriatric patients.
8. Explain how medication therapy should be managed during the different trimesters of pregnancy and considerations for breastfeeding mothers.
9. Describe how drug dosing should be adjusted in patients with acute kidney injury versus chronic kidney disease, including monitoring parameters.
10. Discuss the pharmacist's role in identifying and preventing drug-induced liver injury, including risk assessment and monitoring strategies.

Bibliography

1. Kearns GL, Abdel-Rahman SM, Alander SW, Blowey DL, Leeder JS, Kauffman RE. Developmental pharmacology—drug disposition, action, and therapy in infants and children. N Engl J Med. 2003;349(12):1157-1167.
2. American Geriatrics Society Beers Criteria Update Expert Panel. American Geriatrics Society 2019 updated AGS Beers Criteria for potentially inappropriate medication use in older adults. J Am Geriatr Soc. 2019;67(4):674-694.
3. Koren G, Pastuszak A, Ito S. Drugs in pregnancy. N Engl J Med. 1998;338(16):1128-1137.
4. Sachs HC; Committee on Drugs. The transfer of drugs and therapeutics into human breast milk: an update on selected topics. Pediatrics. 2013;132(3):e796-e809.
5. Matzke GR, Aronoff GR, Atkinson AJ Jr, Bennett WM, Decker BS, Eckardt KU, et al. Drug dosing consideration in patients with acute and chronic kidney disease—a clinical update from Kidney Disease: Improving Global Outcomes (KDIGO). Kidney Int. 2011;80(11):1122-1137.
6. Verbeeck RK. Pharmacokinetics and dosage adjustment in patients with hepatic dysfunction. Eur J Clin Pharmacol. 2008;64(12):1147-1161.
7. van den Anker J, Reed MD, Allegaert K, Kearns GL. Developmental changes in pharmacokinetics and pharmacodynamics. J Clin Pharmacol. 2018;58(Suppl 10):S10-S25.
8. O'Mahony D, O'Sullivan D, Byrne S, O'Connor MN, Ryan C, Gallagher P. STOPP/START criteria for potentially inappropriate prescribing in older people: version 2. Age Ageing. 2015;44(2):213-218.
9. Brouwer KLR, Aleksunes LM, Brandys B, Giacoia GP, Knipp G, Lukacova V, et al. Human ontogeny of drug transporters: review and recommendations of the Pediatric Transporter Working Group. Clin Pharmacol Ther. 2015;98(3):266-287.
10. Qato DM, Alexander GC, Conti RM, Johnson M, Schumm P, Lindau ST. Use of prescription and over-the-counter medications and dietary supplements among older adults in the United States. JAMA. 2008;300(24):2867-2878.

CHAPTER 13

DISEASE MANAGEMENT

Author

Mrs. Indumathy Vemanna, Assistant Professor, PG & Research Department of Biochemistry, Theivanai Ammal College for Women(A), Villupuram, Tamil Nadu, India

Abstract

Disease management applies comprehensive, evidence-based approaches to optimize medication therapy across major therapeutic areas through systematic assessment, intervention, and monitoring strategies. Cardiovascular disorder management encompasses hypertension, dyslipidemia, heart failure, anticoagulation, and coronary syndromes through guideline-directed medication selection, risk stratification, and monitoring protocols addressing both symptomatic control and outcome modification. Endocrine disorder approaches optimize diabetes mellitus, thyroid conditions, adrenal disorders, and metabolic bone diseases through medication regimen individualization, monitoring parameter selection, and complication prevention strategies addressing complex hormonal interactions. Respiratory condition management addresses asthma, COPD, pulmonary infections, and sleep-disordered breathing through appropriate controller and rescue medication selection, device technique optimization, and exacerbation prevention protocols. Infectious disease therapy implements antimicrobial stewardship principles, empiric therapy selection, de-escalation protocols, and transition strategies across bacterial, viral, and fungal infections balancing effective pathogen eradication with resistance prevention. Oncology management encompasses chemotherapy optimization, targeted therapy selection, immunotherapy monitoring, and supportive care integration through molecular biomarker utilization and complex regimen management. Mental health approaches address depression, bipolar disorder, schizophrenia, anxiety, and substance use disorders through appropriate medication selection, therapeutic monitoring, and adherence support addressing both symptomatic control and functional improvement. This systematic approach enables optimal medication management across diverse disease states through specialized therapeutic knowledge and patient-centered application.

Keywords: *Pharmacotherapeutics, Guideline Implementation, Therapy Optimization, Disease Modification, Treatment Algorithms*

Learning Objectives

After completion of the chapter, the learners should be able to:

- Implement evidence-based pharmacotherapy for cardiovascular disorders including hypertension, heart failure, dyslipidemia, and arrhythmias through guideline-directed medical therapy.
- Optimize medication management for endocrine disorders including diabetes mellitus, thyroid conditions, and metabolic bone disease using appropriate therapeutic algorithms.
- Develop comprehensive treatment approaches for respiratory conditions including asthma, COPD, and pulmonary infections addressing both maintenance therapy and exacerbation management.
- Apply antimicrobial stewardship principles to infectious disease management including appropriate empiric selection, de-escalation, and duration optimization.
- Implement specialized medication management strategies for oncology patients including chemotherapy protocols, targeted therapy monitoring, and supportive care optimization.
- Develop therapeutic approaches for mental health conditions including appropriate medication selection, monitoring, and adherence support for depression, anxiety, and serious mental illness.

CARDIOVASCULAR DISORDERS

Hypertension

Initial assessment evaluates secondary causes, target organ damage, and cardiovascular risk factors to establish appropriate treatment goals, typically <130/80 mmHg for most patients based on current guidelines, with consideration of individualized targets for elderly patients (sometimes accepting <140/90 mmHg) or those with significant orthostatic tendencies. First-line agent selection emphasizes thiazide diuretics (chlorthalidone preferred over hydrochlorothiazide due to longer duration of action), ACE inhibitors/ARBs (particularly for those with diabetes, chronic kidney disease, or heart failure), and calcium channel blockers based on compelling indications, demographic considerations, and comorbidities. Combination therapy strategies address resistant hypertension through rational multi-drug approaches addressing complementary mechanisms rather than simply maximizing single-agent doses, with fixed-dose combinations improving adherence compared to multiple individual prescriptions.

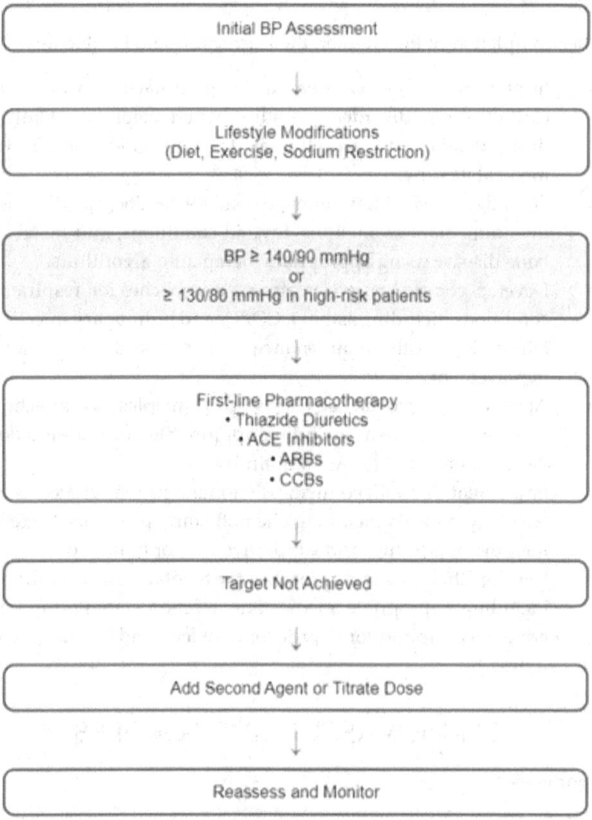

Figure 13.1: Hypertension Management Algorithm

Dyslipidemia

Risk assessment employs validated calculators including the Pooled Cohort Equations to estimate 10-year ASCVD risk, guiding intensity of intervention and treatment goals, with primary prevention typically recommended for those with ≥7.5% 10-year risk plus risk-enhancing factors or ≥20% risk regardless of additional factors. Statin therapy optimization implements appropriate intensity selection based on risk category, with high-intensity statins (atorvastatin 40-80mg, rosuvastatin 20-40mg) for established ASCVD or highest-risk primary prevention, and moderate-intensity statins for intermediate-risk categories, targeting specific LDL reduction percentages (≥50% for high-intensity, 30-49% for moderate-intensity) rather than arbitrary numerical goals.

Non-statin therapy integration addresses residual risk or statin intolerance through evidence-based agents including ezetimibe (10mg daily), PCSK9 inhibitors (evolocumab 140mg every 2 weeks or alirocumab 75-150mg every 2 weeks), bempedoic acid, and icosapent ethyl (4g daily).

Table 13.1: Management of Cardiovascular Disorders

Cardiovascular Condition	Assessment Parameters	Evidence-Based Pharmacotherapy	Monitoring Approach
Hypertension	BP measurement (technique, timing, device), TOD assessment, comorbidity evaluation	ACEI/ARB, CCB, thiazide diuretics, beta-blockers per guideline algorithms	BP target achievement, TOD regression, adverse effect monitoring, adherence assessment
Heart Failure with Reduced EF	NYHA class, volume status, ejection fraction, biomarkers	GDMT (ACEI/ARB/ARNI, beta-blocker, MRA, SGLT2i), diuretics, digoxin, ivabradine	Symptom improvement, hospitalization reduction, biomarker trends, ejection fraction changes
Heart Failure with Preserved EF	Diastolic function, volume status, exercise capacity	Diuretics, blood pressure control, comorbidity management, potentially SGLT2i	Volume status, symptom control, exercise tolerance, hospitalization prevention
Atrial Fibrillation	Rhythm assessment, rate control, stroke risk (CHA_2DS_2-VASc), bleeding risk (HAS-BLED)	Rate control (beta-blockers, CCB, digoxin), rhythm control (antiarrhythmics), anticoagulation	Rate control adequacy, rhythm maintenance, stroke prevention, bleeding avoidance
Coronary Artery Disease	Angina classification, risk factor profile, ischemic burden	Antiplatelet therapy, statins, beta-blockers, nitrates, antianginals	Symptom control, event prevention, risk factor modification, revascularization need

Cardiovascular Condition	Assessment Parameters	Evidence-Based Pharmacotherapy	Monitoring Approach
Dyslipidemia	Lipid panel, ASCVD risk assessment, secondary causes	Statins (intensity based on risk), ezetimibe, PCSK9 inhibitors, other agents	LDL-C reduction goals, ASCVD event prevention, muscle symptoms, liver function
Thromboembolic Disease	VTE risk assessment, bleeding risk, recurrence risk	Anticoagulant selection (DOAC vs. warfarin), duration determination, intensity selection	Clot resolution, recurrence prevention, bleeding avoidance, therapeutic levels if applicable
Peripheral Artery Disease	Functional classification, ABI measurement, symptom assessment	Antiplatelet therapy, statins, cilostazol, risk factor modification	Symptom improvement, walking distance, limb preservation, cardiovascular risk reduction

Heart Failure Management

Stage A/B intervention (patients at risk or with structural heart disease without symptoms) emphasizes risk factor control and neurohormonal blockade to prevent progression, including blood pressure management, diabetes control, and ACE inhibitor/ARB therapy for those with reduced ejection fraction regardless of symptom status. Stage C therapy (symptomatic heart failure) implements comprehensive regimens including RAAS inhibitors (ACE inhibitors, ARBs, or sacubitril/valsartan), beta-blockers (carvedilol, metoprolol succinate, or bisoprolol), aldosterone antagonists (spironolactone or eplerenone), and SGLT2 inhibitors for reduced ejection fraction, with different approaches for preserved ejection fraction focusing on symptom management and comorbidity control. Volume status optimization balances diuretic therapy against electrolyte stability and renal function, with flexible dosing strategies based on congestion assessment including daily weight monitoring, symptom evaluation, and physical examination findings.

Anticoagulation Management

Atrial fibrillation stroke prevention employs risk stratification using CHA_2DS_2-VASc scoring to identify appropriate candidates for anticoagulation (generally recommended for scores ≥2 in men or ≥3 in women), with agent selection between warfarin (target INR 2-3) and direct oral anticoagulants (apixaban, dabigatran, edoxaban, rivaroxaban) based on specific patient factors including renal function, drug interactions, and cost considerations. Venous thromboembolism management implements appropriate acute treatment and secondary prevention durations based on event characteristics, provocation status, and bleeding risk assessment, with provoked events typically treated for 3 months, first unprovoked events for at least 6-12 months, and recurrent unprovoked events often receiving indefinite therapy. Periprocedural management develops bridge therapy protocols addressing thromboembolic risk during temporary anticoagulation interruptions, stratifying patients into low, moderate, and high risk categories with corresponding strategies ranging from simple interruption to full-dose parenteral bridging.

Acute Coronary Syndrome Management

Antiplatelet therapy optimization includes appropriate loading and maintenance strategies for aspirin (162-325mg loading, 81mg daily maintenance) and $P2Y_{12}$ inhibitors (clopidogrel 600mg loading/75mg daily, ticagrelor 180mg loading/90mg twice daily, prasugrel 60mg loading/10mg daily) based on presentation, intervention approach, and bleeding risk. Anticoagulant selection for acute management navigates options including unfractionated heparin, low molecular weight heparins, and direct thrombin inhibitors based on institutional protocols and patient characteristics, with careful attention to appropriate dosing, monitoring, and duration. Secondary prevention implements comprehensive approaches including dual antiplatelet therapy of appropriate duration (typically 12 months after acute coronary syndrome with shorter or longer durations based on individual bleeding and thrombotic risk), high-intensity statin therapy, RAAS inhibition, and risk factor modification addressing smoking cessation, diabetes control, and blood pressure management.

Peripheral Arterial Disease Management

Antiplatelet therapy optimization implements single-agent therapy with aspirin (81mg daily) or clopidogrel (75mg daily) for most patients, with combination therapy in specific high-risk scenarios including recent revascularization or concurrent coronary artery disease with high ischemic and low bleeding risk. Statin therapy employs high-intensity agents based on the established cardiovascular risk equivalent status of peripheral arterial disease, typically atorvastatin 40-80mg or rosuvastatin 20-40mg daily unless contraindicated or poorly tolerated. Claudication symptom management includes structured exercise programs (supervised treadmill exercise 3 times weekly for 30-60 minutes) complemented by pharmacological options including cilostazol (100mg twice daily) for appropriate candidates without heart failure, with revascularization reserved for lifestyle-limiting symptoms despite conservative management or critical limb ischemia.

Pulmonary Hypertension Management

Diagnostic evaluation differentiates between World Health Organization groups 1-5 pulmonary hypertension, with vastly different treatment approaches based on classification determined through comprehensive assessment including echocardiography, right heart catheterization, ventilation-perfusion scanning, pulmonary function testing, and exclusion of left heart disease. Pulmonary arterial hypertension (Group 1) specific therapy employs prostacyclin pathway agents (epoprostenol, treprostinil, selexipag), endothelin receptor antagonists (ambrisentan, bosentan, macitentan), and phosphodiesterase-5 inhibitors (sildenafil, tadalafil) or soluble guanylate cyclase stimulators (riociguat) in sequential combination based on risk stratification. Secondary pulmonary hypertension management focuses on treating underlying causes including left heart disease (optimizing volume status and cardiac output), lung disease (oxygen therapy, treating underlying condition), chronic thromboembolic disease (anticoagulation, surgical thromboendarterectomy, or balloon pulmonary angioplasty), or miscellaneous conditions.

ENDOCRINE DISORDERS

Diabetes Mellitus

Glycemic management implements individualized HbA1c targets based on age, comorbidities, hypoglycemia risk, and disease duration, typically ranging from <7% for most adults to <8% for elderly patients with significant comorbidities or limited life expectancy. Medication selection navigates expanding therapeutic options including metformin (first-line for most patients, 1000-2000mg daily in divided doses), SGLT2 inhibitors (empagliflozin, dapagliflozin, canagliflozin), GLP-1 receptor agonists (semaglutide, dulaglutide, liraglutide), DPP-4 inhibitors (sitagliptin, linagliptin), sulfonylureas (glipizide, glimepiride), thiazolidinediones (pioglitazone), and insulin formulations, with recent guidelines emphasizing cardiovascular and renal protective benefits of SGLT2 inhibitors and GLP-1 receptor agonists independent of glycemic effects. Complication prevention addresses microvascular (retinopathy, nephropathy, neuropathy) and macrovascular (cardiovascular disease) complications through comprehensive risk factor management including blood pressure control (<130/80 mmHg), lipid management (high-intensity statins), and appropriate prophylactic therapies including ACE inhibitors or ARBs for albuminuria.

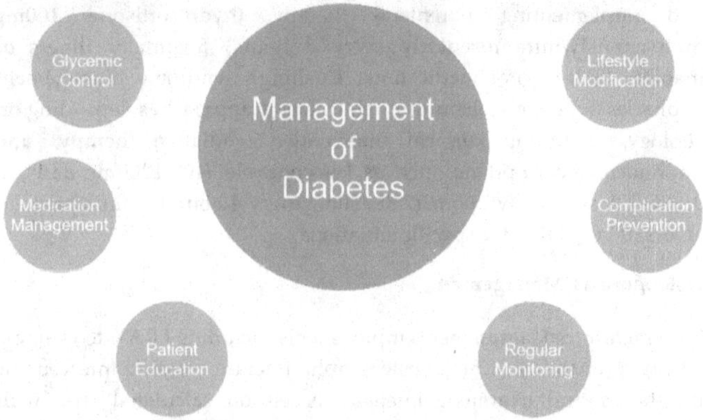

Figure 13.2: Diabetes Management

Thyroid Disorder Management

Hypothyroidism management implements levothyroxine replacement with dosing based on weight, age, pregnancy status, and comorbidities, typically initiating at 1.6 mcg/kg daily for otherwise healthy adults with lower doses (25-50 mcg daily) for elderly patients or those with cardiovascular disease, titrating based on TSH levels measured 6-8 weeks after dose changes. Monitoring strategies evaluate TSH with target ranges based on age and clinical circumstances, typically 0.5-4.0 mIU/L for most adults with different targets for special populations including pregnancy (0.1-2.5 mIU/L in first trimester, 0.2-3.0 mIU/L in second trimester, 0.3-3.0 mIU/L in third trimester). Hyperthyroidism approaches address different etiologies including Graves' disease, toxic nodular goiter, and thyroiditis through appropriate selection between antithyroid medications (methimazole 5-30mg daily or propylthiouracil 100-300mg daily in divided doses), radioactive iodine, and surgical approaches based on patient characteristics, disease type, and treatment goals.

Adrenal Disorder Management

Adrenal insufficiency management implements glucocorticoid replacement with appropriate physiologic dosing, typically hydrocortisone 15-25 mg daily in divided doses (typically 10-15mg on awakening, 5-10mg in afternoon) mimicking natural cortisol rhythms, with mineralocorticoid supplementation using fludrocortisone (0.05-0.2mg daily) when aldosterone deficiency exists. Stress dosing protocols establish clear guidelines for glucocorticoid dose increases during illness, surgery, or other physiological stressors to prevent adrenal crisis, typically doubling or tripling daily hydrocortisone dose for minor illness and implementing parenteral therapy (hydrocortisone 100mg intravenously/intramuscularly every 8 hours) for major illness or inability to take oral medications. Cushing's syndrome management addresses hypercortisolism through different approaches depending on etiology, including surgical intervention, radiation therapy, and pharmacological options such as ketoconazole (400-1200mg daily in divided doses), metyrapone (250-750mg every 4 hours), or mifepristone (300-1200mg daily) for specific situations.

Osteoporosis Management

Fracture risk assessment employs tools including FRAX to estimate 10-year probability of major osteoporotic fracture, guiding intervention thresholds and treatment intensity based on calculated risk, with pharmacologic therapy typically recommended for those with hip or vertebral fractures, T-scores ≤-2.5, or 10-year hip fracture risk ≥3% or major osteoporotic fracture risk ≥20%. Medication selection navigates options including bisphosphonates (alendronate 70mg weekly, risedronate 35mg weekly, zoledronic acid 5mg IV annually), denosumab (60mg subcutaneously every 6 months), selective estrogen receptor modulators (raloxifene 60mg daily), anabolic agents (teriparatide 20mcg subcutaneously daily, abaloparatide 80mcg subcutaneously daily, romosozumab 210mg subcutaneously monthly), and hormone therapy based on specific patient factors, fracture risk, and comorbidities. Duration determination implements appropriate treatment courses with consideration of drug holidays for bisphosphonates based on risk reassessment after initial treatment periods, typically 3-5 years for zoledronic acid and 5-10 years for oral bisphosphonates depending on ongoing fracture risk.

Pituitary Disorder Management

Growth hormone deficiency management implements appropriate replacement with somatropin using weight-based or fixed dosing strategies depending on age and clinical circumstances, typically starting at 0.1-0.3 mg/day for adults and titrating based on IGF-1 levels and clinical response, with higher doses (0.024-0.034 mg/kg/day) for children adjusted regularly based on growth velocity and safety parameters. Hyperprolactinemia treatment employs dopamine agonists including cabergoline (0.25-2mg twice weekly) and bromocriptine (2.5-15mg daily in divided doses) with careful monitoring for both efficacy (prolactin normalization, tumor shrinkage, restoration of gonadal function) and potential adverse effects including cardiac valve changes and impulse control disorders. Diabetes insipidus management implements desmopressin replacement with dosing strategies (oral tablets 0.1-0.8mg daily in divided doses, intranasal spray 5-40mcg daily in divided doses, or sublingual tablets 60-240mcg daily) and monitoring protocols addressing the narrow therapeutic window between symptom control and hyponatremia risk.

Table 13.2: Endocrine Disorder Management

Endocrine Condition	Assessment Parameters	Evidence-Based Pharmacotherapy	Monitoring Approach
Type 1 Diabetes	Glycemic patterns, insulin requirements, hypoglycemia risk, complications	Basal-bolus insulin regimens, carbohydrate counting, insulin pump therapy	A1C targets, TIR, hypoglycemia frequency, complication screening
Type 2 Diabetes	A1C, cardiovascular risk, renal function, hypoglycemia risk	Metformin, SGLT2i, GLP-1 RA, DPP-4i, TZD, insulin based on comorbidities	A1C targets, organ protection, hypoglycemia avoidance, cardiovascular outcomes
Hypothyroidism	TSH, free T4, symptom assessment, special populations	Levothyroxine (dose by weight, age, pregnancy status), combination therapy in select cases	TSH normalization, symptom resolution, dose adjustment for life changes
Hyperthyroidism	TSH, free T4, T3, etiology, symptom burden	Thionamides, beta-blockers, definitive therapy planning	Thyroid function normalization, symptom control, side effect monitoring
Adrenal Insufficiency	Cortisol levels, ACTH stimulation, electrolytes, symptoms	Glucocorticoid replacement, mineralocorticoid if needed, stress dosing education	Symptom control, electrolyte normalization, stress dose implementation
Osteoporosis	BMD measurement, FRAX score, fall risk, secondary causes	Bisphosphonates, RANKL inhibitors, anabolics, SERMs based on risk and characteristics	Fracture prevention, BMD improvement, side effect monitoring, duration decisions
Polycystic Ovary Syndrome	Hyperandrogenism, ovulatory	Combined hormonal contraceptives,	Symptom improvement, menstrual

Endocrine Condition	Assessment Parameters	Evidence-Based Pharmacotherapy	Monitoring Approach
	dysfunction, metabolic status	metformin, anti-androgens, ovulation induction	regulation, metabolic parameter improvement
Male Hypogonadism	Total/free testosterone, symptom assessment, fertility desires	Testosterone replacement (various formulations), alternative approaches for fertility	Symptom improvement, testosterone normalization, adverse effect monitoring

Metabolic Bone Disorders

Paget's disease treatment employs bisphosphonates with higher doses and different regimens than osteoporosis protocols, typically zoledronic acid 5mg as single infusion or oral bisphosphonates for 2-6 months, with treatment goals focusing on normalization of alkaline phosphatase and symptom control rather than bone density improvement. Hyperparathyroidism management addresses different etiologies including primary (surgical referral for symptomatic disease or meeting surgical criteria), secondary (calcium, vitamin D, and phosphate management), and tertiary disease, with pharmacological options including calcimimetics (cinacalcet 30-180mg daily), vitamin D analogs, and phosphate binders based on specific circumstances and underlying causes. Hypophosphatasia approaches employ enzyme replacement with asfotase alfa for severe cases (2mg/kg three times weekly or 1mg/kg six times weekly subcutaneously) or supportive management for milder presentations, addressing bone pain, dental issues, and fracture prevention.

Gender-affirming Hormone Therapy

Feminizing hormone therapy employs estrogen (typically estradiol 2-6mg daily oral, 0.025-0.2mg daily transdermal, or 5-20mg intramuscular valerate every 2 weeks) with or without antiandrogens (spironolactone 100-300mg daily, GnRH agonists, or 5-alpha reductase inhibitors) with dosing strategies balancing desired effects against thromboembolic and other risks, monitoring for efficacy (breast development, body fat redistribution, decreased facial/body hair) and adverse effects (thromboembolism, hyperkalemia with spironolactone, liver effects). Masculinizing hormone therapy implements testosterone administration through various formulations (injections 50-100mg weekly or 200-250mg every 2-3 weeks, gels 50-100mg daily, or patches

2-6mg daily) with dosing titrated to physiologic male range (typically 400-700 ng/dL) while monitoring for erythrocytosis, liver effects, and lipid changes, with particular attention to contraception needs given potential teratogenicity during unintended pregnancy.

RESPIRATORY CONDITIONS

Asthma

Assessment employs standardized tools including the Asthma Control Test or Asthma Control Questionnaire to objectively evaluate symptom control, exacerbation frequency, and impact on activities, with scores guiding treatment adjustments and identifying patients requiring intensification or specialist referral. Pharmacotherapy follows stepwise progression from as-needed relievers alone for intermittent asthma to various combinations of inhaled corticosteroids (low, medium, or high dose), long-acting bronchodilators, biologics, and oral agents for increasing severity levels, with recent guideline changes emphasizing ICS-formoterol as preferred reliever therapy for most patients rather than short-acting beta agonists alone. Inhaler technique optimization addresses the approximately 70-80% error rate with inhaler use through device selection matching patient capabilities, demonstration-based education, and regular technique reassessment, recognizing that poor technique represents a major cause of inadequate asthma control despite appropriate medication selection.

Table 13.3: Respiratory Condition Management

Respiratory Condition	Assessment Parameters	Evidence-Based Pharmacotherapy	Monitoring Approach
Asthma	Symptom frequency, exacerbation history, pulmonary function, phenotype	ICS, LABA, LAMA, LTRA, biologics in stepwise approach	Symptom control, exacerbation reduction, pulmonary function, device technique
COPD	GOLD classification, symptom burden, exacerbation history, phenotype	SABA, LAMA, LABA, ICS combinations based on phenotype and severity	Symptom reduction, exacerbation prevention, functional improvement, inhaler technique

Respiratory Condition	Assessment Parameters	Evidence-Based Pharmacotherapy	Monitoring Approach
Allergic Rhinitis	Symptom pattern, triggers, severity classification	Intranasal corticosteroids, antihistamines, leukotriene modifiers, immunotherapy	Symptom control, quality of life, minimized side effects, comorbidity management
Pulmonary Hypertension	WHO group classification, functional class, hemodynamics	Endothelin receptor antagonists, PDE-5 inhibitors, prostacyclins, sGC stimulators	Functional improvement, hemodynamic changes, exercise capacity, right heart function
Cystic Fibrosis	Pulmonary function, microbiology, nutritional status, CFTR genotype	CFTR modulators, mucolytics, antibiotics, anti-inflammatory therapy	Pulmonary function, exacerbation frequency, nutritional status, quality of life
Obstructive Sleep Apnea	AHI, symptom assessment, comorbidity impact	PAP therapy support, weight management pharmacotherapy, positional therapy	AHI reduction, symptom improvement, comorbidity impact, adherence to therapy
Interstitial Lung Disease	HRCT pattern, pulmonary function, etiology, progression rate	Antifibrotics, immunosuppressants, anti-inflammatories based on specific ILD	Progression rate, pulmonary function, oxygen requirements, quality of life
Pulmonary Infections	Pathogen identification, severity assessment, host factors	Appropriate antimicrobials, adjunctive therapies, prophylactic strategies	Symptom resolution, microbiological eradication, complication prevention

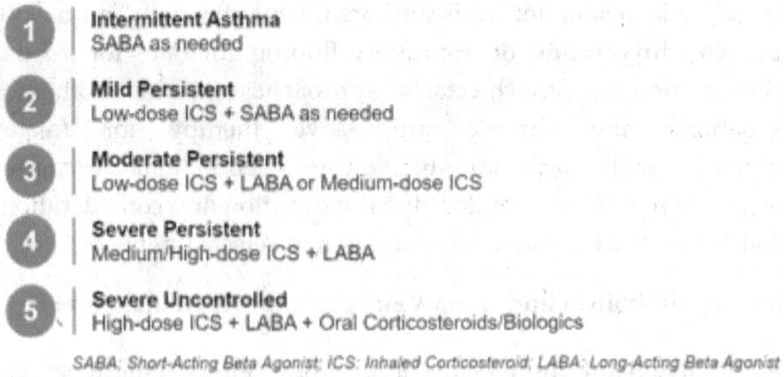

Figure 13.3: Stepwise Approach to Asthma Management

Chronic Obstructive Pulmonary Disease (COPD) Management

Assessment employs tools including the COPD Assessment Test (CAT) and modified Medical Research Council (mMRC) dyspnea scale to evaluate symptom burden and functional limitation, classifying patients into groups based on symptom intensity and exacerbation history to guide appropriate therapy selection. Pharmacotherapy implementation follows GOLD guidelines with treatment selection based on symptom burden and exacerbation history, progressing from single bronchodilators (long-acting muscarinic antagonists preferred initial therapy) to dual bronchodilation (LAMA/LABA combinations), inhaled corticosteroids added for those with blood eosinophils ≥300 cells/μL or history of asthma, and additional agents based on specific phenotypes. Exacerbation management protocols address acute deteriorations through appropriate antibiotic selection based on risk factors for resistant organisms, systemic corticosteroid use (prednisone 40mg daily for 5 days) with appropriate duration limitations, and bronchodilator intensification.

Pulmonary Infection Management

Community-acquired pneumonia treatment implements risk stratification using tools such as CURB-65 or Pneumonia Severity Index to guide site-of-care decisions and antibiotic selection matching coverage to likely pathogens and local resistance patterns, typically employing combinations of beta-lactams (amoxicillin, amoxicillin-clavulanate, ceftriaxone) with macrolides (azithromycin, clarithromycin) or respiratory fluoroquinolone monotherapy (levofloxacin, moxifloxacin) for 5-7 days in most cases. Acute exacerbation of chronic bronchitis management employs antibiotic therapy for patients with increased sputum purulence and either increased dyspnea or increased sputum volume, with agent selection based on risk factors for resistant organisms, typically amoxicillin-clavulanate, doxycycline, or respiratory fluoroquinolones for 5-7 days. Non-cystic fibrosis bronchiectasis approaches address both acute exacerbations and chronic suppressive therapy for frequent exacerbators, with particular attention to Pseudomonas aeruginosa management requiring extended therapy duration and consideration of inhaled antibiotics for chronic suppression in selected patients.

Pulmonary Embolism and Deep Vein Thrombosis Management

Acute treatment implements appropriate anticoagulant selection between unfractionated heparin, low molecular weight heparins (enoxaparin 1mg/kg twice daily or 1.5mg/kg daily), fondaparinux (5-10mg daily based on weight), and direct oral anticoagulants (apixaban 10mg twice daily for 7 days then 5mg twice daily, rivaroxaban 15mg twice daily for 21 days then 20mg daily) based on clinical stability, renal function, bleeding risk, and other patient-specific factors. Long-term anticoagulation determines appropriate duration based on provocation status, recurrence risk, and bleeding risk assessment, with recent guidelines supporting extended therapy for many unprovoked events given continued risk beyond traditional treatment periods, typically 3 months for provoked events, at least 6-12 months for first unprovoked events, and indefinite therapy for recurrent unprovoked events with acceptable bleeding risk. Thrombolytic therapy for massive or submassive pulmonary embolism implements appropriate agent selection, dosing, and monitoring for eligible patients with hemodynamic compromise or right ventricular dysfunction.

Cystic Fibrosis Management

Infection management implements appropriate antibiotic selection for pulmonary exacerbations based on sputum culture results and patient-specific response history, with attention to pharmacokinetic alterations requiring dose optimization for many agents, typically employing combination therapy with extended durations (14-21 days) and higher doses than used for other indications. CFTR modulator therapy employs genotype-specific selection between ivacaftor (150mg every 12 hours for G551D and other gating mutations), lumacaftor/ivacaftor (two tablets containing lumacaftor 200mg/ivacaftor 125mg every 12 hours for F508del homozygous), tezacaftor/ivacaftor (one tablet containing tezacaftor 100mg/ivacaftor 150mg each morning and ivacaftor 150mg each evening), and elexacaftor/tezacaftor/ivacaftor (two tablets containing elexacaftor 100mg/tezacaftor 50mg/ivacaftor 75mg each morning and ivacaftor 150mg each evening) for F508del heterozygous patients. Nutritional support optimizes pancreatic enzyme replacement therapy (typically 1,000-2,500 lipase units/kg/meal), fat-soluble vitamin supplementation, and caloric intake to maintain appropriate growth and nutritional status.

Pulmonary Arterial Hypertension Management

Vasodilator therapy implementation navigates options including phosphodiesterase type 5 inhibitors (sildenafil 20mg three times daily, tadalafil 40mg daily), endothelin receptor antagonists (ambrisentan 5-10mg daily, bosentan 62.5-125mg twice daily, macitentan 10mg daily), prostacyclin analogs (epoprostenol, treprostinil, iloprost), and soluble guanylate cyclase stimulators (riociguat 1-2.5mg three times daily), with initial selection and combination strategies based on risk stratification. Administration optimization addresses the complex delivery requirements for prostacyclin therapies including continuous intravenous infusion (epoprostenol, treprostinil), subcutaneous infusion (treprostinil), and inhaled administration (treprostinil, iloprost) with specific technical requirements, training needs, and monitoring parameters. Supportive therapy manages right heart failure manifestations through appropriate diuretic therapy, oxygen supplementation, and symptom management while avoiding agents with vasodepressor effects potentially worsening pulmonary hypertension.

Sleep-disordered Breathing Management

Primary therapy focuses on continuous positive airway pressure (CPAP) or alternative positive pressure modalities with pharmacist involvement addressing adherence barriers, interface optimization, and complication management, with typical pressure requirements ranging from 5-20 cmH_2O based on titration studies and specific patient factors. Pharmacological approaches address specific aspects including residual sleepiness with wakefulness-promoting agents (modafinil 200mg daily, armodafinil 150-250mg daily) when appropriate adherence is confirmed, adjunctive weight management, and management of medications potentially exacerbating sleep-disordered breathing. Comorbidity management addresses the significant overlap with conditions including hypertension, heart failure, arrhythmias, and metabolic disorders through integrated treatment approaches recognizing the bidirectional relationship between sleep-disordered breathing and these conditions, with particular attention to hypertension management given the significant contribution of obstructive sleep apnea to resistant hypertension.

INFECTIOUS DISEASES

Antimicrobial Stewardship

Empiric therapy selection matches antimicrobial coverage to likely pathogens based on infection site, community or healthcare acquisition, local resistance patterns, and patient risk factors for resistant organisms, balancing appropriate initial coverage against unnecessary broad-spectrum therapy. De-escalation protocols guide therapy narrowing based on culture results, clinical response, and duration appropriateness, converting broad initial regimens to targeted therapy when microbiology data becomes available, typically within 48-72 hours of culture results. Intravenous-to-oral conversion identifies candidates for early transition to oral therapy when appropriate criteria are met, including clinical improvement, functioning gastrointestinal tract, appropriate oral agent availability, and adequate oral absorption, typically implemented after 2-3 days of intravenous therapy for eligible patients.

Table 13.4: Infectious Disease Management

Infection Category	Assessment Approaches	Therapeutic Strategies	Stewardship Elements
Community-Acquired Pneumonia	Severity scoring, pathogen identification, host factors	Empiric therapy based on risk factors, de-escalation, appropriate duration	Timely initiation, guideline concordance, duration limitation, IV-to-PO conversion
Urinary Tract Infections	Classification (uncomplicated vs. complicated), pathogen identification, host factors	Appropriate spectrum coverage, local resistance consideration, duration optimization	Narrow spectrum when possible, appropriate duration, biomarker utilization
Skin/Soft Tissue Infections	Infection type, severity, necrotizing component, host factors	Appropriate coverage for likely pathogens, surgical consideration, duration determination	Appropriate empiric therapy, timely de-escalation, duration optimization

Infection Category	Assessment Approaches	Therapeutic Strategies	Stewardship Elements
Intra-abdominal Infections	Source control evaluation, severity assessment, multidrug-resistant risk	Empiric broad-spectrum coverage, source control facilitation, de-escalation planning	Culture-directed therapy, duration linked to source control, oral conversion
Bloodstream Infections	Source identification, pathogen determination, persistence risk	Source-appropriate coverage, duration based on source and organism, clearance confirmation	Rapid diagnostics utilization, optimal duration, source elimination
Central Nervous System Infections	CSF analysis, pathogen identification, blood-brain barrier considerations	High CNS-penetrating agents, appropriate duration, adjunctive therapies	Therapeutic drug monitoring, penetration optimization, duration appropriateness
Endocarditis	Duke criteria, vegetation characteristics, causative organism	Organism-specific regimens, surgical evaluation, extended therapy consideration	Appropriate combinations, duration optimization, level monitoring when applicable
Fungal Infections	Host risk factors, site of infection, fungal species	Appropriate antifungal selection, therapeutic drug monitoring, duration determination	Species-directed therapy, step-down strategies, host factor modification

Respiratory Tract Infection Management

Upper respiratory infection approaches emphasize appropriate differentiation between viral and bacterial etiologies, with antimicrobial avoidance for conditions including the common cold, most cases of acute bronchitis, and viral pharyngitis, while employing specific testing (rapid streptococcal antigen, throat culture) to identify bacterial pharyngitis requiring treatment. Community-acquired pneumonia treatment implements risk stratification using tools such as CURB-65 or

Pneumonia Severity Index to guide site-of-care decisions and empiric therapy selection covering likely pathogens including Streptococcus pneumoniae, Haemophilus influenzae, and atypical organisms, with additional coverage for Pseudomonas aeruginosa and MRSA in patients with specific risk factors. Hospital-acquired and ventilator-associated pneumonia management addresses healthcare-associated pathogens including gram-negative bacilli and resistant gram-positive cocci through appropriate empiric regimens based on local ecology and patient risk factors.

Urinary Tract Infection Management

Uncomplicated cystitis treatment employs short-course therapy with agents including nitrofurantoin (100mg twice daily for 5 days), trimethoprim-sulfamethoxazole (160/800mg twice daily for 3 days), or fosfomycin (3g single dose) based on local resistance patterns and patient-specific factors. Complicated urinary tract infection management addresses conditions involving structural or functional abnormalities, immunocompromise, or resistant organisms through broader-spectrum therapy and longer treatment courses, typically employing fluoroquinolones, third-generation cephalosporins, or beta-lactam/beta-lactamase inhibitors for 7-14 days depending on specific circumstances. Asymptomatic bacteriuria guidance emphasizes treatment avoidance except in specific circumstances including pregnancy and before urologic procedures, with studies consistently demonstrating harm rather than benefit from treating asymptomatic bacteriuria in most other populations.

Skin and Soft Tissue Infection Management

Uncomplicated cellulitis treatment employs antimicrobials targeting streptococci and methicillin-susceptible Staphylococcus aureus, with specific agent selection based on local resistance patterns and patient risk factors for MRSA, typically cephalexin (500mg four times daily) or dicloxacillin (500mg four times daily) for 5-10 days when MRSA is not suspected, or trimethoprim-sulfamethoxazole (160/800mg twice daily), doxycycline (100mg twice daily), or clindamycin (300-450mg three times daily) when MRSA coverage is necessary. Complicated skin and soft tissue infection management addresses conditions involving deeper tissues, systemic symptoms, or concerning host factors through broader coverage and potential surgical intervention, often requiring hospitalization with intravenous therapy including vancomycin, linezolid, or daptomycin for gram-positive coverage plus gram-negative agents for polymicrobial infections. Diabetic foot infection approaches integrate antimicrobial therapy with appropriate wound care, offloading, and vascular assessment through interdisciplinary management.

Central Nervous System Infection Management

Bacterial meningitis treatment implements empiric therapy with activity against likely pathogens based on age, immunization status, and epidemiological factors, typically including third-generation cephalosporins (ceftriaxone 2g every 12 hours, cefotaxime 2g every 4-6 hours) plus vancomycin (15-20 mg/kg every 8-12 hours) with consideration of ampicillin (2g every 4 hours) for Listeria coverage in vulnerable populations. Adjunctive dexamethasone administration for specific bacterial meningitis scenarios follows evidence-based protocols regarding timing (ideally before or with first antibiotic dose), dosing (0.15 mg/kg every 6 hours for 2-4 days), and eligible patient populations (primarily proven or suspected pneumococcal meningitis). Viral encephalitis management, particularly herpes simplex encephalitis, implements appropriate antiviral therapy with acyclovir (10 mg/kg every 8 hours) while addressing potential mimics and alternative etiologies.

Bloodstream Infection and Endocarditis Management

Empiric therapy for sepsis implements broad-spectrum coverage based on likely sources, healthcare exposure, and patient risk factors, with particular attention to appropriate dosing for optimal pharmacokinetic/pharmacodynamic target attainment in critically ill patients, typically including anti-pseudomonal beta-lactams (piperacillin-tazobactam 4.5g every 6-8 hours, cefepime 2g every 8 hours, or meropenem 1g every 8 hours) plus vancomycin (15-20 mg/kg every 8-12 hours) for most healthcare-associated sepsis. Endocarditis treatment follows pathogen-specific approaches with extended therapy courses (typically 4-6 weeks), synergistic combinations for specific organisms (beta-lactams plus aminoglycosides for enterococci), and careful monitoring for both effectiveness and toxicity. Catheter-related bloodstream infection management addresses both empiric therapy and definitive treatment based on culture results, with decisions regarding catheter removal based on pathogen (mandatory removal for S. aureus, Candida, Pseudomonas, and other virulent organisms), clinical stability, and available vascular access.

Sexually Transmitted Infection Management

Gonorrhea treatment addresses evolving resistance patterns through recommended dual therapy approaches (ceftriaxone 500mg intramuscular single dose plus azithromycin 1g oral single dose or doxycycline 100mg twice daily for 7 days) and alternative regimens for patients with allergies or special circumstances. Syphilis management implements stage-specific treatment with appropriate penicillin formulations and durations, including benzathine penicillin G 2.4 million units intramuscular single dose for primary, secondary, and early latent syphilis, versus three weekly doses for late latent or syphilis of unknown duration, with specific protocols for penicillin-allergic patients including desensitization when appropriate. HIV pre-exposure prophylaxis (PrEP) provides prevention for high-risk individuals through appropriate candidate selection, baseline testing, medication selection between tenofovir disoproxil/emtricitabine (200/300mg daily) and tenofovir alafenamide/emtricitabine (25/200mg daily), and monitoring protocols addressing both effectiveness and potential toxicity.

Fungal Infection Management

Invasive candidiasis treatment implements empiric therapy based on likely species and local epidemiology, with de-escalation based on identification and susceptibility testing, including consideration of echinocandins (caspofungin 70mg loading dose followed by 50mg daily, micafungin 100mg daily, anidulafungin 200mg loading dose followed by 100mg daily), azoles (fluconazole 800mg loading dose followed by 400mg daily), and polyenes (amphotericin B formulations) based on specific circumstances. Invasive aspergillosis management employs voriconazole as primary therapy (6mg/kg every 12 hours for two doses, then 4mg/kg every 12 hours) with appropriate therapeutic drug monitoring (target trough 2-5 mcg/mL), alternative agents for refractory disease, and consideration of combination approaches for specific scenarios. Cryptococcal meningitis treatment follows evidence-based induction, consolidation, and maintenance phases with appropriate agent selection, duration, and intracranial pressure management.

ONCOLOGY

Chemotherapy Management

Protocol implementation ensures accurate dosing based on body surface area, weight, organ function, or other parameters specified in evidence-based regimens, with appropriate dose modifications for toxicity, organ dysfunction, or previous adverse events according to protocol-specific guidelines or institutional standards. Sequencing optimization determines appropriate timing between multiple agents within regimens to maximize efficacy while minimizing overlapping toxicities, particularly important for combinations with specific administration sequence requirements such as rituximab-chemotherapy combinations or platinum-taxane regimens. Supportive care integration coordinates antiemetics, growth factors, hydration, and other adjunctive therapies with chemotherapy administration to prevent or minimize treatment-related complications, following risk-based guidelines for antiemetic selection and growth factor utilization based on regimen emetogenicity and myelosuppression potential.

Targeted Therapy Optimization

Molecular testing coordination ensures appropriate biomarker assessment before targeted therapy initiation, including mutations (EGFR, BRAF, KIT), translocations (ALK, ROS1), and expression patterns (HER2, PD-L1) predicting response to specific agents, with testing methodologies matched to clinical scenarios and available therapies. Drug interaction management addresses the significant interaction potential of many targeted therapies, particularly tyrosine kinase inhibitors metabolized through cytochrome P450 enzymes with numerous clinically significant interactions affecting efficacy and toxicity, requiring systematic screening and management strategies including dose adjustments, administration timing modifications, or alternative agent selection. Adverse effect management implements monitoring and intervention strategies for class-specific and agent-specific toxicities including dermatologic reactions (acneiform rash with EGFR inhibitors), cardiovascular effects (hypertension with VEGF inhibitors), hepatotoxicity, and unique target-related adverse events.

Immunotherapy Management

Immune checkpoint inhibitor therapy implements appropriate agent selection targeting CTLA-4 (ipilimumab), PD-1 (pembrolizumab, nivolumab), or PD-L1 (atezolizumab, durvalumab, avelumab) based on tumor type, biomarker status, and treatment setting, with significant variations in approved indications, dosing, and combination approaches across cancer types. Immune-related adverse event management employs systematic assessment and grading with appropriate intervention strategies including corticosteroids (typically prednisone 1-2 mg/kg/day or equivalent for grade 3-4 toxicities) and additional immunosuppressive agents (infliximab, mycophenolate) for severe or refractory toxicities following established management algorithms specific to each toxicity type. Chimeric antigen receptor T-cell therapy support addresses specialized considerations including cytokine release syndrome management (tocilizumab, corticosteroids), neurologic toxicity assessment, and long-term monitoring for B-cell aplasia and hypogammaglobulinemia following CD19-directed therapies.

Table 13.5: Oncology Pharmacotherapy Management

Oncology Focus	**Assessment Elements**	**Therapeutic Approaches**	**Supportive Care Integration**
Solid Tumor Management	Molecular profiling, staging, performance status	Cytotoxic chemotherapy, targeted therapy, immunotherapy, endocrine therapy	Antiemetics, growth factors, pain management, nutritional support
Hematologic Malignancies	Cell lineage, molecular markers, staging, transplant eligibility	Chemotherapy regimens, targeted agents, immunotherapies, cellular therapies	Infection prophylaxis, transfusion support, tumor lysis prevention
Targeted Therapy	Biomarker testing, resistance mechanisms, line of therapy	Kinase inhibitors, monoclonal antibodies, antibody-drug conjugates, small molecules	Unique toxicity management, drug interaction prevention, adherence support
Immunotherapy	PD-L1 expression, microsatellite status, tumor mutational burden	Checkpoint inhibitors, CAR-T cells, bispecific antibodies, cancer vaccines	Immune-related adverse event management, cytokine release syndrome
Hormonal Therapy	Receptor status, menopausal status, bone health	SERMs, aromatase inhibitors, LH-RH agonists, anti-androgens	Bone health management, menopausal symptom management, cardiovascular risk
Chemotherapy Support	Emetogenic potential, myelosuppression risk, organ function	Antiemetic protocols, colony-stimulating factors, cytoprotective agents	Guideline-based supportive care, prophylaxis appropriateness, symptom management
Oral Antineoplastic Management	Absorption considerations, drug interactions, adherence challenges	Adherence strategies, interaction management, side effect minimization	Financial support, adherence tools, proactive toxicity management

Hormonal Therapy Optimization

Breast cancer hormonal therapy implements appropriate selection between selective estrogen receptor modulators (tamoxifen 20mg daily), aromatase inhibitors (letrozole 2.5mg daily, anastrozole 1mg daily, exemestane 25mg daily), selective estrogen receptor degraders (fulvestrant 500mg intramuscular days 1, 15, 29, then monthly), and ovarian suppression based on menopausal status, recurrence risk, and treatment tolerance. Prostate cancer androgen deprivation approaches address appropriate agent selection between GnRH agonists (leuprolide, goserelin) requiring initial anti-androgen coverage to prevent flare versus GnRH antagonists (degarelix) with immediate testosterone suppression, intermittent versus continuous therapy considerations, and management of adverse effects including bone density loss, metabolic changes, and cardiovascular risk through appropriate monitoring and intervention strategies. Monitoring protocols evaluate both therapeutic efficacy through appropriate disease-specific markers (PSA for prostate cancer, clinical assessment for breast cancer) and adverse effect development with particular attention to bone health, cardiovascular risk, and quality of life impact.

Supportive Care Management

Chemotherapy-induced nausea and vomiting prevention implements risk-stratified antiemetic protocols based on emetogenic potential, with high-risk regimens (cisplatin, AC combination) receiving three-drug prophylaxis with 5-HT3 antagonist (ondansetron 8-16mg or palonosetron 0.25mg), NK1 receptor antagonist (aprepitant 125mg day 1, 80mg days 2-3 or fosaprepitant 150mg day 1), and dexamethasone (12mg day 1, 8mg days 2-4), with appropriate agent selection, timing, and duration to prevent both acute and delayed symptoms. Myelosuppression management addresses neutropenia, anemia, and thrombocytopenia through appropriate growth factor use (filgrastim, pegfilgrastim for neutropenia; erythropoiesis-stimulating agents for chemotherapy-induced anemia), transfusion support, and dose modification strategies following risk-based guidelines from ASCO and NCCN. Oral mucositis prevention and treatment implements systematic approaches including basic oral care, preventive agents for high-risk regimens (palifermin for high-dose therapy with stem cell support), and pain management strategies for established mucositis.

Cancer Pain Management

Nociceptive pain management employs appropriate analgesic selection and titration following the WHO analgesic ladder, with consideration of both around-the-clock and as-needed medications for optimal control, typically beginning with acetaminophen and NSAIDs for mild pain, weak opioids (tramadol, codeine) for moderate pain, and strong opioids (morphine, oxycodone, hydromorphone) for severe pain with appropriate conversion between agents using established equianalgesic tables. Neuropathic pain approaches address nerve injury related to tumor infiltration or treatment effects through adjuvant analgesics including anticonvulsants (gabapentin 300-1200mg three times daily, pregabalin 75-300mg twice daily), antidepressants (duloxetine 30-60mg daily, amitriptyline 10-75mg daily), and NMDA receptor antagonists (ketamine, methadone) for refractory cases. Bone pain management integrates analgesic therapy with bone-targeted agents including bisphosphonates (zoledronic acid 4mg intravenous every 3-4 weeks) and RANK ligand inhibitors (denosumab 120mg subcutaneous every 4 weeks) for metastatic bone disease.

Oncologic Emergencies

Tumor lysis syndrome prevention and management implements risk-stratified approaches including hydration (2-3 L/day), allopurinol (300-600mg daily) or rasburicase (0.1-0.2 mg/kg single dose) for high-risk patients, and electrolyte monitoring and replacement based on tumor type, burden, and renal function, with particularly aggressive prophylaxis for high-cell-turnover malignancies including acute leukemias and high-grade lymphomas. Hypercalcemia of malignancy intervention employs appropriate selection between bisphosphonates (zoledronic acid 4mg, pamidronate 60-90mg), calcitonin (4-8 IU/kg every 12 hours), and denosumab based on severity, onset timing, and renal function, with aggressive hydration (typically normal saline at 200-300 mL/hour initially) as foundational therapy. Spinal cord compression management coordinates corticosteroids (dexamethasone 10mg intravenous followed by 4mg every 6 hours), radiation therapy, and potential surgical intervention with appropriate timing and sequencing based on neurological status, disease characteristics, and overall prognosis.

Hematopoietic Stem Cell Transplantation Support

Conditioning regimen implementation ensures accurate dosing and scheduling of high-intensity chemotherapy and/or radiation therapy preparing the recipient for cell infusion, with particular attention to pharmacokinetic monitoring for agents including busulfan (target AUC 900-1500 μmol·min/L daily) where individual dose adjustment significantly reduces toxicity and graft failure risks. Graft-versus-host disease prophylaxis and treatment employs combinations of calcineurin inhibitors (cyclosporine, tacrolimus), methotrexate, mycophenolate, antithymocyte globulin, and corticosteroids with patient-specific selection and monitoring based on transplant type (autologous vs. allogeneic), stem cell source (peripheral blood, bone marrow, cord blood), and HLA matching status. Infection prophylaxis implements comprehensive antimicrobial strategies addressing bacterial, viral, and fungal pathogens with agent selection and duration based on transplant type, graft source, and patient-specific risk factors, including fluconazole or posaconazole for fungal prophylaxis, acyclovir or valacyclovir for herpes virus prevention, and trimethoprim-sulfamethoxazole or atovaquone for Pneumocystis jirovecii pneumonia prophylaxis.

MENTAL HEALTH

Depression Management

Initial therapy selection navigates options including selective serotonin reuptake inhibitors (sertraline 50-200mg daily, escitalopram 10-20mg daily), serotonin-norepinephrine reuptake inhibitors (venlafaxine 75-225mg daily, duloxetine 30-120mg daily), atypical antidepressants (bupropion 150-450mg daily, mirtazapine 15-45mg daily), and other classes based on symptom profile, comorbidities, previous response, and adverse effect considerations. Dosing optimization ensures adequate trial duration (typically minimum 4-6 weeks) and appropriate dose titration before concluding treatment failure, with particular attention to common underdosing of agents including sertraline (target 100-200mg daily), escitalopram (target 20mg daily for adults), and venlafaxine (target 150-225mg daily). Treatment resistance protocols address inadequate response through strategies including optimization of initial therapy (ensuring adequate dose and duration), augmentation with complementary agents (typically second-generation antipsychotics, lithium, or thyroid hormone), combination approaches with multiple primary antidepressants, or switching to alternative mechanisms including monoamine oxidase inhibitors.

Bipolar Disorder Management

Acute mania treatment implements appropriate selection between lithium (target levels 0.8-1.2 mEq/L), anticonvulsants (valproate 750-2000mg daily, carbamazepine 400-1600mg daily), and second-generation antipsychotics (olanzapine 10-20mg daily, risperidone 2-6mg daily, quetiapine 400-800mg daily) based on symptom severity, previous response, and comorbidity profile. Bipolar depression approaches navigate limited effective options including quetiapine (300-600mg daily), lurasidone (20-120mg daily), cariprazine (1.5-3mg daily), olanzapine-fluoxetine combination, and lamotrigine (target 200mg daily with slow titration), with caution regarding traditional antidepressant monotherapy due to potential mood destabilization and switch risk. Maintenance therapy selection identifies appropriate long-term agents based on predominant episode polarity, treatment during acute phases, and tolerability considerations, with lithium particularly effective for suicide prevention and classical presentations, while anticonvulsants or atypical antipsychotics may better address mixed features or rapid cycling.

Table 13.6: Mental Health Pharmacotherapy

Mental Health Condition	**Assessment Approaches**	**Evidence-Based Pharmacotherapy**	**Monitoring Elements**
Major Depressive Disorder	PHQ-9, symptom profile, previous response, suicide risk	SSRIs, SNRIs, bupropion, mirtazapine, TCAs, MAOIs, augmentation strategies	Symptom improvement, side effect management, suicide risk, functional recovery
Bipolar Disorder	Mood episode type, cycling pattern, suicide risk, comorbidities	Lithium, valproate, lamotrigine, atypical antipsychotics, combination approaches	Mood stability, episode prevention, side effect monitoring, therapeutic levels
Schizophrenia	Positive/negative symptoms, cognitive impact, functional status	First and second-generation antipsychotics, long-acting injectables, clozapine	Symptom control, metabolic monitoring, movement disorders, treatment resistance
Anxiety Disorders	Specific disorder type, symptom pattern, functional impact	SSRIs, SNRIs, buspirone, benzodiazepines (limited), pregabalin	Symptom reduction, functional improvement, dependence avoidance, side effects
Attention-Deficit/Hyperactivity Disorder	Symptom profile, comorbidities, functional impact, age	Stimulants, atomoxetine, alpha-2 agonists, bupropion	Symptom control, growth monitoring, cardiovascular effects, substance misuse

Mental Health Condition	Assessment Approaches	Evidence-Based Pharmacotherapy	Monitoring Elements
Post-Traumatic Stress Disorder	Symptom clusters, trauma history, functional impact	SSRIs, SNRIs, prazosin, mood stabilizers, atypical antipsychotics	Symptom reduction, nightmare control, functional improvement, comorbidity management
Substance Use Disorders	Specific substance, withdrawal risk, comorbidities, readiness	Medication-assisted treatment, craving reduction agents, deterrent medications	Abstinence/reduction, withdrawal management, craving control, recovery support
Insomnia	Sleep patterns, contributing factors, daytime functioning	Cognitive behavioral therapy plus targeted pharmacotherapy, appropriate agent selection	Sleep improvement, daytime functioning, dependence avoidance, cognitive effects

Schizophrenia Spectrum Disorder Management

Initial therapy selection navigates options among second-generation antipsychotics based on efficacy considerations, metabolic risk profiles, extrapyramidal side effect potential, and specific symptom targets including positive, negative, and cognitive symptoms, with commonly used agents including risperidone (2-6mg daily), olanzapine (10-20mg daily), aripiprazole (10-30mg daily), and quetiapine (300-800mg daily). Long-acting injectable antipsychotic implementation addresses adherence challenges through appropriate candidate selection, initiation protocols including oral overlapping requirements, and monitoring schedules based on specific agent pharmacokinetics, with options including paliperidone palmitate (monthly or every 3 months), aripiprazole monohydrate (monthly), aripiprazole lauroxil (monthly, every 6 weeks, or every 2 months), and risperidone microspheres (every 2 weeks). Clozapine management addresses this uniquely effective agent for treatment-resistant schizophrenia through appropriate initiation protocols (starting 12.5-25mg daily with gradual titration to 300-450mg daily), required monitoring programs (REMS), therapeutic drug monitoring (target trough 350-600 ng/mL), and adverse effect management including agranulocytosis risk, metabolic effects, seizure prophylaxis, and myocarditis surveillance.

Anxiety Disorder Management

First-line therapy implementation typically employs selective serotonin reuptake inhibitors or serotonin-norepinephrine reuptake inhibitors at appropriate dosing for anxiety indications, which often differ from depression dosing targets, including sertraline (50-200mg daily), escitalopram (10-20mg daily), paroxetine (20-50mg daily), venlafaxine (75-225mg daily), or duloxetine (30-120mg daily) with gradual titration to minimize activation side effects common in anxiety disorders. Benzodiazepine appropriate use addresses legitimate short-term roles while implementing strategies to prevent long-term dependence, including limited duration (ideally <2-4 weeks), scheduled rather than as-needed dosing, and planned tapering protocols employing gradual dose reduction (typically 10-25% every 1-2 weeks) to minimize withdrawal symptoms. Augmentation strategies for partial response or treatment resistance navigate options including buspirone (15-60mg daily in divided doses), pregabalin (150-600mg daily in divided doses), hydroxyzine (25-100mg three to four times daily), and specific antipsychotics with evidence in anxiety disorders (quetiapine 25-300mg daily).

Post-traumatic Stress Disorder (PTSD) Management

First-line therapy typically employs selective serotonin reuptake inhibitors or venlafaxine at doses often higher than depression targets, with sertraline (50-200mg daily) and paroxetine (20-60mg daily) having specific FDA approval for this indication, while fluoxetine (20-80mg daily) and venlafaxine (75-300mg daily) have strong evidence despite lacking specific regulatory approval. Symptomatic treatment addresses specific manifestations including nightmares (prazosin 1-15mg at bedtime, with gradual titration based on response and tolerability), hyperarousal (propranolol 20-80mg daily in divided doses), and insomnia (non-benzodiazepine approaches including trazodone 25-200mg at bedtime or low-dose doxepin 3-6mg at bedtime) when core symptoms remain despite primary treatment. Comorbidity management addresses the high rates of co-occurring depression, substance use disorders, and other anxiety conditions requiring integrated treatment approaches, with careful attention to selecting primary agents addressing multiple comorbidities when possible to minimize polypharmacy.

Substance Use Disorder Management

Alcohol use disorder pharmacotherapy implements appropriate selection between naltrexone (50mg daily oral or 380mg monthly intramuscular), acamprosate (666mg three times daily), and disulfiram

(250-500mg daily) based on treatment goals, comorbidities, and patient preferences, with naltrexone particularly useful for reducing heavy drinking, acamprosate supporting abstinence, and disulfiram serving as a deterrent for highly motivated patients. Opioid use disorder management employs evidence-based approaches including buprenorphine induction and maintenance (typically 16-24mg daily), methadone through specialized programs (typically 80-120mg daily), or extended-release naltrexone (380mg intramuscular monthly) for patients achieving initial abstinence, with selection based on individual factors, treatment availability, and patient preference. Withdrawal management implements appropriate protocols for different substances including benzodiazepine tapers for alcohol withdrawal (typically diazepam or chlordiazepoxide with symptom-triggered or fixed-schedule approaches), buprenorphine or methadone for opioid withdrawal, and supportive approaches for stimulant and other substance discontinuation.

Sleep Disorder Management

Cognitive-behavioral therapy for insomnia (CBT-I) support emphasizes this first-line treatment through patient education, motivational approaches, and appropriate resource connection, focusing on stimulus control, sleep restriction, relaxation techniques, sleep hygiene, and cognitive restructuring as core components. Pharmacological management for short-term or refractory insomnia navigates options including melatonin receptor agonists (ramelteon 8mg at bedtime), orexin receptor antagonists (suvorexant 5-20mg at bedtime, lemborexant 5-10mg at bedtime), and sedating antidepressants (trazodone 25-100mg at bedtime, doxepin 3-6mg at bedtime), with cautious use of benzodiazepine receptor agonists (zolpidem 5-10mg, eszopiclone 1-3mg, zaleplon 5-10mg at bedtime) and traditional benzodiazepines due to adverse effect concerns, dependence potential, and limited evidence for long-term efficacy. Circadian rhythm disorder approaches address conditions including delayed sleep phase syndrome through appropriate timing of melatonin (0.5-5mg 2-3 hours before desired sleep onset), light therapy, and sleep scheduling interventions based on individual circadian pattern assessment.

Neurocognitive Disorder Management

Cognitive enhancer therapy implements appropriate selection and use of cholinesterase inhibitors (donepezil 5-10mg daily, rivastigmine 1.5-6mg twice daily oral or 4.6-13.3mg/24 hours transdermal, galantamine 8-24mg daily) and memantine (10mg twice daily or 28mg extended-release daily) based on dementia type, disease stage, and tolerability considerations, with attention to contraindications including significant bradycardia or conduction abnormalities for cholinesterase inhibitors. Behavioral and psychological symptom management employs non-pharmacological approaches as first-line intervention, with cautious use of pharmacotherapy including antipsychotics (risperidone 0.25-1mg daily, quetiapine 25-200mg daily), antidepressants (citalopram 10-20mg daily, sertraline 25-100mg daily), or mood stabilizers (valproate 250-1000mg daily) for specific symptom clusters when non-drug approaches prove insufficient, employing the lowest effective dose with regular reassessment for continued necessity. Medication optimization for cognitively impaired patients includes systematic review to eliminate unnecessary medications, minimize anticholinergic burden, and simplify regimens to support adherence.

Summary

- Cardiovascular disorder management focuses on evidence-based pharmacotherapy for hypertension, heart failure, dyslipidemias, and anticoagulation with emphasis on guideline-directed medical therapy and risk factor modification.

- Endocrine disorder management centers on glycemic control in diabetes mellitus, thyroid disorders, and adrenal conditions, requiring careful monitoring of metabolic parameters and individualized therapy goals.

- Respiratory condition management includes stepwise approaches to asthma and COPD therapy, with attention to proper inhaler technique, trigger avoidance, and prevention of exacerbations.

- Infectious disease management requires appropriate antimicrobial selection based on likely pathogens, local resistance patterns, patient factors, and principles of antimicrobial stewardship to optimize outcomes while minimizing resistance.

- Oncology pharmacy practice involves complex chemotherapy regimen management, supportive care for side effects, drug interaction prevention, and specialized handling of hazardous medications.

- Mental health disorder management includes medication selection and monitoring for depression, anxiety, bipolar disorder, and schizophrenia, with attention to adherence challenges and metabolic monitoring.

- Patient-specific goals of therapy should be established for each disease state, considering comorbidities, quality of life, prognosis, and alignment with patient preferences and values.

Multiple Choice Questions

1. A 62-year-old patient with heart failure with reduced ejection fraction (HFrEF) is currently taking lisinopril and metoprolol. Which of the following represents the MOST appropriate next agent to add to optimize guideline-directed medical therapy?
   A) Amlodipine
   B) Spironolactone
   C) Digoxin
   D) Hydralazine
2. A patient with type 2 diabetes has an A1C of 8.2% despite maximum tolerated metformin therapy. The patient has established coronary artery disease. Which of the following agents would be MOST appropriate to add based on current evidence?
   A) Sulfonylurea
   B) DPP-4 inhibitor
   C) SGLT2 inhibitor
   D) Thiazolidinedione
3. When managing a patient with community-acquired pneumonia, which of the following represents the MOST appropriate application of antimicrobial stewardship principles?
   A) Using the broadest spectrum antibiotic available to ensure coverage
   B) Selecting an appropriate empiric regimen based on guidelines, then de-escalating based on culture results
   C) Always using multiple antibiotics to prevent resistance
   D) Continuing antibiotics for 14 days regardless of patient response
4. A patient with asthma reports using their albuterol inhaler daily for symptom control despite regular use of a low-dose inhaled corticosteroid. According to step-wise management, the MOST appropriate next step would be:
   A) Adding a long-acting beta-agonist (LABA)
   B) Doubling the dose of inhaled corticosteroid
   C) Adding a leukotriene receptor antagonist
   D) Starting oral corticosteroid therapy
5. Which of the following medication regimens is MOST appropriate for a patient with newly diagnosed schizophrenia?
   A) Lithium monotherapy

B) Second-generation antipsychotic monotherapy

C) SSRI antidepressant monotherapy

D) Benzodiazepine monotherapy

6. A 58-year-old patient with non-small cell lung cancer is found to have an EGFR mutation. The MOST appropriate initial therapy would be:

   A) Platinum-based chemotherapy

   B) EGFR tyrosine kinase inhibitor

   C) Immune checkpoint inhibitor

   D) Radiation therapy alone

7. For a patient with atrial fibrillation and a CHA_2DS_2-VASc score of 4, which of the following is the MOST appropriate antithrombotic approach?

   A) Aspirin monotherapy

   B) No antithrombotic therapy due to bleeding risk

   C) Oral anticoagulation with warfarin or a direct oral anticoagulant

   D) Dual antiplatelet therapy

8. A patient with moderate COPD (GOLD Group B) is experiencing shortness of breath despite using a short-acting bronchodilator as needed. The MOST appropriate next step in therapy would be:

   A) Adding an inhaled corticosteroid

   B) Starting a long-acting bronchodilator

   C) Adding oral corticosteroid therapy

   D) Starting oxygen therapy

9. When selecting an initial treatment regimen for a patient with newly diagnosed HIV infection, which of the following is the MOST important consideration?

   A) Cost of therapy only

   B) Pill burden only

   C) Results of resistance testing and patient-specific factors

   D) Using the oldest proven regimen first

10. A patient with bipolar I disorder is experiencing acute mania. The MOST appropriate initial pharmacotherapy would be:

    A) SSRI antidepressant monotherapy

    B) Benzodiazepine monotherapy

    C) Mood stabilizer or second-generation antipsychotic

    D) Tricyclic antidepressant monotherapy

Self-Assessment Questions

1. Compare and contrast the pharmacological management of heart failure with reduced ejection fraction (HFrEF) versus heart failure with preserved ejection fraction (HFpEF), including specific medication classes and their mechanisms of benefit.
2. Explain the role of SGLT2 inhibitors in the management of type 2 diabetes, including their cardiovascular and renal benefits beyond glycemic control.
3. Describe the step-wise approach to asthma management according to current guidelines, including controller and rescue medications and criteria for stepping up or stepping down therapy.
4. Discuss the principles of antimicrobial stewardship in the management of infectious diseases, including strategies to optimize antimicrobial selection, dosing, and duration.
5. Explain the pharmacist's role in managing medication-related toxicities in patients receiving cancer chemotherapy, including preventive strategies and management approaches.
6. Compare and contrast the pharmacological management of major depressive disorder and bipolar disorder, including medication selection considerations and monitoring parameters.
7. Describe the comprehensive approach to managing a patient with atherosclerotic cardiovascular disease, including pharmacological and non-pharmacological interventions.
8. Explain the concept of targeted therapy in oncology, including how molecular testing guides treatment selection and the role of pharmacists in managing these therapies.
9. Discuss the pharmacological management of COPD, including the appropriate use of inhaled bronchodilators, corticosteroids, and strategies to prevent exacerbations.
10. Explain the considerations for selecting antiretroviral therapy for HIV, including regimen composition, resistance testing, and monitoring parameters.

Bibliography

1. Whelton PK, Carey RM, Aronow WS, Casey DE Jr, Collins KJ, Dennison Himmelfarb C, et al. 2017 ACC/AHA/AAPA/ABC/ACPM/AGS/APhA/ASH/ASPC/NMA/PCNA guideline for the prevention, detection, evaluation, and management of high blood pressure in adults: a report of the American College of Cardiology/American Heart Association Task Force on Clinical Practice Guidelines. Hypertension. 2018;71(6):e13-e115.
2. Yancy CW, Jessup M, Bozkurt B, Butler J, Casey DE Jr, Colvin MM, et al. 2017 ACC/AHA/HFSA focused update of the 2013 ACCF/AHA guideline for the management of heart failure: a report of the American College of Cardiology/American Heart Association Task Force on Clinical Practice Guidelines and the Heart Failure Society of America. Circulation. 2017;136(6):e137-e161.
3. American Diabetes Association. Standards of medical care in diabetes—2021. Diabetes Care. 2021;44(Suppl 1):S1-S232.
4. Global Initiative for Chronic Obstructive Lung Disease. Global strategy for the diagnosis, management, and prevention of chronic obstructive pulmonary disease: 2021 report. Available from: https://goldcopd.org/
5. Global Initiative for Asthma. Global strategy for asthma management and prevention, 2021. Available from: https://ginasthma.org/
6. Metlay JP, Waterer GW, Long AC, Anzueto A, Brozek J, Crothers K, et al. Diagnosis and treatment of adults with community-acquired pneumonia. An official clinical practice guideline of the American Thoracic Society and Infectious Diseases Society of America. Am J Respir Crit Care Med. 2019;200(7):e45-e67.
7. Arnett DK, Blumenthal RS, Albert MA, Buroker AB, Goldberger ZD, Hahn EJ, et al. 2019 Circulation. 2019;140(11):e596-e646.
8. NCCN Clinical Practice Guidelines in Oncology. Available from: https://www.nccn.org/guidelines/
9. American Psychiatric Association. The American Psychiatric Association practice guideline for the treatment of patients with schizophrenia. 3rd ed. Washington, DC: American Psychiatric Association Publishing; 2021.
10. Gelenberg AJ, Freeman MP, Markowitz JC, Rosenbaum JF, Thase ME, Trivedi MH, et al. Practice guideline for the treatment of patients with major depressive disorder. 3rd ed. Arlington, VA: American Psychiatric Association; 2010

CHAPTER 14

MEDICATION SAFETY

Author

Dr. Anurag Sahu, Clinical Pharmacist, Department of Clinical Pharmacology, Apollo SAGE Hospital, Bhopal, Madhya Pradesh, India

Abstract

Medication safety systems provide comprehensive frameworks for preventing, identifying, and mitigating medication-related harm through integrated approaches addressing system vulnerabilities throughout the medication use process. Error prevention strategies employ human factors engineering, high-alert medication safeguards, technology utilization, and standardized communication techniques creating multiple layers of protection against medication misadventures. Risk management methodologies implement proactive assessment through failure mode analysis, medication use evaluation, root cause investigation, and simulation training identifying system weaknesses before patient harm occurs. Quality assurance programs develop performance indicators, compliance monitoring systems, peer review processes, and continuous improvement methodologies ensuring consistent adherence to safe medication practices across diverse healthcare settings. Reporting systems establish voluntary and mandatory event notification mechanisms, just culture implementation, aggregate data analysis, and systematic learning dissemination transforming individual incidents into system-wide improvement opportunities. Safety initiatives target high-risk medications including anticoagulants, insulin, opioids, and chemotherapy through specialized protocols, technology implementation, and process redesign addressing known vulnerability points. This comprehensive approach shifts focus from individual blame to system improvement through standardization, simplification, automation, and education creating resilient medication systems capable of preventing errors despite human fallibility and complex healthcare environments.

Keywords: *Medication Error Prevention, System Reliability, Safety Culture, Risk Mitigation, Adverse Event Reduction*

Learning Objectives

After completion of the chapter, the learners should be able to:

- Implement error prevention strategies including tall-man lettering, sound-alike/look-alike safeguards, and high-alert medication protocols to enhance medication safety.
- Apply risk management methodologies including failure mode effects analysis and root cause analysis to identify and address system vulnerabilities.
- Develop quality assurance programs incorporating performance indicators, compliance monitoring, and continuous improvement methodologies.
- Implement effective medication error reporting systems that encourage reporting, facilitate analysis, and promote system-wide learning.
- Design targeted safety initiatives addressing high-risk medications, vulnerable populations, and transition points in the medication use process.
- Foster a culture of safety that promotes non-punitive reporting, system improvement, and proactive risk identification throughout the medication use process.

ERROR PREVENTION

Human Factors Engineering

Cognitive load reduction designs systems acknowledging limited working memory capacity, particularly during stressful situations or with interruptions common in healthcare environments, through strategies including standardized order sets, clinical decision support tools, and simplified processes requiring fewer mental calculations or memory-dependent steps. Forcing functions create physical constraints preventing dangerous actions, such as incompatible connections between epidural and intravenous tubing preventing wrong-route administration, non-interchangeable gas line connections preventing delivery of incorrect medical gases, or electronic systems preventing concurrent orders for interacting medications without explicit override. Standardization reduces unnecessary variation in processes, concentrations, and ordering practices, limiting decision points where errors commonly occur through approaches including standard concentrations for intravenous medications, uniform prescribing terminology, and consistent placement of information on medication labels.

Table 14.1: Medication Error Prevention Strategies

Error Type	Contributing Factors	Preventive Measures
Prescribing Errors	Knowledge deficits, communication issues, alert fatigue	Clinical decision support, standardized orders, CPOE systems
Transcription Errors	Illegible handwriting, verbal order miscommunication, abbreviation misinterpretation	Electronic prescribing, standardized communication, prohibited abbreviation lists
Dispensing Errors	Look-alike/sound-alike drugs, interruptions, confirmation bias	Barcode verification, tall man lettering, separated storage, double-checks
Administration Errors	Distractions, calculation errors, pump programming errors	Barcode medication administration, smart pumps, independent double-checks
Monitoring Errors	Missed follow-up, documentation gaps, communication failures	Structured monitoring plans, closed-loop systems, automated alerts
High-Alert Medication Errors	Narrow therapeutic index, complex dosing, high harm potential	Special protocols, enhanced verification, restricted access
Transition of Care Errors	Information gaps, multiple providers, reconciliation challenges	Medication reconciliation, standardized handoffs, transition pharmacists
Technology-Related Errors	Design flaws, workarounds, alert fatigue	Human factors engineering, usability testing, appropriate alert thresholds

High-Alert Medication Management

Identification and designation uses resources including ISMP's high-alert medication lists to identify agents requiring special handling, including insulin, anticoagulants, opioids, neuromuscular blockers, and concentrated electrolytes, creating organization-specific protocols based on both published recommendations and local experience with medication incidents. Storage and access limitations include separation of look-alike products, restricted access to concentrated electrolytes, and segregation of neuromuscular blockers from other medications, with particular attention to emergency medications, pediatric preparations, and critical care drugs where dosing errors can rapidly cause serious harm. Independent double-check requirements mandate verification by two qualified individuals for high-risk processes including preparation and administration of chemotherapy, pediatric medications, and patient-controlled analgesia programming, with specific protocols defining check procedures, documentation requirements, and appropriate timing relative to medication administration.

Technology Utilization

Computerized provider order entry (CPOE) with clinical decision support incorporates safety features including dose range checking, allergy screening, duplicate therapy alerts, and clinical contraindication warnings, though requiring careful implementation to prevent alert fatigue from excessive or clinically insignificant warnings, with tiered alert presentation strategies prioritizing highest-risk interactions for interruptive alerts while providing non-interruptive information for lower-risk situations. Barcode medication administration systems verify the "five rights" through electronic matching of patient, medication, dose, route, and time, with studies demonstrating 50-80% reductions in administration errors following implementation, particularly effective when integrated with electronic medication administration records documenting actual administration times rather than scheduled times alone. Smart infusion pumps with drug libraries incorporate medication-specific safety limits, requiring override acknowledgment when programmed doses exceed typical parameters, ideally with wireless connectivity allowing library updates, utilization tracking, and integration with electronic health records.

Pharmacy Preparation Safety

Sterile compounding protocols implement USP <797> standards including appropriate engineering controls, aseptic technique, environmental monitoring, and beyond-use dating to ensure both product sterility and accuracy, with particular attention to hazardous medication handling following USP <800> requirements for personal protective equipment, containment strategies, and waste management. Calculation double-checks require independent verification of critical calculations including pediatric doses, chemotherapy, and high-risk medications using standardized documentation, ideally employing different calculation methods or approaches between primary and verification calculations to prevent replication of the same error. Ready-to-use product utilization replaces manual preparation with commercially available or pharmacy-prepared standardized products whenever possible, reducing manipulation points where errors occur through commercially available premixed infusions, unit-dose packaging, and standardized concentrations requiring minimal preparation before administration.

Look-alike/Sound-alike Medication Error Prevention

Name confusion countermeasures include tall-man lettering (highlighting distinguishing parts of similar names such as DOPamine and DOBUTamine), separating similar products in storage areas, and including both brand and generic names on labels, with systematic assessment of new products for potential confusion with existing inventory before formulary addition. Packaging differentiation employs strategies including auxiliary labels, storage separation, and purchasing from different manufacturers when possible to create visual distinctions between similar products, with particular attention to products with similar packaging within the same therapeutic category where wrong drug errors may go undetected due to similar clinical effects. Order clarification protocols require verbal confirmation of unusual doses, verification of indication for medications with multiple uses, and spelling of drug names during verbal orders, with specific procedures for high-risk sound-alike situations such as morphine/hydromorphone or methotrexate/metronidazole.

Verbal and Telephone Order Safety

Read-back verification requires the recipient to read back the complete order including patient name, drug, dose, route, and frequency, with the prescriber confirming accuracy before implementation, replacing ineffective "repeat-back" practices where information may be incorrectly heard twice rather than verified. Limitation policies restrict verbal orders to urgent situations where written or electronic ordering is impractical, rather than convenience or routine practice, with specific documentation requirements noting the emergent circumstances necessitating verbal communication rather than standard ordering processes. Standardized terminology employs protocols prohibiting dangerous abbreviations and requiring spelling of medication names, full expression of doses, and explicit leading zeros for decimal doses, with particular attention to numbers where misheard digits could result in ten-fold dosing errors.

Handoff Communication Improvement

Standardized handoff tools including SBAR (Situation-Background-Assessment-Recommendation) or I-PASS (Illness severity, Patient summary, Action list, Situation awareness, Synthesis) provide structured frameworks ensuring complete information transfer, with medication-specific elements highlighted as critical components requiring explicit communication rather than assumed knowledge. Medication reconciliation processes systematically compare medication regimens across transitions to identify and resolve discrepancies before causing harm, with particular attention to high-risk transitions including hospital admission, transfer between units, and discharge to different care levels. Documentation standardization creates consistent formats for medication information across care settings, electronic systems, and departments to prevent misinterpretation, including standardized medication histories, administration records, and discharge instructions with explicit sections addressing medication changes, monitoring requirements, and follow-up expectations.

Patient Engagement Strategies

Medication education provides information about medication purposes, appearance, expected effects, and potential adverse reactions, enabling patients to question unexpected medications, with teach-back verification ensuring comprehension beyond passive information provision or simple acknowledgment of instructions. Self-management tools including medication lists, administration schedules, and symptom diaries support patient participation in safety monitoring, with updated information provided following medication changes and specific guidance about which symptoms warrant immediate contact versus routine follow-up. Reporting encouragement empowers patients to speak up about potential errors, medication concerns, or unexpected effects without fear of negative consequences, with specific mechanisms including bedside reporting systems, direct communication pathways to pharmacy departments, and inclusion of safety reporting options in patient education materials.

RISK MANAGEMENT

Failure Mode and Effects Analysis (FMEA)

Process mapping creates detailed flowcharts documenting each step in high-risk medication processes, identifying decision points, handoffs, and complexity that increase error vulnerability, typically beginning with broad process outlines and progressively adding detail to capture all substeps, responsible parties, and information transfers within complex medication systems. Failure identification systematically examines each process step to determine potential failure modes, considering human factors, environmental variables, and system weaknesses through structured team discussion including representatives from all disciplines involved in the medication process. Severity and probability scoring assigns numerical ratings to each potential failure based on likelihood of occurrence and potential consequences, creating prioritization for improvement efforts, typically using 1-10 scales for both dimensions with combined scores or matrices determining overall risk ranking.

Medication Use Evaluation (MUE)

Criteria development establishes explicit standards for appropriate medication use based on evidence-based guidelines, institutional protocols, or best practice recommendations, creating objective measures against which actual practice can be evaluated without relying on individual judgment or variable standards.

Table 14.2: Risk Management Methodologies

Risk Management Approach	Application Methodology	Implementation Requirements	Outcome Measures
Failure Mode and Effects Analysis (FMEA)	Proactive process analysis, failure identification, mitigation development	Multidisciplinary team, process mapping, risk scoring, action planning	Risk reduction scores, process improvement, prevented failures
Root Cause Analysis (RCA)	Retrospective event investigation, contributing factor identification, system improvement	Event reporting, investigation team, causal factor identification, action plans	Recurrence prevention, system changes, contributing factor reduction
Medication Use Evaluation (MUE)	Targeted drug use assessment, criteria development, performance measurement	Drug selection criteria, data collection methodology, performance comparison	Practice alignment with criteria, intervention development, improvement trends
Medication Error Reporting Analysis	Aggregate data review, pattern identification, system vulnerability detection	Reporting system, taxonomy standardization, trend analysis methodology	Error category trends, intervention effectiveness, reporting culture measures
Probabilistic Risk Assessment	Mathematical modeling, failure probability calculation, risk quantification	Statistical expertise, comprehensive data sources, model validation	Risk probability reduction, intervention prioritization, resource allocation

Risk Managemen t Approach	Application Methodology	Implementation Requirements	Outcome Measures
Hazard Analysis	Systematic hazard identification, severity assessment, mitigation prioritization	Hazard identification methodology, severity classification, priority matrix	Hazard elimination/mitigatio n, severity reduction, control effectiveness
Safety Culture Assessment	Staff perception evaluation, communicatio n assessment, just culture analysis	Validated survey tools, psychological safety promotion, leadership engagement	Culture scores, reporting willingness, perception of response to errors
High Reliability Organizatio n Principles	Preoccupation with failure, sensitivity to operations, commitment to resilience	Leadership commitment, mindfulness development, process reliability	Reliability metrics, recovery effectiveness, failure anticipation measures

Data collection methods include retrospective chart review, concurrent assessment during therapy, and database analysis of prescribing patterns, with sampling strategies balancing comprehensive evaluation against resource constraints through random selection, focused high-risk targeting, or triggered review based on specific events. Intervention design addresses identified gaps through system changes, education, clinical decision support tools, or policy modifications based on specific findings, with follow-up measurement demonstrating whether implemented changes successfully improved practice patterns compared to baseline assessment.

Root Cause Analysis (RCA)

Multidisciplinary investigation assembles representatives from all involved disciplines to examine events without individual blame, focusing on system vulnerabilities rather than personal fault, typically including direct participants in the event alongside those with process expertise who can provide objective assessment without defensive responses. Causal factor identification distinguishes between proximate causes (immediate actions or conditions) and underlying system causes (policies, procedures, environmental factors) contributing to the event, using techniques including "five whys" questioning, fishbone diagrams, or causal trees to identify fundamental issues rather than superficial factors. Contributing factor classification organizes identified causes into categories including communication, training, fatigue, environment, policies, and barriers, facilitating pattern recognition across multiple events and directing improvement efforts toward systematic rather than isolated issues.

High-Risk Population Safeguards

Pediatric safety systems address weight-based dosing risks through required independent calculations, standardized concentrations, and specialized references appropriate for children, with particular attention to decimal point errors, unit conversion mistakes, and dose range verification spanning the wide weight range from neonates through adolescents. Geriatric medication management employs screening tools including Beers Criteria and STOPP/START to identify potentially inappropriate medications requiring additional review before use in older adults, with automated alerts, pharmacist review protocols, or mandatory geriatric consultation for high-risk prescribing. Renal and hepatic impairment protocols implement systematic screening and dosage adjustment for medications affected by organ dysfunction, preventing toxicity from impaired clearance through automated calculation of renal function with corresponding dosage recommendations, default substitutions, or required pharmacist review before dispensing.

Simulation Training

High-fidelity simulations recreate complex medication emergencies including anaphylaxis, malignant hyperthermia, or opioid overdose with mannequins simulating physiological responses to interventions, allowing teams to practice critical medication administration, dose calculation, and emergency response without patient risk. Procedural simulations focus on high-risk tasks including chemotherapy preparation, epidural medication management, or emergency medication preparation under pressure, identifying workflow vulnerabilities, knowledge gaps, and system weaknesses in controlled environments where errors become learning opportunities rather than patient harm. Debriefing sessions following simulations identify knowledge gaps, system vulnerabilities, and improvement opportunities revealed during scenarios, using structured facilitation techniques to explore both technical performance and team communication factors contributing to successful outcomes or potential errors.

Risk Assessment Tools

Self-assessment instruments including the ISMP Medication Safety

Self Assessment guide systematic evaluation of medication systems against established best practices, identifying gaps requiring attention through structured review of key safety domains including patient information, drug information, communication, labeling, environment, staff competency, and quality processes. Trigger tool methodology employs specific clinical markers suggestive of adverse drug events (abnormal laboratory values, antidote use, abrupt medication discontinuation) to efficiently identify potential medication harm for further investigation, providing more comprehensive detection than spontaneous reporting while requiring less resource investment than comprehensive chart review. Proactive risk rounds conduct regular multidisciplinary assessments of clinical areas, identifying environmental factors, workflow issues, and practice variations creating safety vulnerabilities before errors occur, using structured checklists or observational protocols to ensure consistent evaluation across different units and time periods.

Safety Culture Assessment and Improvement

Assessment tools including the AHRQ Hospital Survey on Patient Safety Culture measure staff perceptions regarding safety priorities, communication openness, error response, and leadership commitment, providing baseline data and improvement targets through standardized measurement across organizations with national benchmarking capabilities. Just culture implementation establishes balanced approaches to error response, distinguishing between human error (requiring system redesign rather than punishment), at-risk behavior (requiring coaching and process improvement), and reckless conduct (requiring appropriate accountability) with clear organizational policies defining each category and corresponding responses. Psychological safety development creates environments where staff feel comfortable speaking up about concerns, questioning potential errors, and suggesting improvements without fear of negative consequences, through leadership modeling, positive reinforcement of safety communication, and appropriate response to raised concerns demonstrating organizational commitment to error prevention over hierarchical authority.

Formulary Management as Risk Mitigation

Class consolidation limits unnecessary therapeutic duplication within medication classes, reducing look-alike/sound-alike risks and cognitive burden associated with managing multiple similar agents, while maintaining sufficient options to address specific patient needs, contraindications, or specialized clinical scenarios. High-alert medication restrictions implement additional safeguards for particularly dangerous medications, including limited formulary options within high-risk classes, special ordering requirements, or mandatory pharmacist review before dispensing, balancing medication access against safety considerations through evidence-based selection of preferred agents within high-risk categories. Novel therapy introduction protocols require structured safety evaluation before adding new medications to formulary, including error potential assessment, look-alike/sound-alike evaluation, and implementation planning addressing training needs, monitoring requirements, and integration with existing systems and workflows.

QUALITY ASSURANCE

Performance Indicator Development

Structure measures assess the foundation for safe medication use including staffing adequacy, technology implementation, policy comprehensiveness, and physical environment characteristics, focusing on system capabilities and resources rather than actual practices or outcomes, with examples including pharmacist-to-patient ratios, percentage of units using barcode medication administration, or availability of standardized concentrations for high-risk medications. Process measures evaluate adherence to safe medication practices including independent double-checks, barcode scanning compliance, hand-off communication completeness, and medication reconciliation performance, typically reported as percentage compliance with established protocols based on direct observation, documentation review, or electronic system data. Outcome measures assess actual or potential patient impact including adverse drug events, medication errors reaching patients, and harm categorization when events occur, with severity classification using standardized frameworks such as NCC MERP categories or AHRQ harm scales.

Dashboard Development

Metric selection focuses measurement on high-risk processes, problem-prone medications, and key safety practices most critical to patient protection, balancing comprehensive monitoring against excessive data collection that dilutes attention to priority areas, typically selecting 8-12 key indicators representing different aspects of medication safety spanning various process steps and medication classes. Threshold establishment defines expected performance levels with alert triggers when metrics deviate from acceptable ranges requiring investigation or intervention, typically using statistical process control methods, benchmark comparisons, or expert consensus to establish appropriate targets and variance parameters. Trend analysis examines data longitudinally to identify gradual changes that might not be apparent in isolated time periods, distinguishing random variation from meaningful shifts requiring attention through statistical techniques including run charts, control charts, or regression analysis identifying significant patterns beyond month-to-month fluctuations.

Compliance Monitoring

Policy and procedure evaluation assesses alignment with current evidence, regulatory requirements, and professional standards, with regular revision cycles maintaining relevance, typically conducting comprehensive review every 1-3 years with interim updates as needed for significant practice changes, new regulations, or identified safety concerns. Direct observation studies measure actual practice conformance with established safety procedures, identifying gaps between policy and frontline implementation through structured observation protocols, tracer methodology, or work sampling techniques providing objective assessment beyond self-reported compliance. Tracer methodology follows specific medications through the entire use process from ordering through administration, evaluating system performance for representative high-risk agents or recently identified problem areas, with multidisciplinary teams observing and documenting each process step against established standards.

Table 14.3: Quality Assurance for Medication Systems

Quality Assurance Categories	Assessment	Performance Indicators	Improvement Approaches
Medication Process Standards	Policy/procedure compliance audits, workflow analysis, competency assessment	Compliance rates, workflow efficiency, error reduction metrics	Standards revision, workflow redesign, competency development
Technology Performance Monitoring	Override analysis, alert firing patterns, system utilization metrics	Override rates, alert acceptance, system utilization patterns	Alert redesign, system optimization, user interface improvement
Clinical Pharmacy Service Quality	Intervention documentation, clinical impact assessment, recommendation acceptance	Intervention rates, clinical significance, acceptance percentages	Service redesign, impact enhancement, documentation improvement

Quality Assurance Categories	Assessment	Performance Indicators	Improvement Approaches
Dispensing Accuracy Assessment	Random sample verification, error detection methodologies, near-miss analysis	Error rates by type, near-miss frequencies, accuracy percentages	Process redesign, verification enhancement, automation optimization
Staff Competency Evaluation	Knowledge assessment, simulation performance, peer review	Competency scores, performance metrics, continuous education completion	Targeted education, simulation training, peer coaching
High-Risk Process Evaluation	Process-specific audits, outcome measurement, risk assessment	Error rates in high-risk processes, near-miss frequencies, harm events	Protocol enhancement, verification processes, specialized training
Medication Storage and Security	Environment audits, temperature monitoring, access control evaluation	Compliance with storage requirements, security breach incidents, temperature excursions	Environmental modifications, access system enhancement, monitoring improvement
Regulatory Compliance Assessment	Readiness surveys, mock inspections, standard compliance review	Compliance rates, deficiency identification, regulatory readiness	Gap closure, standard implementation, continuous compliance monitoring

Peer Review Processes

Medication order review evaluates prescribing patterns, adherence to protocols, and appropriate clinical decision-making with structured feedback to prescribers, using random sampling, focused review of high-risk medications, or triggered evaluation following identified concerns to balance comprehensive oversight with practical resource limitations. Clinical documentation assessment examines pharmacist interventions, monitoring practices, and therapeutic recommendations against established standards with peer feedback for improvement, ensuring consistent application of pharmaceutical care processes across different practitioners and clinical areas. Practice evaluation employs structured assessment tools measuring performance in core competency areas including medication reconciliation, patient education, and high-risk medication management, with results guiding individual improvement plans, targeted educational initiatives, or system changes addressing common deficiencies.

Regulatory Readiness

Regulatory standard monitoring tracks evolving requirements from organizations including The Joint Commission, CMS, state boards of pharmacy, and other oversight entities, ensuring timely implementation of new or revised standards through systematic review of regulatory publications, participation in professional organizations, and dedicated compliance oversight responsibilities. Gap analysis compares current practices against regulatory requirements, identifying discrepancies requiring correction before external review through structured self-assessment, mock surveys, or consultant evaluation using the same standards and methodology employed by regulatory surveyors. Survey preparation implements mock evaluations, tracer activities, and focused reviews of high-risk areas commonly scrutinized during regulatory visits, familiarizing staff with survey processes while identifying improvement opportunities before official inspections.

Staff Competency Assessment

Competency validation tools establish objective assessment methods for critical safety skills including high-alert medication management, chemotherapy preparation, pediatric dosing, and emergency medication use, using direct observation, knowledge testing, simulation scenarios, or chart audit methodologies to verify both theoretical understanding and practical application capability. Simulation-based assessment evaluates performance in realistic scenarios replicating high-risk situations, identifying both technical and decision-making competencies requiring development through standardized cases with objective scoring criteria addressing both procedure completion and critical thinking elements. Remediation protocols establish structured approaches for addressing identified competency gaps, including additional training, supervised practice, and reassessment before independent practice, with progressive intervention intensity based on deficiency severity and repeated assessment results.

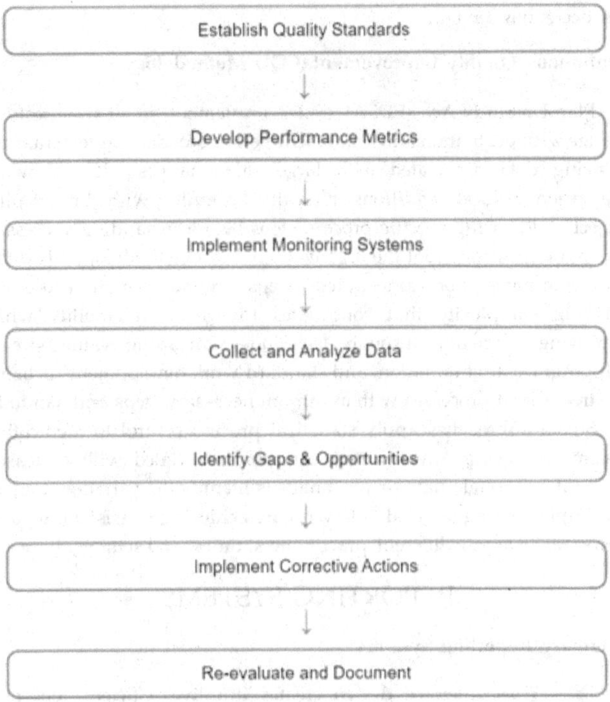

Figure 14.1: Pharmacy Quality Assurance Process

Audit and Feedback Systems

Targeted audits focus on high-risk processes including insulin management, anticoagulation, chemotherapy, and pediatric medications with structured tools measuring compliance with safety requirements, concentrating limited resources on areas with greatest potential for serious harm rather than attempting equal oversight across all medication processes. Random sampling methodologies evaluate representative processes across departments and shifts, preventing predictable audit patterns that may distort typical practice assessment, with sample size determination balancing statistical validity against resource constraints through appropriate power calculations or established quality assurance sampling standards. Constructive feedback provides specific, actionable information to involved staff and leadership, focusing on system improvement rather than individual criticism, with timely communication, recognition of positive practices alongside improvement opportunities, and clear recommendations for practice enhancement.

Continuous Quality Improvement (CQI) Methodology

Plan-Do-Study-Act (PDSA) cycles implement small-scale tests of change with evaluation and refinement before broader implementation, reducing risks associated with large-scale changes while allowing adaptation to local conditions, typically beginning with limited pilot projects addressing specific process steps before expanding successful interventions throughout the organization. Lean methodology identifies and eliminates non-value-added steps in medication processes, reducing complexity that contributes to error vulnerability while improving efficiency through techniques including value stream mapping, waste elimination, and standard work development focusing on streamlined processes with minimum necessary steps and handoffs. Six Sigma approaches apply statistical process control to medication systems, reducing unwarranted variation associated with increased error rates through data-driven analysis identifying variation sources and implementing targeted interventions achieving consistent, reliable performance across different practitioners, times, and settings.

REPORTING SYSTEMS

Voluntary Reporting Systems

User interface design creates intuitive, efficient reporting tools minimizing documentation burden while capturing essential information for meaningful analysis, balancing comprehensive data collection against time requirements that discourage reporting, typically employing branching logic, pre-populated fields, and streamlined workflows requiring less than 5 minutes for routine report completion. Anonymity and confidentiality provisions protect reporters from inappropriate disclosure or potential retaliation, encouraging reporting of events that might otherwise remain hidden through policy guarantees, technical safeguards, and cultural reinforcement emphasizing information use for system improvement rather than individual accountability. Classification taxonomies provide standardized categorization of event types, contributing factors, and severity levels, enabling pattern identification across multiple reports through consistent terminology, hierarchical classification structures, and standardized definitions ensuring reports from different sources can be meaningfully aggregated and analyzed.

Just Culture Implementation

Human error recognition addresses unintentional mistakes occurring despite good intentions, focusing on system improvement rather than individual punishment when errors result from system vulnerabilities including confusing interfaces, look-alike medications, interruption-prone environments, or excessive workload, with response emphasizing consolation, support, and environmental modification rather than disciplinary action. At-risk behavior management addresses conscious decisions to deviate from safe practices, typically motivated by perceived efficiency or workload pressures rather than malicious intent, requiring coaching and system examination rather than disciplinary response, with focus on understanding why circumvention seemed necessary and addressing underlying system issues making compliance difficult. Reckless conduct response addresses conscious disregard for substantial risk, appropriately involving corrective action while remaining proportional to circumstances, reserved for situations involving deliberate protocol violations without mitigating factors, substance abuse affecting performance, or falsification of documentation.

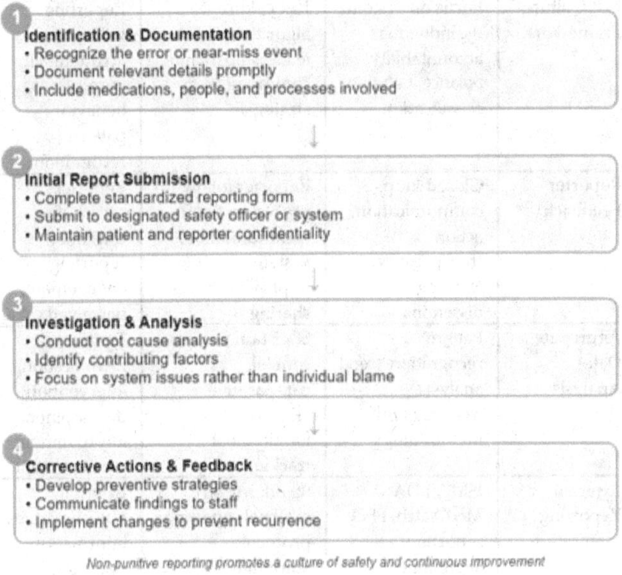

Figure 14.2: Medication Error Reporting Process

Table 14.4: Medication Error Reporting Systems

Reporting System Element	Design Features	Implementation	Effectiveness Measures
Reporting Process	User-friendly interface, appropriate anonymity options, multiple access methods	Simplified forms, electronic submission, 24/7 availability	Reporting rates, report quality, user satisfaction
Event Classification	Standardized taxonomy, harm categorization, contributing factor identification	NCC MERP classification, standardized definitions, structured fields	Classification consistency, contributing factor identification, trend analysis capability
Just Culture Framework	Focus on system vs. individual, accountability balance, behavior classification	Just culture algorithm, leadership training, communication strategies	Reporting willingness, accountability perceptions, behavior pattern recognition
Reporter Feedback	Closed-loop communication, action transparency, learning dissemination	Reporter follow-up process, action communication, system improvement sharing	Reporter satisfaction, continued reporting engagement, perceived value
Aggregate Data Analysis	Pattern recognition, trend analysis, prioritization methodology	Statistical process control, comparative analysis, longitudinal tracking	Trend identification, intervention development, improvement measurement
External Reporting Integration	ISMP, FDA MedWatch, PSO reporting alignment	Standardized external reporting protocols, automated submissions where possible	External reporting rates, information sharing contribution, system improvement
Learning System Integration	Error analysis to education connection, system change implementation, shared learning	Case-based education, system modification processes, interdepartmental sharing	Knowledge improvement, system enhancement

Reporting System Element	Design Features	Implementation	Effectiveness Measures
Near-Miss Capture	Special near-miss focus, positive reinforcement, learning emphasis	Near-miss specific forms, recognition for reporting, proactive analysis	Near-miss reporting rates, proactive intervention development, prevention effectiveness

Mandatory Reporting Requirements

Sentinel event protocols define specific serious occurrences requiring thorough investigation and corrective action, including medication errors resulting in death or serious harm, according to regulatory definitions from The Joint Commission or similar oversight bodies, with specific timelines for investigation completion, corrective action implementation, and formal report submission to appropriate authorities. External reporting obligations address requirements to notify agencies including FDA (for medication and device-related events), state departments of health, or accrediting bodies depending on event type and severity, with clear organizational policies defining which events require external reporting, responsible parties for submission, and appropriate documentation maintenance. Timeframe compliance ensures appropriate urgency in reporting based on event severity, with clear delineation of which events require immediate notification versus routine documentation, typically including 24-hour reporting requirements for deaths or serious injuries and longer timeframes for less severe or potential harm situations.

Aggregate Data Analysis

Trend analysis examines data longitudinally to identify increasing or decreasing event types, revealing emerging problems or improvement opportunities not apparent from isolated reports, using statistical techniques including run charts, control charts, or regression analysis to distinguish significant patterns from random variation. Contributing factor analysis identifies common elements across multiple events, revealing system issues affecting diverse error types and clinical areas through structured coding of environmental, procedural, communication, and training factors associated with reported incidents, allowing identification of fundamental system weaknesses requiring intervention. Severity-weighted analysis balances event frequency against potential harm, ensuring appropriate prioritization of lower-frequency but higher-consequence error types through rating matrices combining occurrence rates with actual or potential harm levels to identify highest-risk areas requiring immediate attention.

Feedback and Learning Systems

Reporter feedback provides specific information to individuals submitting reports about analysis findings and resulting improvement actions, closing the loop to demonstrate report impact through automated acknowledgments, investigation status updates, and eventual communication about system changes resulting from reported concerns. Organizational learning dissemination shares key findings and safety improvements across departments and disciplines, expanding learning beyond those directly involved in specific events through safety newsletters, educational alerts, case-based discussions, or formal communication systems ensuring widespread awareness of identified risks and implemented safeguards. Safety alert communications distribute time-sensitive information about emerging risks or critical safety issues identified through reporting systems, enabling rapid intervention before additional occurrences through standardized alert formats, clear action recommendations, and verification mechanisms ensuring critical information reaches frontline practitioners.

Near-miss Analysis

Barrier identification examines what protective systems successfully intercepted errors, highlighting effective safeguards deserving reinforcement or expansion to other areas, with particular attention to both technical barriers (alerts, forcing functions, verification systems) and human factors (situational awareness, knowledge application, team communication) contributing to successful error prevention. Recovery analysis studies how near-misses were detected and corrected, identifying successful error recognition patterns that can be formalized or taught to others, including cues triggering suspicion, verification behaviors confirming concerns, and intervention techniques effectively addressing potential errors before patient impact. Potential harm assessment evaluates what consequences might have occurred without successful interception, maintaining appropriate urgency despite absence of actual injury through structured analysis of likely outcomes based on medication characteristics, patient factors, and error type, ensuring near-misses receive attention proportional to their prevention value rather than actual outcome.

Patient Reporting Systems

Patient portal integration creates accessible electronic reporting options through existing patient communication platforms, reducing barriers to reporting concerns through familiar interfaces, simplified reporting formats, and seamless integration with healthcare communication systems already used for appointments, messages, and health information access. Structured assessment tools employ patient-friendly language to gather information about possible medication experiences, distinguishing between expected effects and potential errors through guided questions addressing timing, appearance, effects, and relationship to medication administration rather than requiring patients to determine what constitutes a reportable event. Investigation protocols establish consistent approaches to evaluating patient-reported concerns, ensuring appropriate follow-up while maintaining respect for patient perspectives, including acknowledgment timelines, investigation standards, and communication expectations providing meaningful response regardless of whether reported concerns ultimately represent actual errors.

Inter-organizational Sharing

Patient safety organization participation provides federal confidentiality protections encouraging transparent sharing of safety information between organizations without litigation concerns, enabling more comprehensive learning than possible through isolated institutional experience while maintaining appropriate privacy protections through specialized entities established under the Patient Safety and Quality Improvement Act. Collaborative learning networks establish structured mechanisms for sharing de-identified safety events, analysis findings, and improvement strategies across multiple organizations, creating communities of practice through regular meetings, shared databases, or formal collaboratives addressing common medication safety challenges through collective experience and diverse perspectives. Emerging risk alerts disseminate time-sensitive information about new safety threats identified through aggregate analysis across multiple facilities, enabling proactive intervention before similar events occur elsewhere through standardized alert formats, evidence-based recommendations, and wide distribution networks reaching diverse healthcare settings.

SAFETY INITIATIVES

Anticoagulation Safety Programs

Protocol standardization establishes consistent approaches to dosing, monitoring, reversal, and periprocedural management based on current evidence and guidelines, with specific protocols addressing different anticoagulants (warfarin, direct oral anticoagulants, heparins), indications (atrial fibrillation, venous thromboembolism, mechanical valves), and clinical scenarios (initiation, maintenance, interruption, bleeding). Specialized management services implement dedicated anticoagulation clinics or pharmacy-managed programs with specialized expertise and structured follow-up systems, demonstrating approximately 70% time in therapeutic range for warfarin compared to 40-50% in usual care, with corresponding reductions in thrombotic and bleeding complications. Patient education enhancement develops standardized materials, teach-back verification, and ongoing support addressing the complexities of anticoagulant therapy and monitoring requirements, including specific guidance on diet interactions, medication effects, monitoring importance, and bleeding recognition appropriate to health literacy level and specific anticoagulant characteristics.

Table 14.5: Medication Safety Initiatives

Safety Initiative	Implementation Components	Resource Requirements	Outcome Evaluation
Anticoagulation Safety Program	Standardized protocols, specialized monitoring, reversal agent availability	Dedicated personnel, monitoring systems, patient education materials	Adverse event rates, therapeutic goal achievement, reversal agent utilization
High-Alert Medication Management	Identification system, enhanced safeguards, specialized protocols	Comprehensive list, visual identifiers, protocol development	High-alert medication event rates, protocol compliance, near-miss reduction
Insulin Safety Initiative	Standardized concentrations, dedicated devices, hypoglycemia protocols	Standardized order sets, specialized administration devices, monitoring systems	Hypoglycemia rates, administration error reduction, protocol compliance

Safety Initiative	Implementation Components	Resource Requirements	Outcome Evaluation
Opioid Stewardship Program	Appropriate prescribing guidelines, monitoring protocols, naloxone availability	Prescribing tools, monitoring systems, education resources	Appropriate utilization rates, adverse event reduction, naloxone utilization
Antimicrobial Stewardship	Appropriate selection protocols, duration optimization, resistance monitoring	Clinical decision support, tracking systems, interdisciplinary team	Appropriate utilization rates, resistance patterns, clinical outcomes
Pediatric Medication Safety	Weight-based protocols, calculation verification, pediatric formulations	Specialized calculators, verification systems, pediatric-specific resources	Pediatric-specific error rates, calculation accuracy, harm prevention
Chemotherapy Safety Program	Prescribing templates, independent verification, specialized handling	Chemotherapy-specific systems, specialized training, verification protocols	Chemotherapy error rates, exposure incidents, verification compliance
Transition of Care Medication Safety	Standardized reconciliation, high-risk medication focus, follow-up systems	Reconciliation tools, discharge protocols, follow-up mechanisms	Transition-related errors, post-discharge adverse events, reconciliation compliance

Insulin Safety Initiatives

Concentration and product standardization limits unnecessary variety that contributes to selection errors, with protocols specifying standard concentrations, formulations, and delivery devices, typically limiting formulary to one rapid-acting analog, one long-acting analog, one human regular, and one human NPH product rather than multiple options within each category, while implementing consistent concentration (U-100) unless specifically justified. Hypoglycemia management protocols establish standardized approaches to prevention, recognition, and treatment of low blood glucose, including rescue medication availability and standardized response procedures, with specific guidelines for treatment based on glucose ranges (typically oral carbohydrates for alert patients with glucose 50-70 mg/dL, intravenous dextrose or glucagon for severe hypoglycemia or unconscious patients). Independent double-check requirements mandate verification of insulin doses, particularly for high-risk situations including pediatric patients, insulin infusions, and high-dose requirements, with explicit check processes addressing both dose calculation and product selection.

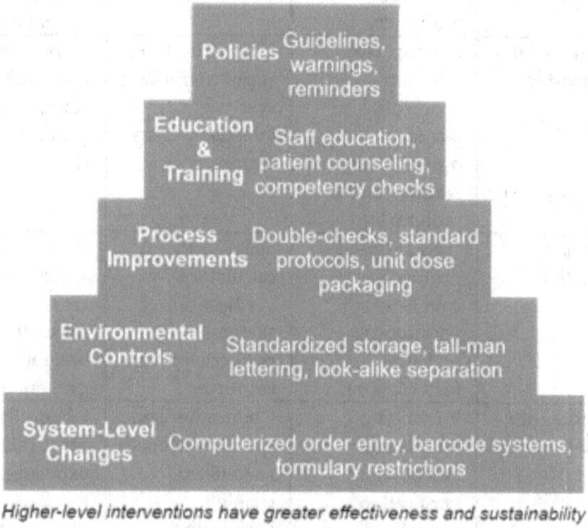

Figure 14.3: Hierarchy of Medication Safety Initiatives

Opioid Stewardship Programs

Prescribing guideline development establishes evidence-based standards for appropriate indication, initial dosing, titration parameters, and duration limitations based on procedure, condition, and patient factors, with particular attention to opioid-naïve patients, elderly individuals, and those with respiratory risk factors including sleep apnea or concurrent central nervous system depressants. Monitoring protocol standardization creates consistent approaches to respiratory depression assessment, sedation evaluation, and appropriate use of monitoring technology including capnography and pulse oximetry, with clear parameters defining monitoring frequency, assessment tools, and intervention thresholds based on patient risk factors and specific opioid characteristics. Naloxone accessibility initiatives ensure appropriate availability of this rescue medication with clear administration protocols for patients receiving opioid therapy, including standardized ordering linked to high-risk prescribing patterns, automated dispensing cabinet placement, and nursing education regarding appropriate use and administration technique.

Pediatric Medication Safety Initiatives

Dose range checking implements automated or manual verification systems comparing calculated doses against age-appropriate reference ranges before dispensing or administration, with specific alerts for doses exceeding maximum recommendations or falling below therapeutic thresholds, ideally using weight-based calculations with hard stops preventing extreme deviations without appropriate override documentation. Standardized concentrations establish consistent formulation strengths for high-risk medications including opioids, sedatives, and electrolytes, eliminating the need for complex calculations during emergency situations through pre-defined standard dilutions, preparation protocols, and administration guidelines specific to neonatal, infant, and pediatric populations. Pediatric-specific resources develop specialized references, protocols, and clinical decision support systems addressing the unique medication needs of children rather than adapting adult systems, with dedicated pediatric formularies, weight-based dosing calculators, and specialized clinical guidelines accounting for developmental differences across age groups.

Chemotherapy Safety Initiatives

Standardized ordering implements protocol-based prescribing with pre-defined regimens, explicit dose calculation methods, and required supportive care components, typically employing electronic systems with built-in safety features including BSA calculation verification, cumulative dose tracking, and automated checks against standard protocols rather than free-text or verbal chemotherapy ordering. Specialized verification procedures require independent double-checks of calculations, preparation, and final product verification by qualified personnel before dispensing, with documented verification of critical elements including drug selection, dose calculation, concentration appropriateness, and compatibility with administration fluids. Administration safety protocols establish consistent practices for patient identification, infusion pump programming, extravasation management, and monitoring requirements, with specialized training requirements, competency verification, and environment controls minimizing distractions during critical administration steps.

Transitions of Care Medication Safety Initiatives

Medication reconciliation standardization establishes consistent processes for comparing medication regimens across transitions, with clear responsibility assignment and documentation requirements, implementing structured forms, electronic tools, or dedicated personnel ensuring comprehensive capture of pre-admission medications, in-hospital changes, and discharge plans with explicit documentation of intentional changes versus discrepancy resolution. Discharge medication management implements systematic approaches to ensure accurate information transfer, appropriate prescription provision, and adequate patient education before leaving controlled healthcare environments, with particular attention to high-risk medications, therapy changes, and monitoring requirements requiring specific patient understanding verification. High-risk patient identification establishes criteria for enhanced transition support, including medication therapy management referrals, post-discharge phone follow-up, or early primary care appointments based on medication regimen complexity and risk factors, typically targeting patients with polypharmacy, recent high-risk medication changes, or limited support systems.

Smart Infusion Technology Implementation

Drug library development creates comprehensive databases of medications with standardized concentrations, dosing units, and appropriate dose ranges based on patient population and clinical setting, with specific libraries tailored to different care areas including adult critical care, general medical-surgical, pediatrics, and neonatal units reflecting different medication usage patterns and acceptable dosing ranges. Dose limit establishment defines soft limits (requiring override confirmation) and hard limits (preventing programming) for high-risk medications based on clinical appropriateness and safety considerations, with limits typically set capturing 95-98% of appropriate doses while preventing extreme outliers potentially representing decimal point errors or unit confusion. Compliance monitoring tracks override patterns, limit violations, and library utilization to identify improvement opportunities and potential workarounds requiring intervention, with regular data analysis identifying medications with frequent overrides requiring limit adjustment or education regarding appropriate dosing practices.

Medication Reconciliation Improvement Initiatives

Role definition clarifies specific responsibilities for obtaining medication histories, identifying discrepancies, and resolving differences, with appropriate assignment based on setting, staffing, and patient risk, typically involving pharmacy technicians or pharmacists for high-risk patients while using nurses or other providers for lower-risk situations with defined escalation pathways for complex cases. Best possible medication history techniques implement structured interview approaches, multiple source verification, and standardized documentation to enhance information accuracy, employing open-ended questioning, visual aids, focused probing about easily forgotten medications (inhalers, patches, injections), and routine verification against dispensing records when available. Discrepancy resolution protocols establish clear procedures for addressing identified differences between medication lists, including communication pathways, documentation requirements, and escalation processes for unresolved issues, with explicit attribution of intentional changes versus corrections of unintended discrepancies.

Non-punitive Reporting Culture Initiatives

Leadership commitment demonstration includes visible executive support for just culture principles, appropriate response to errors focusing on learning rather than blame, and resource allocation for safety improvement, with senior leaders participating in safety rounds, publicly acknowledging and discussing errors, and demonstrating personal commitment to safety principles through consistent messaging and action alignment. Staff safety champion development identifies and supports frontline advocates promoting safety culture within work units, facilitating bidirectional communication between leadership and staff, with formal roles, protected time, and specific responsibilities for promoting reporting, disseminating safety information, and identifying local improvement opportunities. Recognition programs acknowledge and reward error reporting, near-miss identification, and safety improvement suggestions rather than exclusively focusing on error-free performance, creating positive reinforcement for safety-promoting behaviors through both formal awards and informal appreciation consistently demonstrating organizational valuing of transparency over perfectionism.

Summary

- Error prevention strategies include standardization of processes, use of technology (CPOE, barcoding), tall man lettering, separation of look-alike/sound-alike drugs, and independent double-checks for high-alert medications.

- Risk management involves proactive identification of potential failure points in medication systems, implementing preventive measures, and creating a culture that prioritizes safety over blame.

- Quality assurance programs systematically monitor medication use processes, measure outcomes, identify trends, and implement improvement initiatives to enhance safety and effectiveness.

- Reporting systems for medication errors and near-misses should be non-punitive, confidential, accessible, and designed to capture sufficient detail for meaningful analysis and improvement.

- Safety initiatives include national programs (ISMP, NPSG), institutional policies, technology implementation, and team-based approaches to create multiple layers of protection against medication errors.

- Just culture principles balance individual accountability with system responsibility, focusing on behavioral choices rather than outcomes and encouraging reporting without fear of inappropriate punishment.

- High-alert medications require special safeguards due to their elevated risk of causing significant patient harm when used in error, including concentrated electrolytes, anticoagulants, insulin, and chemotherapy.

Multiple Choice Questions

1. Which of the following best represents a system-based approach to medication error prevention?
   A) Disciplining staff members who make errors
   B) Implementing tall-man lettering for look-alike drug names
   C) Requiring staff to be more careful with high-risk medications
   D) Posting lists of error-prone abbreviations in workspaces
2. When conducting a root cause analysis after a medication error, which of the following approaches is MOST effective?
   A) Focusing primarily on identifying which individual was responsible
   B) Conducting a thorough analysis using a structured methodology to identify system failures
   C) Implementing immediate solutions before analyzing the causes
   D) Limiting the investigation to the pharmacy department only
3. Which of the following represents the MOST effective use of technology in preventing medication errors?
   A) Implementing technology without workflow consideration
   B) Using technology to replace all manual double-checks
   C) Integrating barcode medication administration with electronic health records
   D) Implementing as many technological solutions as possible simultaneously
4. In a "Just Culture" approach to medication errors, which of the following is the MOST appropriate response to an error resulting from a process violation?
   A) Automatic termination of employment
   B) Ignoring the violation if no patient harm occurred
   C) Evaluating the reason for the violation and addressing system issues
   D) Publicly identifying the individual responsible to prevent recurrence
5. Which of the following is the MOST effective strategy for preventing errors with high-alert medications?
   A) Labeling all high-alert medications with warning stickers
   B) Implementing standardized concentrations, order sets, and independent double-checks

C) Requiring pharmacist verification after administration

D) Restricting high-alert medications to certain prescribers

7. The MOST important characteristic of an effective medication error reporting system is:

   A) Mandatory reporting of all errors regardless of severity

   B) Anonymous reporting without any identifiers

   C) Non-punitive environment focused on system improvement

   D) Detailed investigation of the individual's background

8. When conducting a Failure Mode and Effects Analysis (FMEA) for a medication process, which of the following is the MOST appropriate approach?

   A) Waiting until errors occur to analyze the process

   B) Focusing only on catastrophic failure modes

   C) Proactively identifying potential failure points and their effects

   D) Limiting the analysis to pharmacy processes only

9. Which of the following represents the BEST approach to medication reconciliation during transitions of care?

   A) Relying solely on the patient's electronic health record

   B) Obtaining a comprehensive medication history from multiple sources

   C) Having patients self-report their medications without verification

   D) Focusing only on prescription medications

10. Which of the following medication safety initiatives would be MOST effective in reducing adverse drug events in pediatric patients?

   A) Using adult dosing references with mathematical conversions

   B) Implementing weight-based dosing protocols with independent double-checks

   C) Rounding all doses to the nearest whole number

   D) Using the same medication concentrations as for adult patients

11. When measuring the impact of a medication safety initiative, which of the following represents the MOST comprehensive approach?

   A) Tracking the number of reported errors

   B) Measuring staff compliance with the new process

C) Evaluating multiple outcome measures including process measures, error rates, and harm events

D) Conducting a one-time assessment after implementation

Self-Assessment Questions

1. Describe three system-based approaches to medication error prevention and explain why they are more effective than focusing on individual performance.
2. Explain the concept of "Just Culture" in medication safety and how it promotes error reporting while maintaining accountability.
3. Discuss the process of conducting a Root Cause Analysis (RCA) following a serious medication error, including key steps and potential outcomes.
4. Describe the role of technology (such as computerized provider order entry, barcode medication administration, and smart pumps) in preventing medication errors, including both benefits and limitations.
5. Explain three strategies for preventing errors with high-alert medications, providing specific examples for different medication classes.
6. Discuss the importance of medication error reporting systems, including characteristics of effective systems and barriers to reporting.
7. Describe how Failure Mode and Effects Analysis (FMEA) can be used proactively to identify potential medication safety issues before errors occur.
8. Explain how pharmacists should approach medication reconciliation to prevent errors during transitions of care, including key elements of an effective process.
9. Discuss three initiatives that can improve medication safety in vulnerable populations (e.g., pediatrics, geriatrics), explaining the specific risks in these populations.
10. Explain how quality improvement methodologies can be applied to medication safety initiatives, including how to measure the impact of safety interventions.

Bibliography

1. Institute of Medicine (US) Committee on Quality of Health Care in America; Kohn LT, Corrigan JM, Donaldson MS, editors. To err is human: building a safer health system. Washington (DC): National Academies Press (US); 2000.
2. Reason J. Human error: models and management. BMJ. 2000;320(7237):768-770.
3. Agency for Healthcare Research and Quality. PSNet: Patient Safety Network. Medication errors and adverse drug events. Available from: https://psnet.ahrq.gov/primer/medication-errors-and-adverse-drug-events
4. Institute for Safe Medication Practices. ISMP list of high-alert medications in acute care settings. Available from: https://www.ismp.org/recommendations/high-alert-medications-acute-list
5. Bates DW, Cullen DJ, Laird N, Petersen LA, Small SD, Servi D, et al. Incidence of adverse drug events and potential adverse drug events. Implications for prevention. ADE Prevention Study Group. JAMA. 1995;274(1):29-34.
6. Aspden P, Wolcott J, Bootman JL, Cronenwett LR, editors. Preventing medication errors: quality chasm series. Washington (DC): National Academies Press (US); 2007.
7. Marx D. Patient safety and the "just culture": a primer for health care executives. New York: Columbia University; 2001.
8. Leape LL, Berwick DM. Five years after To Err Is Human: what have we learned? JAMA. 2005;293(19):2384-2390.
9. Nuckols TK, Smith-Spangler C, Morton SC, Asch SM, Patel VM, Anderson LJ, et al. The effectiveness of computerized order entry at reducing preventable adverse drug events and medication errors in hospital settings: a systematic review and meta-analysis. Syst Rev. 2014;3:56.
10. The Joint Commission. Sentinel event alert: using medication reconciliation to prevent errors. Issue 35, January 25, 2006. Available from: https://www.jointcommission.org/resources/patient-safety-topics/sentinel-event/sentinel-event-alert-newsletters/sentinel-event-alert-issue-35-using-medication-reconciliation-to-prevent-errors/

ANSWERS TO THE MCQS

Chapter 1: 1.B 2.B 3.B 4.B 5.B 6.C 7.B 8.B 9.B 10.C

Chapter 2: 1.B 2.C 3.C 4.B 5.C 6.B 7.B 8.B 9.C 10.C

Chapter 3: 1.D 2.B 3.D 4.B 5.C 6.C 7.C 8.C 9.B 10.C

Chapter 4: 1.C 2.C 3.B 4.C 5.C 6.B 7.B 8.C 9.B 10.C

Chapter 5: 1.B 2.C 3.B 4.B 5.D 6.A 7.B 8.B 9.C 10.A

Chapter 6: 1.B 2.C 3.C 4.B 5.B 6.A 7.B 8.B 9.C 10.B

Chapter 7: 1.B 2.C 3.B 4.B 5.C 6.C 7.D 8.B 9.C 10.D

Chapter 8: 1.C 2.B 3.B 4.C 5.B 6.D 7.C 8.B 9.B 10.C

Chapter 9: 1.B 2.B 3.C 4.A 5.B 6.C 7.B 8.B 9.D 10.B

Chapter 10: 1.C 2.C 3.B 4.C 5.B 6.B 7.B 8.B 9.B 10.B

Chapter 12: 1.C 2.B 3.B 4.B 5.B 6.B 7.C 8.C 9.B 10.C

Chapter 13: 1.B 2.C 3.B 4.A 5.B 6.B 7.C 8.B 9.C 10.C

Chapter 14: 1.B 2.B 3.C 4.C 5.B 6.C 7.C 8.B 9.B 10.C

APPENDIX

A: Clinical Documentation Templates and Examples

SOAP Note Template

Subjective

Patient: Age: Sex:

Date:

Chief complaint:

History of present illness:

- Onset/duration:
- Alleviating/aggravating factors:
- Related symptoms:
- Previous treatments:

Medication history:

- Current medications:
- Adherence:
- Allergies:

Past medical history:

Social history:

Family history:

Review of systems:

Objective

Vital signs: BP: HR: RR:

Temp: SpO2: Pain:

Physical exam findings:

Laboratory results:

Medication profile review:

Assessment

Problem list:

1.
2.

Drug therapy problems:

1.
2.

Comprehensive Medication Review Documentation

Patient: ______ **Date:** ______

Reason for Review: ______

Current Medications

Medication, Dose, Frequency	Indication	Effectiveness	Safety	Adherence
______	______	______	______	______
______	______	______	______	______
______	______	______	______	______
______	______	______	______	______

OTC/Supplements: ______

Allergies: ______

Drug Therapy Problems Identified

1. **Problem:** ______
   Description: ______
   Recommendation: ______
2. **Problem:** ______
   Description: ______
   Recommendation: ______

Action Plan

1. ______
2. ______
3. ______

Patient Education Provided

- ______
- ______

Follow-up Plan: ______

Pharmacist: ______ **Date:** ______

____

Pharmacist Signature, Credentials

Intervention Documentation Format

Date/Time: ……

Patient Identifier: ……

Setting: ……

Intervention Category: ……

Drug(s) Involved: ……

Description of Situation

……

……

……

Intervention

……

……

Rationale

1. ……
2. ……
3. ……

Recommendation Acceptance: □ Yes □ No □ Partial

Outcome

……

……

Time Spent: …… minutes

____

Pharmacist Signature, Credentials

Care Plan Template for Hypertension Management

Patient Name: ____

Medical Record Number: ____

Date of Care Plan: ____

Current BP: ____ mmHg

BP Goal: ____ mmHg

Comorbidities Affecting Treatment Plan

- ____
- ____

Current Antihypertensive Therapy

- ____
- ____

Assessment of Current Therapy

- ____
- ____
- ____

Therapeutic Goals

1. ____
2. ____

Interventions

1. **Medication Adjustments:**
   - ____
   - ____
2. **Monitoring Plan:**
   - ____
   - ____
3. **Lifestyle Modifications:**
   - ____

Appendix B: Laboratory Value Reference Guide

Reference Ranges for Common Laboratory Tests

Hematology

Test	Reference Range (Adult)	Critical Values
Hemoglobin	Male: 13.5-17.5 g/dL Female: 12.0-16.0 g/dL	<7.0 or >20.0 g/dL
Hematocrit	Male: 41-53% Female: 36-46%	<20% or >60%
WBC	4,500-11,000/mm³	<2,000 or >30,000/mm³
Platelet Count	150,000-450,000/mm³	<20,000 or >1,000,000/mm³
INR	0.8-1.2 (no anticoagulation) 2.0-3.0 (standard anticoagulation)	>5.0
Absolute Neutrophil Count	1,800-7,800/mm³	<500/mm³

Chemistry

Test	Reference Range (Adult)	Critical Values
Sodium	135-145 mEq/L	<120 or >160 mEq/L
Potassium	3.5-5.0 mEq/L	<2.5 or >6.5 mEq/L
Chloride	98-108 mEq/L	<80 or >120 mEq/L
CO_2	22-29 mEq/L	<10 or >40 mEq/L
BUN	7-20 mg/dL	>100 mg/dL
Creatinine	Male: 0.7-1.3 mg/Dl Female: 0.6-1.1 mg/dL	>7.0 mg/dL
Glucose (fasting)	70-99 mg/dL	<40 or >500 mg/dL
Calcium	8.5-10.5 mg/dL	<6.5 or >13.0 mg/dL
Magnesium	1.5-2.5 mEq/L	<1.0 or >4.5 mEq/L
Phosphorus	2.5-4.5 mg/dL	<1.0 or >9.0 mg/dL

Liver Function

Test	Reference Range (Adult)	Critical Values
ALT	7-56 units/L	>1000 units/L
AST	5-40 units/L	>1000 units/L
Alkaline Phosphatase	44-147 units/L	>1000 units/L
Total Bilirubin	0.1-1.2 mg/dL	>15.0 mg/dL
Direct Bilirubin	0.0-0.3 mg/dL	>10.0 mg/dL
Albumin	3.5-5.0 g/dL	<1.5 g/dL

Lipid Panel

Test	Desirable Range	Borderline	High Risk
Total Cholesterol	<200 mg/dL	200-239 mg/dL	≥240 mg/dL
LDL Cholesterol	<100 mg/dL	100-159 mg/dL	≥160 mg/dL
HDL Cholesterol	>60 mg/dL	40-59 mg/dL	<40 mg/dL
Triglycerides	<150 mg/dL	150-199 mg/dL	≥200 mg/dL

Cardiac Markers

Test	Reference Range	Critical Values
Troponin I	<0.04 ng/mL	≥0.5 ng/mL
Troponin T	<0.01 ng/mL	≥0.1 ng/mL
CK-MB	<3.0 ng/mL	>25.0 ng/mL
BNP	<100 pg/mL	>5000 pg/mL
NT-proBNP	<125 pg/mL (age <75) <450 pg/mL (age ≥75)	>10,000 pg/mL

Endocrine

Test	Reference Range	Critical Values
TSH	0.4-4.0 mIU/L	>50 mIU/L
Free T4	0.8-1.8 ng/dL	<0.4 or >5.0 ng/dL
HbA1c	<5.7% (normal) 5.7-6.4% (prediabetes) ≥6.5% (diabetes)	N/A
Cortisol (AM)	5-23 mcg/dL	<2.0 mcg/dL

Drug-Specific Monitoring Parameters

Antiepileptics

Drug	Therapeutic Range	Monitoring Parameters	Frequency
Carbamazepine	4-12 mcg/mL	CBC, electrolytes, LFTs, drug levels	Baseline, monthly for 3 months, then every 6-12 months
Phenytoin	10-20 mcg/mL	CBC, LFTs, drug levels, albumin	Baseline, then every 6-12 months
Valproic Acid	50-100 mcg/mL	CBC, LFTs, platelets, drug levels	Baseline, monthly for 3 months, then every 6-12 months
Lamotrigine	3-14 mcg/mL	CBC, LFTs	Baseline, then annually

Cardiovascular Drugs

Drug	Therapeutic Range	Monitoring Parameters	Frequency
Digoxin	0.8-2.0 ng/mL	Digoxin level, K^+, Mg^{2+}, SCr, HR	Baseline, 7-14 days after initiation or dose change, then every 6-12 months
Amiodarone	0.5-2.5 mcg/mL	TFTs, LFTs, chest X-ray, ECG, ophthalmic exam	Baseline, every 6 months
Warfarin	INR 2.0-3.0 or 2.5-3.5 (depending on indication)	INR, signs of bleeding	2-3 times weekly until stable, then monthly
DOACs	N/A	CBC, SCr, LFTs	Baseline, then annually

Immunosuppressants

Drug	Therapeutic Range	Monitoring Parameters	Frequency
Cyclosporine	Varies by indication and time post-transplant	Cyclosporine level, SCr, K^+, Mg^{2+}, BP, LFTs	Weekly for 3 months, then monthly
Tacrolimus	Varies by indication and time post-transplant	Tacrolimus level, SCr, K^+, Mg^{2+}, glucose, BP, LFTs	Weekly for 3 months, then monthly
Sirolimus	Varies by indication and time post-transplant	Sirolimus level, CBC, lipids, LFTs, SCr	Weekly for 3 months, then monthly
Mycophenolate	N/A	CBC, SCr, LFTs	Weekly for 1 month, then monthly

Psychotropics

Drug	Therapeutic Range	Monitoring Parameters	Frequency
Lithium	0.6-1.2 mEq/L	Lithium level, SCr, electrolytes, TSH, ECG	5-7 days after initiation or dose change, then every 3-6 months
Clozapine	350-600 ng/mL	WBC, ANC, metabolic panel, weight, BP	Weekly for 6 months, then every 2-4 weeks
Valproic Acid	50-100 mcg/mL	Drug level, CBC, LFTs, weight, ammonia if altered mental status	Baseline, monthly for 3 months, then every 6-12 months

Laboratory Test Interpretation Guides

Interpreting Renal Function Tests

Creatinine Clearance (CrCl)

- Normal: 90-140 mL/min (males), 80-125 mL/min (females)
- Mild impairment: 60-89 mL/min
- Moderate impairment: 30-59 mL/min
- Severe impairment: 15-29 mL/min
- Kidney failure: <15 mL/min

eGFR

- Normal: ≥90 mL/min/1.73m^2
- Mild impairment: 60-89 mL/min/1.73m^2
- Moderate impairment: 30-59 mL/min/1.73m^2
- Severe impairment: 15-29 mL/min/1.73m^2
- Kidney failure: <15 mL/min/1.73m^2

BUN:Creatinine Ratio:

Normal: 10:1 to 20:1
20:1 may indicate:

- Prerenal azotemia (dehydration, heart failure)
- GI bleeding
- Steroid use
- Increased catabolism

<10:1 may indicate:

- Low protein intake
- Liver disease
- SIADH
- Pregnancy

Interpreting Liver Function Tests

- Hepatocellular pattern: Predominant elevation of ALT and AST
- Cholestatic pattern: Predominant elevation of ALP and GGT
- Mixed pattern: Proportional elevation of both patterns

AST:ALT Ratio:

- <1: Viral hepatitis, medication-induced liver injury
- 2: Alcoholic liver disease, cirrhosis
- 1-2: Nonalcoholic fatty liver disease, other causes

Elevated Bilirubin:

- Direct (conjugated): Hepatocellular or biliary disease
- Indirect (unconjugated): Hemolysis, Gilbert's syndrome

Interpreting Electrolyte Abnormalities

Sodium Abnormalities

Hyponatremia (Na^+ <135 mEq/L):

Assess volume status:

- Hypervolemic: Heart failure, cirrhosis, nephrotic syndrome
- Euvolemic: SIADH, hypothyroidism, psychogenic polydipsia
- Hypovolemic: Diuretics, vomiting, diarrhea, adrenal insufficiency

Drug causes: Diuretics, SSRIs, carbamazepine, oxcarbazepine

Hypernatremia (Na^+ >145 mEq/L):

- Typically indicates water deficit
- Causes: Inadequate water intake, diabetes insipidus, excessive water loss
- Drug causes: Lithium, demeclocycline, mannitol

Potassium Abnormalities

Hypokalemia (K^+ <3.5 mEq/L):

- Causes: Diuretics, GI losses, alkalosis, hyperaldosteronism
- Drug causes: Thiazide and loop diuretics, insulin, beta-agonists, amphotericin B

Hyperkalemia (K^+ >5.0 mEq/L):

- Causes: Renal failure, acidosis, tissue breakdown, hypoaldosteronism
- Drug causes: ACEIs, ARBs, K^+-sparing diuretics, NSAIDs, trimethoprim

Considerations for Special Populations

Pediatric Laboratory Values

Test	Neonate	Infant	Child	Adolescent
Hemoglobin	14.0-24.0 g/dL	10.0-17.0 g/dL	11.0-16.0 g/dL	Male: 13.0-16.0 g/dL Female: 12.0-16.0 g/dL
WBC	9,000-30,000/mm³	6,000-17,500/mm³	5,000-14,500/mm³	4,500-13,500/mm³
Creatinine	0.3-1.0 mg/dL	0.2-0.5 mg/dL	0.3-0.7 mg/dL	0.5-1.0 mg/dL
Glucose	40-90 mg/dL	50-90 mg/dL	60-100 mg/dL	70-110 mg/dL
Calcium	7.6-10.4 mg/dL	9.0-11.0 mg/dL	8.8-10.8 mg/dL	8.4-10.2 mg/dL

Geriatric Laboratory Values

Test	Geriatric Considerations
Creatinine	May be normal despite significant decrease in renal function due to decreased muscle mass
eGFR	More accurate measure of renal function in elderly; calculate with appropriate formula
Albumin	Often lower in elderly; affects drug binding and free drug concentration
ALP	May be naturally elevated due to bone remodeling or vitamin D deficiency
TSH	Reference range may be slightly higher in elderly without pathology
Hemoglobin	May be lower due to chronic disease, nutritional deficiencies

Considerations:

- Age-related changes in pharmacokinetics affect drug dosing and monitoring
- Polypharmacy increases risk of drug-lab interactions
- Renal function decline may not be reflected in creatinine due to reduced muscle mass
- Hepatic metabolism typically decreases with age
- Albumin may be decreased, affecting highly protein-bound drugs
- Fluid and electrolyte balance may be more tenuous

Pregnancy Laboratory Values

Test	First Trimester	Second Trimester	Third Trimester	Postpartum
Hemoglobin	Slight decrease	Decrease by 0.5-1.0 g/dL	Further decrease	Return to baseline
WBC	5,000-12,000/mm³	6,000-16,000/mm³	6,000-16,000/mm³	Leukocytosis during labor
Platelets	Normal to slight decrease	Further decrease	Further decrease	Return to baseline
Creatinine	Decrease by ~0.2 mg/dL	Decrease	Decrease	Return to baseline
Albumin	Slight decrease	Decrease by 0.5-1.0 g/dL	Further decrease	Return to baseline
ALP	Increase (placental production)	Significant increase	2-4x normal	Return to baseline
Glucose	Slight decrease	Variable	Variable	Return to baseline

Considerations:

- Plasma volume expands by 40-50%, causing dilutional effect on laboratory values
- Glomerular filtration rate increases by 40-65% during pregnancy
- Hepatic enzyme changes affect drug metabolism
- Decreased albumin affects drug binding
- Increased cardiac output and blood flow alter drug distribution and elimination
- Physiologic anemia of pregnancy is normal due to plasma volume expansion
- Screening for gestational diabetes requires specialized glucose targets

Hepatic Impairment Assessment

Child-Pugh Classification:

Parameter	1 point	2 points	3 points
Bilirubin (mg/dL)	<2	2-3	>3
Albumin (g/dL)	>3.5	2.8-3.5	<2.8
PT (seconds prolonged)	<4	4-6	>6
Ascites	None	Mild	Moderate-Severe
Encephalopathy	None	Grade 1-2	Grade 3-4

Classification:

- Class A: 5-6 points (mild hepatic impairment)
- Class B: 7-9 points (moderate hepatic impairment)
- Class C: 10-15 points (severe hepatic impairment)

Drug Dosing Considerations:

- Class A: No dosage adjustment for most drugs
- Class B: Consider 25-50% dose reduction for hepatically metabolized drugs
- Class C: Consider 50-75% dose reduction for hepatically metabolized drugs or avoid if possible

Appendix C: Drug Interaction and Compatibility Tables

High-Priority Drug Interactions by Therapeutic Class

Anticoagulants and Antiplatelets

Drug	Interacting Agents	Potential Effect	Severity	Management
Warfarin	NSAIDs	↑ Bleeding risk	Major	Avoid combination or use lowest effective NSAID dose with close INR monitoring
Warfarin	Antibiotics (fluoroquinolones, macrolides, metronidazole)	↑ INR, ↑ bleeding risk	Major	Monitor INR closely, consider warfarin dose reduction
Warfarin	Amiodarone	↑ INR, ↑ bleeding risk	Major	Reduce warfarin dose by 30-50%, monitor INR frequently
Warfarin	Phenytoin, carbamazepine, rifampin	↓ Warfarin effect	Major	Monitor INR closely, may need increased warfarin dose
DOACs	P-gp inhibitors (amiodarone, verapamil, dronedarone)	↑ DOAC levels, ↑ bleeding risk	Major	Consider DOAC dose reduction or alternate agent
Antiplatelet agents	NSAIDs	↑ Bleeding risk	Moderate	Minimize duration, consider gastroprotection
Clopidogrel	PPIs (especially omeprazole)	↓ Clopidogrel activation	Moderate	Consider pantoprazole instead of omeprazole if PPI needed

Antimicrobials

Drug	Interacting Agents	Potential Effect	Severity	Management
Macrolides	QT-prolonging agents	↑ QT prolongation risk	Major	Avoid combination if possible or monitor ECG
Macrolides	Statins	↑ Statin levels, ↑ myopathy risk	Major	Hold statin during short-term macrolide treatment or use non-interacting statin
Fluoroquinolones	Antacids, multivitamins, iron	↓ Fluoroquinolone absorption	Moderate	Separate administration by 2 hours before or 4 hours after
Rifampin	Multiple drugs (oral contraceptives, warfarin, HIV medications)	↓ Effect of interacting drugs	Major	Avoid combination or increase dose of affected medication
Azole antifungals	QT-prolonging agents	↑ QT prolongation risk	Major	Avoid combination if possible or monitor ECG
Azole antifungals	Benzodiazepines, statins	↑ Levels of interacting drugs	Major	Use lower doses of interacting drugs or choose alternatives

Cardiovascular Agents

Drug	Interacting Agents	Potential Effect	Severity	Management
Statins	Gemfibrozil	↑ Statin levels, ↑ myopathy risk	Major	Avoid combination, consider fenofibrate instead
Simvastatin, Lovastatin	Strong CYP3A4 inhibitors	↑ Statin levels, ↑ myopathy risk	Major	Avoid combination or switch to non-CYP3A4 dependent statin
Amiodarone	Multiple drugs (warfarin, digoxin, statins)	↑ Levels of interacting drugs	Major	Reduce dose of interacting drugs, monitor levels
Beta-blockers	Verapamil, diltiazem	↑ Bradycardia, heart block	Major	Avoid combination or monitor closely
ACEIs/ARBs	K^+-sparing diuretics, K^+ supplements	↑ Hyperkalemia risk	Major	Monitor K^+ levels, avoid if possible in high-risk patients
ACEIs/ARBs	NSAIDs	↓ Antihypertensive effect, ↑ renal dysfunction	Moderate	Monitor BP and renal function, use lowest effective NSAID dose

CNS Agents

Drug	**Interacting Agents**	**Potential Effect**	**Severity**	**Management**
MAOIs	SSRIs, SNRIs, TCAs	Serotonin syndrome	Major	Allow 2-week washout when switching
MAOIs	Sympathomimetics, tyramine-rich foods	Hypertensive crisis	Major	Avoid combination, follow dietary restrictions
Lithium	NSAIDs, thiazide diuretics	↑ Lithium levels, toxicity	Major	Monitor lithium levels, adjust dose if necessary
Carbamazepine	Multiple CYP inducers	↓ Effect of interacting drugs	Major	Avoid combination or adjust doses
Lamotrigine	Valproic acid	↑ Lamotrigine levels, ↑ toxicity	Major	Reduce lamotrigine dose by 50%
Benzodiazepines	Opioids	↑ CNS depression, respiratory depression	Major	Avoid combination if possible or use lowest effective doses

Cytochrome P450 Substrate, Inhibitor, and Inducer Charts

CYP1A2

Substrates	Inhibitors	Inducers
Amitriptyline	Ciprofloxacin	Carbamazepine
Clozapine	Fluvoxamine	Cigarette smoking
Duloxetine	Methoxsalen	Phenobarbital
Olanzapine	Mexiletine	Rifampin
Theophylline	Oral contraceptives	Ritonavir
Warfarin (R-isomer)	Zileuton	St. John's wort

CYP2C9

Substrates	Inhibitors	Inducers
Celecoxib Glipizide Ibuprofen Losartan Phenytoin Warfarin (S-isomer)	Amiodarone Fluconazole Metronidazole Sulfamethoxazole Voriconazole Zafirlukast	Carbamazepine Phenobarbital Rifampin St. John's wort

CYP2C19

Substrates	Inhibitors	Inducers
Citalopram Clopidogrel (activation) Diazepam Lansoprazole Omeprazole Voriconazole	Esomeprazole Fluconazole Fluvoxamine Omeprazole Ticlopidine Voriconazole	Carbamazepine Rifampin St. John's wort

CYP2D6

Substrates	Inhibitors	Inducers
Amitriptyline Codeine (activation) Metoprolol Ondansetron Risperidone Tamoxifen (activation) Tramadol (activation)	Bupropion Duloxetine Fluoxetine Paroxetine Quinidine Ritonavir Terbinafine	Carbamazepine Phenobarbital Rifampin

CYP3A4/5

Substrates	Inhibitors	Inducers
Alprazolam	Clarithromycin	Carbamazepine
Atorvastatin	Erythromycin	Phenobarbital
Cyclosporine	Grapefruit juice	Phenytoin
Fentanyl	Itraconazole	Rifampin
Midazolam	Ketoconazole	St. John's wort
Nifedipine	Ritonavir	
Simvastatin	Verapamil	
Tacrolimus	Voriconazole	

IV Compatibility Matrix

Compatible Combinations (Y-site)

Drug	Compatible With
Amikacin	Cefepime, ciprofloxacin, furosemide, heparin, insulin (regular), metronidazole, piperacillin-tazobactam
Calcium gluconate	Ceftriaxone (in adults only), dopamine, heparin, insulin, morphine
Dexamethasone	Ciprofloxacin, famotidine, furosemide, heparin, insulin, metoclopramide
Dopamine	Calcium gluconate, dobutamine, heparin, insulin, lorazepam, midazolam
Furosemide	Amikacin, ciprofloxacin, dexamethasone, heparin, morphine
Heparin	Most IV medications except for aminoglycosides in high concentrations
Insulin (regular)	Amikacin, calcium gluconate, dopamine, heparin, potassium chloride
Morphine	Calcium gluconate, furosemide, heparin, lorazepam, midazolam

Incompatible Combinations (Y-site)

Drug	Incompatible With
Ampicillin	Aminoglycosides, calcium-containing solutions, dopamine, gentamicin
Calcium (any salt)	Ceftriaxone (in neonates/infants), phosphate-containing solutions, sodium bicarbonate
Diazepam	Most other IV drugs due to propylene glycol vehicle
Midazolam	Albumin, amphotericin B, diazepam, furosemide, phenytoin
Phenytoin	Most other IV medications - requires dedicated line
Sodium bicarbonate	Calcium-containing solutions, catecholamines, dobutamine, dopamine
Vancomycin	Albumin, aminoglycosides, ceftriaxone, heparin (high concentration)

QT-Prolonging Medications

Known Risk of Torsades de Pointes

Drug Class	Examples
Antiarrhythmics	Amiodarone, disopyramide, dofetilide, procainamide, quinidine, sotalol
Antibiotics	Azithromycin, clarithromycin, erythromycin, moxifloxacin
Antipsychotics	Chlorpromazine, haloperidol, thioridazine, ziprasidone
Antiemetics	Ondansetron, droperidol
Others	Cisapride*, methadone, ranolazine

*Not available in many countries due to QT prolongation risk

Possible Risk of Torsades de Pointes

Drug Class	Examples
Antibiotics	Ciprofloxacin, levofloxacin, trimethoprim-sulfamethoxazole
Antidepressants	Citalopram, escitalopram, fluoxetine, venlafaxine
Antifungals	Fluconazole, voriconazole
Antivirals	Atazanavir, lopinavir/ritonavir
Others	Domperidone, famotidine, lithium, tacrolimus

Risk Factors for Drug-Induced QT Prolongation

- Female sex
- Age >65 years
- Bradycardia
- Hypokalemia, hypomagnesemia, hypocalcemia
- Heart failure
- Congenital long QT syndrome
- Renal or hepatic impairment
- Multiple QT-prolonging medications
- Rapid IV administration of QT-prolonging drugs

Food-Drug and Herb-Drug Interaction Guide

Food-Drug Interactions

Food	Interacting Drugs	Effect	Recommendation
Grapefruit juice	Statins (atorvastatin, simvastatin, lovastatin), calcium channel blockers, cyclosporine, tacrolimus	↑ Drug levels, ↑ toxicity risk	Avoid grapefruit juice with affected medications
High-vitamin K foods	Warfarin	↓ Anticoagulant effect	Maintain consistent vitamin K intake
Dairy products	Tetracyclines, fluoroquinolones	↓ Drug absorption	Take 2 hours before or 4 hours after dairy
Tyramine-rich foods	MAOIs	Hypertensive crisis	Avoid tyramine-rich foods with MAOIs
Alcohol	CNS depressants, metronidazole, sulfonylureas	↑ CNS depression, disulfiram-like reaction, hypoglycemia	Avoid alcohol with interacting medications
High-fat meals	Some HIV medications, some statins	↑ or ↓ absorption depending on drug	Follow specific administration recommendations

Herb-Drug Interactions

Herb	Interacting Drugs	Effect	Recommendation
St. John's wort	Oral contraceptives, antiretrovirals, cyclosporine, tacrolimus, warfarin, antidepressants	↓ Drug levels and efficacy due to CYP3A4 induction	Avoid St. John's wort with affected medications
Ginkgo biloba	Anticoagulants, antiplatelets	↑ Bleeding risk	Avoid combination or monitor closely
Garlic suppleme nts	Anticoagulants, antiplatelets	↑ Bleeding risk	Monitor for increased bruising or bleeding
Echinacea	Immunosuppressa nts, CYP1A2 substrates	↓ Immunosuppress ant effect, altered metabolism	Avoid with immunosuppressa nts, monitor other drugs
Valerian	CNS depressants	↑ Sedation	Avoid combination or use with caution
Saw palmetto	5-alpha reductase inhibitors	Additive effects	Monitor for increased side effects
Black cohosh	Hepatotoxic drugs	↑ Hepatotoxicity risk	Monitor liver function tests
Green tea extract	Warfarin	↓ Anticoagulant effect due to vitamin K content	Maintain consistent intake or avoid

Appendix D: Clinical Assessment Tools and Scales

Numeric Pain Rating Scale (NPRS)

Ask the patient: "On a scale from 0 to 10, where 0 means no pain and 10 means the worst possible pain, how would you rate your pain right now?"

0	1	2	3	4	5	6	7	8	9	10
No Pain		Mild Pain		Moderate Pain			Severe Pain			Worst Possible Pain

Interpretation

- **0:** No pain
- **1-3:** Mild pain (nagging, annoying, interfering little with ADLs)
- **4-6:** Moderate pain (interferes significantly with ADLs)
- **7-10:** Severe pain (disabling; unable to perform ADLs)

Documentation

Patient Name: ______________________________ Date: ______________

Pain Score: _____ Location: _______________ Time: ______________

Clinician: ____

Visual Analog Scale (VAS)

Ask the patient to mark on the line below the point that represents their pain intensity. Measure the distance from "No pain" to the mark in millimeters (0-100mm) to quantify pain.

Patient Instructions: Please mark on the line below to indicate how bad your pain is right now:

No pain ____________________ Worst possible pain

Interpretation

- **0-4mm:** No pain
- **5-44mm:** Mild pain
- **45-74mm:** Moderate pain
- **75-100mm:** Severe pain

Advantages of VAS: High sensitivity to change, continuous scale, avoids use of descriptive terms.

Documentation

Patient Name: ______________________ Date: ____________

Pain Score: _____ mm Location: ____________ Time: ____________

Clinician: ______________________________

FACES Pain Scale-Revised (FPS-R)

Used primarily for children (ages 4-12) or patients with communication difficulties. Point to each face and explain the scale to the patient.

Patient Instructions: "These faces show how much pain a person can feel. The face on the left shows no pain. Each face shows more and more pain, up to the face on the right which shows the worst pain possible. Point to the face that shows how much pain you have right now."

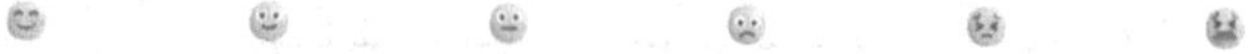

0	2	4	6	8	10

Interpretation

- **0:** No pain
- **2-4:** Mild pain
- **6:** Moderate pain
- **8-10:** Severe pain

Documentation

Patient Name: ______________________________ Date: ______________

Pain Score: ______ Location: _______________ Time: _______________

Clinician: ____

Pain Assessment in Advanced Dementia (PAINAD) Scale

For patients with advanced dementia or cognitive impairment who cannot self-report pain. Observe the patient for 5 minutes during activity/movement.

Behavior	0	1	2	Score
Breathing	Normal	Occasional labored breathing or short hyperventilation	Noisy labored breathing, long hyperventilation, Cheyne-Stokes	☐
Negative vocalization	None	Occasional moan/groan, low-level speech with negative quality	Repeated troubled calling out, loud moaning/groaning, crying	☐
Facial expression	Smiling or inexpressive	Sad, frightened, frown	Facial grimacing	☐
Body language	Relaxed	Tense, distressed pacing, fidgeting	Rigid, fists clenched, knees pulled up, pulling/pushing away, striking out	☐
Consolability	No need to console	Distracted or reassured by voice or touch	Unable to console, distract or reassure	☐
			TOTAL SCORE:	☐

Interpretation

- **0-1:** No pain
- **2-3:** Mild pain
- **4-6:** Moderate pain
- **7-10:** Severe pain

Documentation

Patient Name: ______________________________ Date: ______________

PAINAD Score: ______ Time: ________ Activity: __________________

Clinician: ____

Mini-Mental State Examination (MMSE)

A brief 30-point questionnaire used to screen for cognitive impairment. It takes approximately 10 minutes to administer.

Assessment Items

Domain	Questions/Tasks	Max Points	Score
Orientation	What is the (year) (season) (date) (day) (month)?	5	☐
	Where are we: (country) (state) (county) (city) (place/building)?	5	☐
Registration	Name 3 objects. Give 1 second to say each. Then ask patient to repeat all 3. Give 1 point for each correct answer. Repeat until patient learns all 3.	3	☐
Attention & Calculation	Serial 7s: Subtract 7 from 100, then 7 from that, etc. Stop after 5 answers. Alternative: Spell "WORLD" backwards.	5	☐
Recall	Ask for the 3 objects repeated above. Give 1 point for each correct answer.	3	☐
Language	Name a pencil and watch. Repeat "No ifs, ands, or buts." Follow 3-stage command: "Take paper in right hand, fold in half, put on floor."	5	☐
Visual-Spatial	Read and obey: "Close your eyes." Write a sentence. Copy a design (intersecting pentagons).	4	☐
	TOTAL SCORE:	30	☐

Interpretation

- **24-30:** No cognitive impairment
- **19-23:** Mild cognitive impairment
- **10-18:** Moderate cognitive impairment
- **≤9:** Severe cognitive impairment

Consider educational level, prior level of functioning, and other factors that may affect performance.

Montreal Cognitive Assessment (MoCA)

A 30-point test that assesses multiple cognitive domains. More sensitive than MMSE for detecting mild cognitive impairment. Takes approximately 10-15 minutes to administer.

Assessment Domains

Domain	Tasks	Max Points	Score
Visuospatial/ Executive	Trail-making, cube copy, clock drawing (contour, numbers, hands)	5	☐
Naming	Identify 3 animals (lion, rhino, camel)	3	☐
Memory	Registration of 5 words, delayed recall (no points for registration)	5	☐
Attention	Digit span, vigilance task, serial 7 subtractions	6	☐
Language	Sentence repetition, verbal fluency	3	☐
Abstraction	Similarities (e.g., train-bicycle, watch-ruler)	2	☐
Orientation	Date, month, year, day, place, city	6	☐
	TOTAL SCORE:	30	☐

Interpretation

- **26-30:** Normal cognition
- **18-25:** Mild cognitive impairment
- **10-17:** Moderate cognitive impairment
- **≤9:** Severe cognitive impairment

Add 1 point for individuals with ≤12 years of education. Available in multiple languages at www.mocatest.org

Patient Health Questionnaire-9 (PHQ-9)

A 9-item self-report questionnaire to screen for and measure depression severity.

Patient Instructions: Over the last 2 weeks, how often have you been bothered by any of the following problems?

Problem	Not at all (0)	Several days (1)	More than half the days (2)	Nearly every day (3)	Score
1. Little interest or pleasure in doing things	☐	☐	☐	☐	☐
2. Feeling down, depressed, or hopeless	☐	☐	☐	☐	☐
3. Trouble falling/staying asleep, or sleeping too much	☐	☐	☐	☐	☐
4. Feeling tired or having little energy	☐	☐	☐	☐	☐
5. Poor appetite or overeating	☐	☐	☐	☐	☐
6. Feeling bad about yourself or that you're a failure	☐	☐	☐	☐	☐
7. Trouble concentrating	☐	☐	☐	☐	☐
8. Moving/speaking slowly OR being fidgety/restless	☐	☐	☐	☐	☐
9. Thoughts of self-harm or that you'd be better off dead	☐	☐	☐	☐	☐
			TOTAL SCORE:		☐

Interpretation

- **0-4:** Minimal or no depression
- **5-9:** Mild depression
- **10-14:** Moderate depression
- **15-19:** Moderately severe depression
- **20-27:** Severe depression

ASCVD Risk Calculator

Estimates 10-year risk of atherosclerotic cardiovascular disease based on the Pooled Cohort Equations (2013 ACC/AHA).

Patient Variables

Age:	________ years (40-79)	**Sex:**	◻ Male ◻ Female
Race:	◻ African American ◻ White/Other		
Total Cholesterol:	________ mg/dL	**HDL Cholesterol:**	________ mg/dL
Systolic BP:	________ mmHg	**On BP medication?**	◻ Yes ◻ No
Diabetes?	◻ Yes ◻ No	**Smoker?**	◻ Yes ◻ No

Interpretation of 10-Year ASCVD Risk

- **<5%**: Low risk
- **5-7.4%**: Borderline risk
- **7.5-19.9%**: Intermediate risk
- **≥20%**: High risk

Statin Recommendations

- **High Intensity Statin:** ≥20% 10-year ASCVD risk, LDL ≥190 mg/dL, or diabetes with multiple risk factors
- **Moderate Intensity Statin:** 7.5-19.9% 10-year ASCVD risk or diabetes without multiple risk factors
- **Consider Statin:** 5-7.4% 10-year ASCVD risk with risk-enhancing factors

Note: This calculator may overestimate or underestimate risk in certain populations. Clinical judgment is required for final treatment decisions.

ABOUT THE EDITORS

Mr. SRI VENKATESH URITI

Mr. Sri Venkatesh Uriti is an Associate Professor in the Department of Pharmacology at Sri Sivani College of Pharmacy, Srikakulam, Andhra Pradesh. With over eight years of experience in academia, he has published 30 research articles, secured four patents, and contributed to two book chapters. He actively participates in faculty development programs, ATAL workshops, and UGC-MMTC short-term courses. He holds lifetime memberships in professional organizations including APTI, IPA, OPF, and SPER. In 2024, he received the "Outstanding Liaison in Community Engagement Award" from the Council for Skills and Competencies.

Mr. VENKATESWARLU GARLA

Mr. Venkateswarlu Garla is working as an Assistant Professor in the School of Pharmacy at Sharda University, specializing in Pharmaceutical Chemistry. He holds a B. Pharm and M. Pharm from JNTUA and achieved an impressive AIR 4652 in GPAT 2019. He is currently pursuing doctoral research at DIPSAR (Delhi) under the AICTE QIP program. His published research includes significant studies on anticancer therapies, herbal antioxidant properties, and nanotechnology applications in cancer treatment. He also serves as the President of the Nava Jyothi Youth Organization in Podalakur, Andhra Pradesh, where he champions educational upliftment for underprivileged children.

Miss. PRATIKSHA P. ALABADE

Miss Pratiksha P. Alabade is currently serving as an Assistant Professor (Pharmacology) at D.K. Patil Institute of Pharmacy, Loha, Maharashtra, India. She completed her graduation from School of Pharmacy, S.R.T.M University, Nanded, and pursued her post-graduation from Nanded Pharmacy College, Maharashtra. With two years of teaching experience and two years of industrial experience in the Discovery Preclinical Department in Delhi, she has established herself in both academic and industrial sectors. She has published 4 research papers and 4 review papers in Scopus-indexed and peer-reviewed journals. She holds certifications in Good Clinical Practice (GCP) and Good Laboratory Practice (GLP) awarded by WHO and the GMP association committee.

Dr. SRIDHAR BABU GUMMADI

Dr. Sridhar Babu Gummadi, M. Pharmacy, Ph.D., is Professor and Principal in the Department of Pharmaceutical Chemistry at Sri Shivani College of Pharmacy, Warangal, Telangana, India. He is a highly accomplished researcher and educator with over 22 years of experience in pharmaceutical sciences. After earning his doctorate from Kakatiya University, Warangal, he has made significant contributions to both academics and research. He published more than 54 publications in reputed national and international journals, holds 6 patents, and authored 3 books. He has presented his work at 15 conferences and has successfully guided over 80 M. Pharmacy students, 90 B. Pharmacy students, and 5 Ph.D. scholars. He actively contributes to the scholarly community as a member of the Editorial Board for the International Journal of Pharmacy and Biological

Sciences (IJPBS) and other international journals.

Dr. SHIVKUMAR SHETE

Dr. Shivkumar Shete, Pharm.D., Ph.D., is a Professor in the Department of Pharmacy Practice with 11 years of distinguished experience in academia and research. He has rich expertise in clinical pharmacy education and pharmaceutical research methodology. Throughout his career, he has shown excellence in teaching pharmacy practice and has been instrumental in developing clinical pharmacy programs. He has contributed significantly to the field through his research publications and has guided numerous pharmacy students in their academic pursuits. His commitment to pharmacy education and practice has made him a respected figure in the pharmaceutical academic community, where he continues to bridge the gap between theoretical knowledge and practical application in pharmacy practice.

INDEX

www.ingramcontent.com/pod-product-compliance
Lightning Source LLC
Chambersburg PA
CBHW061344230926
51848CB00004B/523
* 9 7 8 8 1 9 8 7 6 5 7 0 3 *